Non-Neoplastic Diseases
of the Anorectum

An Interdisciplinary Approach

FALK SYMPOSIUM 118

Non-Neoplastic Diseases of the Anorectum

An Interdisciplinary Approach

Edited by

P. Frühmorgen

*Medizinische Klinik I
(Schwerpunkt Gastroenterologie/Hepatologie)
Klinikum Ludwigsburg
Posilipostr. 4
D-71640 Ludwigsburg
Germany*

H.-P. Bruch

*Universitätsklinikum Lübeck
Ratzeburger Allee 160
D-23562 Lübeck
Germany*

*Proceedings of Falk Symposium 118 held in Freiburg, Germany,
October 1–2, 2000*

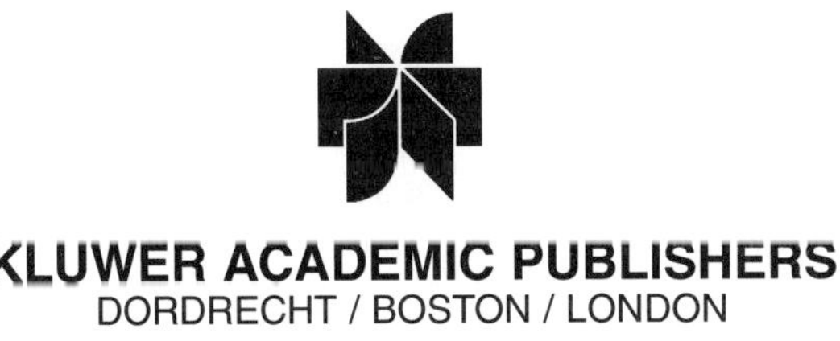

KLUWER ACADEMIC PUBLISHERS
DORDRECHT / BOSTON / LONDON

Library of Congress Cataloging-in-Publication Data is available.

ISBN 0–7923–8766–X

Published by Kluwer Academic Publishers, BV
P.O. Box 17, 3300 AA Dordrecht, The Netherlands.

Sold and distributed in North, Central and South America
by Kluwer Academic Publishers,
101 Philip Drive, Norwell, MA 02061, USA.

In all other countries, sold and distributed
by Kluwer Academic Publishers, Distribution Center,
P.O. Box 322, 3300 AH Dordrecht, The Netherlands.

Printed on acid-free paper

Contents

List of Principal Contributors

S. Bar-Meir
Department of Gastroenterology
Chaim Sheba Medical Center
Sackler School of Medicine
IL-52621 Tel Hashomer
Israel

G. Bianchi Porro
Gastrointestinal Unit
"L. Sacco" University Hospital
Via G.B. Grassi, 74
I-20157 Milano
Italy

J.-U. Bock
Beselerallee 67
D-24105 Kiel
Germany

H.-P. Bruch
Universitätsklinikum Lübeck
Ratzeburger Allee 160
D-23562 Lübeck
Germany

P. Buchmann
Chirurgische Klinik
Stadtspital Waid
Tièchestr. 99
CH-8037 Zürich
Switzerland

A. Forbes
St Mark's Hospital
Watford Road
Harrow
Middlesex
HA1 3UJ
UK

P. Fornara
Universitätsklinik u. Poliklinik f.
Urologie
Martin-Luther-Universität
Halle-Wittenberg
Magdeburger straße 16
D-06112 Halle/Saale

H. Fritsch
Institut für Anatomie und Histologie
Universität Innsbruck
Müllerstr. 59
A-6010 Innsbruck
Austria

P. Frühmorgen
Medizinische Klinik I
(Schwerpunkt Gastroenterologie/
  Hepatologie)
Klinikum Ludwigsburg
Posilipostr. 4
D-71640 Ludwigsburg
Germany

A. Fuerst
Klinik für Chirurgie
Universitätsklinik
D-93042 Regensburg
Germany

P. Gast
Endoscopies Digestives
Centre Hospitalier
Universitaire de Department de
  Médecine Liège
BP 35 Policlinique 2
B-4020 Liège
Belgium

LIST OF PRINCIPAL CONTRIBUTORS

D. Geile
Proktologisches Institut
München-Ost
Chirurgische Privatklinik
Denninger Str. 44
D-81679 München
Germany

T. C. Hicks
Ochsner Clinic
1514 Jefferson Highway
New Orleans, LA 70121
USA

H. Hinninghofen
Universitätsklinikum Tübingen
Abteilung für Allgemeine Chirurgie
Hoppe-Seylerstr. 3
D-72076 Tübingen
Germany

W. H. Jost
Deutsche Klinik für Diagnostik
FB Neurologie und Klinische
  Neurophysiologie
Aukammallee 33
D-65191 Wiesbaden
Germany

H.-J. Krammer
IV. Medizinische Universitätsklinik
Theodor-Kutzer-Ufer 1-3
D-68135 Mannheim
Germany

A. Lienemann
Institut für diagnostische Radiologie
Universitäts-Klinikum Großhadern
Marchioninistr. 15
D-81377 München
Germany

M. Niewald
Department of Radiotherapy
University Hospital of Saarland
D-66421 Homburg/Saar
Germany

D. H. Present
Mount Sinai Medical Center
12 East, 86th Street
New York, NY 10028-0517
USA

T. H. K. Schiedeck
Universitätsklinikum Lübeck Chirurgie
Ratzeburger Allee 160
D-23538 Lübeck
Germany

J. Schmidt
Chirurgische Universitäts-Klinik
Im Neuenheimer Feld 110
D-69120 Heidelberg
Germany

S. Schreiber
I. Medizinische Universitäts-Klinik für
  Allgemeine Innere Medizin
Schittenhelmstr. 12
D-24015 Kiel
Germany

R. A. Silva
Serviço de Gastroenterologia do
  Instituto Português de Oncologia
Rua Dr. António Bernardino de
  Almeida
P-4200-072 Porto
Portugal

A. Stallmach
Innere Medizin II
Medizinische Klinik und Poliklinik
Universität des Saarlandes
Kirrberger Str.
D-66421 Homburg
Germany

E. F. Stange
Zentrum Innere Medizin
Abt. Innere Medizin I
Robert-Bosch-Krankenhaus GmbH
Auerbachstrasse 110
D-70376 Stuttgart
Germany

S. A. Strong
Cleveland Clinic Desk A 111
9500 Euclid Avenue
Cleveland, OH 44195-5044
USA

E. A. Trowers
Department of Internal Medicine
Division of Gastroenterology
Texas Technical University Health
  Sciences Center
3601, 4th Street, MS 9410
Lubbock, TX 79430
USA

V. Wienert
Universitäts-Hautklinik
Klinikum der RWTH Aachen
Paulwelsstr. 30
D-52074 Aachen
Germany

Preface

Hardly any other part of the human body is of such interdisciplinary interest as the anal, perianal and rectal region. Gastroenterologists, dermatologists, urologists, general practitioners and surgeons specializing in proctology, phlebology and coloproctological surgery are involved in this region between the ectoderm, transitional zone and entoderm.

Diagnostic procedures such as endoscopy, radiology, sonography, manometry, electromyography and histopathology are even more diverse, in particular where the differential diagnosis of non-neoplastic conditions of the anorectal region is concerned.

The 118th Falk Symposium, which was accompanied by a poster exhibition, focused on the morphology and function of the pelvic floor and its dysfunction, radiation damage in proctology, haemorrhoidal complaints, and chronic inflammatory rectal diseases, as well as conditions of the anal and perianal region.

The symposium gathered research physicians and colleagues working at hospitals or in their own practice who are involved in the diagnosis and treatment of anorectal pathologies, so that they could be made aware of and discuss the established facts and new developments. This clearly represents the incentive and the challenge of this symposium.

These proceedings demonstrate the enormous progress that has been made since the 64th Falk Symposium, which was organized by Professor L. Demling, MD, and Professor P. Frühmorgen, MD, in 1991.

P. Frühmorgen
H.-P. Bruch

Section I
Pelvic floor disorders

1
The pelvic floor – morphology

H. FRITSCH

INTRODUCTION

The anatomy and physiology of the pelvic floor are of burning clinical interest. Defects in the ventral or dorsal compartment of the pelvic floor may cause urinary or faecal incontinence in elderly patients. Though the anatomy of the pelvic floor is intrinsically related to its function the anatomical concepts of the pelvic floor are mainly based on separate, and to some degree single-minded, studies of gross anatomists, histologists and clinicians. Though the morphological descriptions are rather detailed, they are confusing. Several connective tissue spaces[1-3], fasciae[4,5] and ligaments[6,7] are supposed to exist. The pelvic diaphragm[8-12], the anal and urethral sphincter complexes[13-17] have been subjects of intensive studies, yet much appears to remain unsettled.

An accurate and reasonable account of pelvic floor anatomy will emerge only when it is studied using a multidisciplinary approach.

For the past decade we have therefore studied pelvic floor anatomy in undisturbed morphological sections[18,19] and we have compared our findings with the results of modern imaging techniques[20-22] as well as with those of the pelvic surgeons[23,24]. Thus we have made a first attempt towards interdisciplinary work on the pelvic floor that provides many new details of human pelvic floor anatomy, but always presents them in a clinical and functional context.

MATERIALS AND METHODS

Anatomical sections

The sectional anatomy of the adult pelvic floor was studied in 11 (six female and five male) specimens from persons who were 58–81 years old. The pelves were frozen at $-80°C$ and then serially cut into sections in the transverse, sagittal, or coronal plane with a bandsaw. The thickness of the sheets ranged between 3 and 5 mm. The sawdust was carefully removed from the sheets, which were then dehydrated with acetone at $-25°C$ for 5 weeks, defatted in methylene chloride at room temperature for 2 weeks, and then impregnated with an epoxy resin mixture[18]. Finally, the sheets were placed into a chamber composed of glass plates, filled with epoxy resin, and were cured at 50°C.

Sections of the fetal pelvis

The pelvic floor was studied in seven newborn children and 79 fetuses, which were all obtained followed legal abortion or miscarriage, and which showed no signs of maceration or macroscopic abnormality. The fetuses and newborn children had been fixed by immersion and stored in a 4% formaldehyde solution for at least 3 months. The crown–rump (CR) length of the fetuses ranged between 34 and 351 mm, corresponding to a gestational age of 9–37 weeks p.c.

The fetal pelves and the pelves of the newborn children were taken for plastination histology[19], and had therefore been impregnated with the epoxy resin Biodur® E12 and serially sectioned with a diamond-wire saw (Well®) either in the transverse, coronal or sagittal plane. The thickness of the sections ranged from 300 to 700 μm. After mounting and polishing, the sections were stained with azure II/methylene blue and counterstained with basic fuchsin. The stained sections were examined and photographed with a macroscope (Wild, Heerbrugg) at magnifications of 4–80×.

Macroscopic preparations

Additionally, the anal sphincter and the pelvic diaphragm were dissected in four embalmed specimens of adult pelves.

RESULTS

From a clinical point of view it is commonly accepted to subdivide the pelvic cavity into a ventral and a dorsal compartment. As the dorsal compartment is of great importance for proctologists, our results from this compartment will be described in detail, and those of the ventral compartment only as far as they are necessary for an integrative understanding.

Connective tissue structures

The dorsal compartment of the pelvic cavity is subdivided into two definite connective tissue compartments. A small presacral space is situated in front of the sacrum and the coccyx (Fig. 1); it is demarcated by the parietal pelvic fascia ventrally and it contains loose connective tissue, adipose tissue and a number of vessels. The larger perirectal compartment is situated circularly around the rectal wall. In the adult it is situated in front of the presacral space (Fig. 1). It is composed of the rectal adventitia, also called the mesorectum in the literature[25], and it contains the superior rectal vessels and their branches, as well as branches of the medial rectal artery, the rectal lymph nodes and the rectal nerves. The localization of the rectal lymph nodes is clearly different from that of the neighbouring pelvic lymph nodes accompanying the iliac vessels. The outer connective tissue lamella of the rectal adventitia may be regarded as rectal fascia or border lamella. It can be seen in histological preparations and it can be touched during

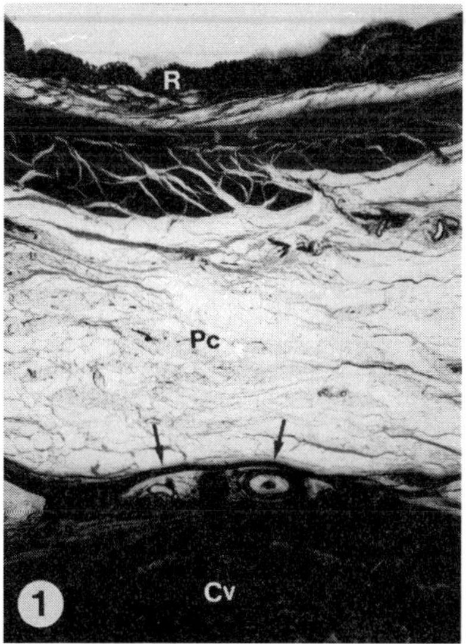

Figure 1 Transverse section (500 μm) through the precoccygeal region of an adult (original magnification × 5); R, rectum; Cv, coccygeal vertebra; Pc, perirectal compartment; arrows: pelvic parietal fascia

surgical procedures. In the adult female pelvis the sacrouterine ligaments (Fig. 2) constitute a visible border between the perirectal compartment and the structures that are adjacent laterally. In the male pelvis the nerves of the inferior hypogastric (pelvic) plexus border the perirectal compartment laterally.

The extent of the perirectal compartment depends on the branching pattern of the superior rectal vessels. Thus the compartment constitutes a thick layer at the lateral and dorsal rectal wall. However, it only constitutes a thin layer ventrally, where it is connected with the capsule of the prostate to form the fascia of Denonvillier in the male, and where it is connected with the adventitia of the vagina to form the rectovaginal fascia in the female. The extent of the perirectal compartment decreases in size in the craniocaudal direction.

The ventral compartment of the pelvic cavity contains a large paravisceral compartment that fills the space between the lateral walls of the urogenital organs and the lateral pelvic wall (Fig. 3). This compartment is mainly filled with adipose tissue in the adult, and the only ligaments that have been detected in between are the puboprostatic (Fig. 4) or the pubovesical ligaments. No borders of specialized connective tissue structures between the prevesical, para-vesical, paracervical, paravaginal or paraseminal portion have been found. The medial border between dorsal and ventral pelvic compartments is delineated by the fascia of Denonvillier in the male and the rectovaginal fascia in the female. Dorsomedially the big vessels and nerves supplying the urogenital organs separate the two pelvic compartments.

Furthermore it can be stated that no visceral pelvic fasciae ensheathing the pelvic organs have been detected.

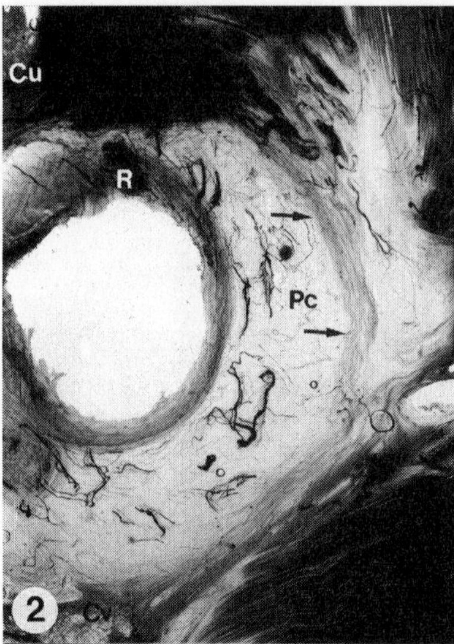

Figure 2 Transverse section (5 mm) through the pelvis of a 77-year-old female at a level with the sacrouterine ligament (arrows) (original magnification × 0.7); Cu, cervix uteri; R, rectum; Cv, coccygeal vertebra; Pc, perirectal compartment

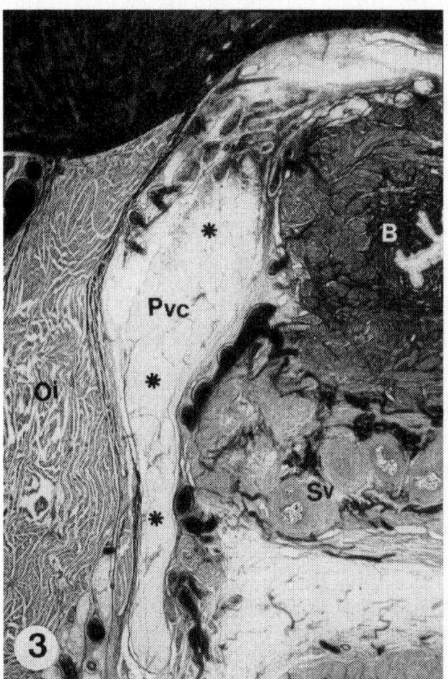

Figure 3 Transverse section (400 μm) through the pelvis of a newborn male at a level with the seminal vesicle. The paravisceral compartment is filled with fat lobules (asterisks) (original magnification × 10); B, bladder; Sv, seminal vesicle; Oi, obturator internus; Pvc, paravisceral compartment

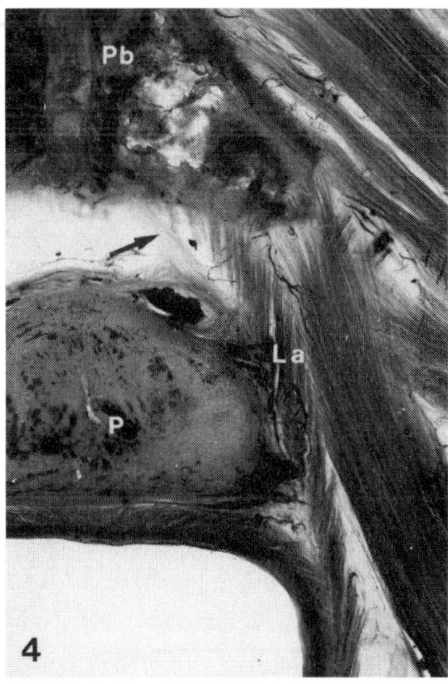

Figure 4 Transverse section (3 mm) through the pelvis of a 56-year-old male at a level with the pubo-prostatic ligament (arrow) (original magnification × 1); Pb, pubic bone; P, prostate; La, levator ani

Muscles

The caudal borders of both paravisceral and perirectal compartments abut on the cranial border of the levator ani muscle. This muscle can be subdivided into the three classical portions: pubococcygeus, iliococcygeus and puborectalis (Fig. 5). Whereas the pubococcygeus and iliococcygeus form a muscular plate for the pelvic organs, and are connected to the coccyx dorsally, the puborectalis portion forms a muscular sling around the rectal wall at a level with the anorectal flexure. It is not connected to the coccyx dorsally. There are no muscular fibres intermingling between the wall of the pelvic organs and the portions of the levator ani muscle.

At the anorectal flexure the puborectalis is continuous with the external anal sphincter that is attached to the coccyx by the anococcygeal ligament. Whereas macroscopically the anal sphincter complex appears as a continuous sheet covering the anal canal, in sectional anatomy and microscopically it can be subdivided into a thickened internal sphincter, a medical longitudinal layer and a striated external sphincter. The external sphincter can clearly be subdivided into a caudal portion that is intermingled with the longitudinal muscle fibres and a cranial portion that is not. The external sphincter is not completely circular. Its cranial portion is not circular ventrally, but it is intimately intermingled with fibres of the puborectalis laterally (Fig. 6). This portion is strong and thick in the female and thin and elongated in the male. At a level with the anal fold the caudal portion of the external anal sphincter is not circular dorsally (Fig. 7). Here the

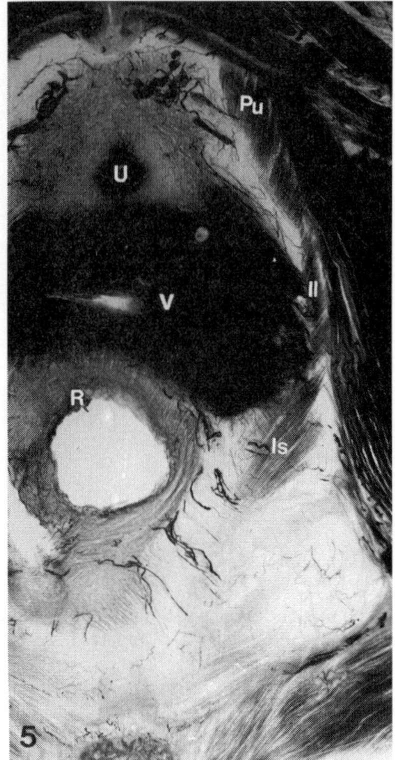

Figure 5

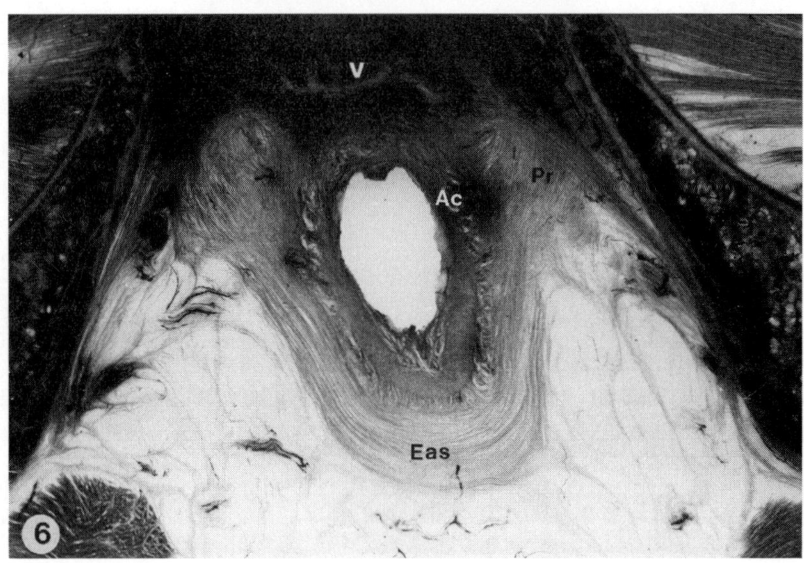

Figure 6

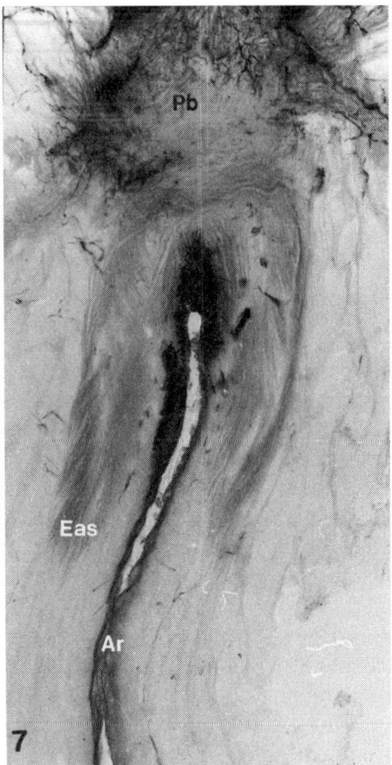

Figures 5–7   Transverse sections through the pelvis of a 77-year-old female. **Figure 5** at a level of the levator ani portions (original magnification × 1.3); U, urethra; V, vagina, R, rectum, Pu, pubococcygeus, Il, ilicoccygeus; Is, ischiococcygeus. **Figure 6** at the level with the external anal sphinter (original magnification × 1.6); V, vagina; Ac, anal canal; Eas, External anal sphincter; Pr, puborectalis. **Figure 7** at a level with the perineum (original magnification × 2.6); Ar, anal rim; Eas, external anal sphincter; Pb, perineal body

external sphincter turns over internally and is continuous with the internal sphincter. Ventrally the caudal portion of the external sphincter is circular and it is connected to the perineal body. This portion is shorter in the female than in the male.

DISCUSSION

Our comparative study of the sectional anatomy of the fetal and the adult pelvis shows that the classical concepts concerning the connective tissue as well as the muscles need to be revised.

According to the literature different spaces are supposed to be arranged around the pelvic organs[1,3] We propose to drop the term 'space' and only to speak of connective tissue compartments, for the following reasons. From the point of view of the surgeon, 'spaces' are empty. They are only filled with a delicate connective tissue and contain neither large vessels nor nerves. We have shown in a previous study[18] that the existence and topography of such spaces can be understood only during early fetal life when the so-called spaces are filled only with mesenchyme. From a morphological point of view empty 'spaces' normally do not exist within the pelvic cavity of the adult. According to our results we propose to subdivide the connective and adipose tissue of the adult pelvis into presacral, perirectal and paravisceral compartments. This subdivision is in accordance with clinical requirements. The perirectal compartment is most important for the surgeon[23,25]. As it contains the rectal adventitia with vessels and lymph nodes, it must be entirely removed in the case of carcinoma. The guiding pathway during the operation is the thin rectal fascia.

In the anatomical and clinical literature a visceral pelvic fascia has been described for each pelvic organ. The parietal pelvic fascia is supposed to reflect to the different visceral fasciae at a level with the pelvic floor. We have shown in fetuses that the connective tissue sheath has to be defined separately for each pelvic organ, and we proposed to speak of a fascia only in the case of the border lamella of the rectal adventitia. There are capsules for the prostate and the seminal vesicle and an adventitial layer for the bladder, the uterus and the vagina. Thus we propose to drop the term 'visceral pelvic fascia'.

Our studies demonstrate that the so-called supportive ligaments of the pelvic organs must be denied apart from the sacrouterine and the puboprostatic/pubovesical ligaments. Most important structures for the support of the pelvic viscera are those parts of the levator ani that constitute a muscular plate. We have shown that uterus, vagina and rectum are situated above the levator plate and not upon the urogenital hiatus[23]. The puborectalis portion of the levator ani constitutes a sling around the rectal wall and is therefore important for rectal continence. Contraction of the levator ani causes the puborectalis to draw the anorectal flexure as well as the vagina ventrally and against the perineal body. On the whole, the contraction of the levator ani prevents descent of the pelvic viscera and closes the pelvic floor aperture.

Furthermore our data point to the fact that the external anal sphincter is not completely circular. In both sexes it is open dorsocaudally at a level with the anal rim. Here the external sphincter is double-folded and intimately connected with both layers of the smooth musculature. Thus the whole complex works as a circular sphincter. Damage at this level may be caused by the stapler during rectal surgery and may even lead to rupture of the smooth internal sphincter muscle. Above a level of the perineal body the external sphincter is not circular ventrally, but it constitutes a muscle sling with the puborectalis and thus also functions as a circular muscle. This is the most important morphological speciality in the female pelvis, where the anal sphincter portions are able to make way for the child during delivery. Ruptures at this level may affect the internal sphincter as well as the external sphincter and the puborectalis portion of the levator ani.

In addition, we have recently shown that morphologically the external urethral sphincter is not completely circular either, but it also functions as a circular muscle.

In many respects our results are controversial compared with most of the classical concepts of pelvic floor anatomy, as well as with most of the classical operative techniques. Our results yield for interdisciplinary studies with the aim of ameliorating operative concepts in urology, gynaecology and proctology.

References

1. Pernkopf E. Topographische Anatomie, Bd 2, 1 and 2. Hälfte. Berlin: Urban & Schwarzenberg, 1941.
2. Tandler J. Lehrbuch der systematischen Anatomie. Die Eingeweide, Bd 2. Leipzig: Vogel, 1923.
3. Waldeyer W. Das Becken. Bonn: Cohen, 1899.
4. Holl M. Fascien des Beckenausgangs. In: Bardeleben K von, editor. Handbuch der Anatomie des Menschen, Bd 7, Teil 2, Abteilung 2. Jena: Fischer, 1897:279–300.
5. Ulenhuth E, Nolley GW. Vaginal fascia, a myth? Obstet Gynecol. 1957;4:349–58.
6. Bastian D, Lassau JP. The suspensory mechanism of the uterus. Anat Clin. 1982;4:147–60.
7. Mackenrodt A. Über die Ursachen der normalen und pathologischen Lage des Uterus. Arch Gynaekol. 1895;48:393–421.
8. Ayoub SF. The anterior fibres of the levator ani muscle in man. J Anat. 1979;128:571–80.
9. Holl M. Die Muskeln im Beckenausgang des Menschen. Ergeb Anat Entwicklungsgesch. 1901;11:1115–73.
10. Lawson JON. Pelvic anatomy. I. Pelvic floor muscles. Ann R Coll Surg Engl. 1974;54:244–52.
11. Shafik A. A new concept of the anatomy of the anal sphincter mechanism and the physiology of defecation. II. Anatomy of the levator ani muscle with the special reference to puborectalis. Invest Urol. 1975;13:175–82.
12. Zacharin RF. Pelvic Floor Anatomy and the Surgery of Pulsion Enterocoele. New York: Springer, 1985:31–63.
13. Ayoub SF. Anatomy of the external anal sphincter in men. Acta Anat. 1979;105:25–36.
14. Dalley AF. The riddle of the sphincters. The morphophysiology of the anorectal mechanism reviewed. Am Surg. 1987;53:298–308.
15. Dorschner W. Der Streit um den Muskulus sphincter urethrae. Histomorphologische Untersuchungen. Akt Urol. 1992;23:163–8.
16. Oh C, Kark AE. Anatomy of the external anal sphincter. Br J Surg. 1972;59:717–23.
17. Oelrich TM. The urethral sphincter muscle in the male. Am J Anat. 1980;158:2229–46.
18. Fritsch H. Development changes in the retrorectal region of the human fetus. Anat Embryol. 1988;177:513–22.
19. Fritsch H. Staining of the different tissues in thick epoxy resin impregnated sections of human fetuses. Stain Technol. 1989;64:75–9.
20. Fritsch H, Hötzinger H. Tomographical anatomy of the pelvis, visceral pelvic connective tissue, and its compartments. Clin Anat. 1995;8:17–24.
21. Fröhlich B, Hötzinger H, Fritsch H. Tomographical anatomy of the pelvis, pelvic floor, and related structures. Clin Anat. 1997;10:223–30.
22. Peschers UM, De Lancey JOL, Fritsch H, Quint LE, Prince MR. Cross-sectional imaging anatomy of the anal sphincters. Obstet Gynecol. 1997;90:839–44.
23. Fritsch H, Kühnel W, Stelzner F. Entwicklung und klinische Anatomie der Adventitia recti. Bedeutung für die Radikaloperation eines Mastdarmkrebses. Langenbecks Arch Chir. 1996;381:237–43.
24. Ludwikowski B, Oesch HI, Brenner E, Fritsch H. Development of the external urethral sphincter in humans. Br J Urol. 2000 (In press).
25. Heald RJ, Husband EM, Ryall RD. The mesorectum in rectal cancer surgery—the clue to pelvic recurrence? Br J Surg. 1982;69:613–16.

2
Pathophysiology of the pelvic floor

P. BUCHMANN and S. MISHRA

INTRODUCTION

The anatomy and physiology of the pelvic floor are extremely complex. Although, in the past few years, every effort has been undertaken to investigate the function, morphology and microscopical structure, they are to this day not completely understood[1-3].

The same applies to the pathophysiology[4]; many symptoms are directly related to its manifestations, although the causality is often not known. For example, an enterocele is a widened pouch of Douglas which contains intestine. This can cause a compression of the rectum against the sacrum, which in turn causes a defaecation obstruction. This is often observed in women after hysterectomy. However, the conclusion that an enterocele is often observed after a hysterectomy is not true. It is not known what causes the pouch of Douglas to develop into a enterocele. It is also unclear whether the pelvic peritoneum reaches down between rectum and vagina to the pelvic floor congenitally or if an acquired alteration is present.

For teaching purposes 'pelvic floor disorders' can be assigned either to incontinence or defaecation disorders. During the development of the disorder the symptoms can change from one category to the other. For example, a rectocele causes disturbed defaecation if above the sphincter apparatus; however, if the sacculation extends caudally and encloses the anterior sphincter, then an incontinence arises during squeezing.

ANAL INCONTINENCE

Faecal incontinence has many causes. Detailed information can be found in refs 5 and 6. Causes that arise from the pelvic floor are either the result of trauma (e.g. perineal tear, postoperative sphincter lesion, impalement injury) or from descending perineum syndrome. An incontinence caused by a rectocele has already been mentioned, and will be discussed later.

Neurogenic incontinence, especially pudendal nerve neuropathy, was for a long time regarded as the main cause of the descending perineum. Pudendal nerve neuropathy is considered as a late effect of the overstretching of the pudendal nerve during the expulsion period in labour. In a recent paper[7] it was demonstrated that incontinence in elderly women was due to the ageing of the sphincter and pelvic floor muscles, and was not of neurogenic origin.

The causes of traumatic incontinence appear to be obvious. However, many women with birth trauma are initially continent and have complete control of the rectum. The complaints arise with advancing age, which in turn leads to a medical consultation. The compensation mechanism which guarantees continence becomes insufficient. It is still unclear whether pudendal nerve neuropathy or muscle ageing is responsible. The aim of biofeedback training with incontinent patients is to improve the compensation capabilities; therefore this is also partially successful with patients with sphincter lesions.

'Idiopathic incontinence' of elderly women is often a combination of degenerative and mechanical damage and must be worked up as such. An endosonography should be performed to document the state of the sphincter muscles (Fig. 1). If necessary the reconstruction should be discussed even if a descending perineum is present. The aim of the operation is not to attain perfect continence but to reduce incontinence[8].

The importance of the anorectal angle for the maintenance of continence is not judged the same by all. Sir Allen Parks strove to reconstruct the anorectal angle with his postanal repair in patients with descending perineum[9]. The early results led to some optimism. However, after years of follow-up the technique was discarded due to a high percentage of recurrent incontinence[10]. Whatever the cause is for the descensus, either muscle ageing or pudendus neuropathy, surgical intervention cannot prevent the progression of muscle fibre degeneration. It is not surprising that a surgical procedure has no effect on muscle fibre degeneration, as this is a biological process. The procedure has been unjustly abandoned by many. In patients with a partial muscle contractility the operation can improve continence, at least for a few years. The procedure is unsuccessful and pointless with a descended pelvic floor[11]. Again an endosonography of the anal canal must be performed before the intervention, in order to identify the extent of any additional defects.

The aim of surgery for incontinence is to restore the initial morphological state and achieve the best physiological benefits. The prospect of a long-lasting improvement should be considered in the choice of therapy.

The anal canal does not, strictly speaking, belong to the pelvic floor, but alterations may interfere with continence. Scarring, enlarged internal haemorrhoidal plexus, hypertrophic papilla, fissure-in-ano or tumour influences the continence because they create an asymmetric anal canal through which discharge flows causing a perianal dermatitis. If the epithelium is destroyed below the dentate line discrimination in the quality of bowel contents (solid, loose, gas) is then no longer possible, and continence is therefore impaired.

DEFAECATION DISORDERS

Defaecation disorders have many causes. Patients complain most often about constipation, and do not differentiate between inertia coli or distal alterations.

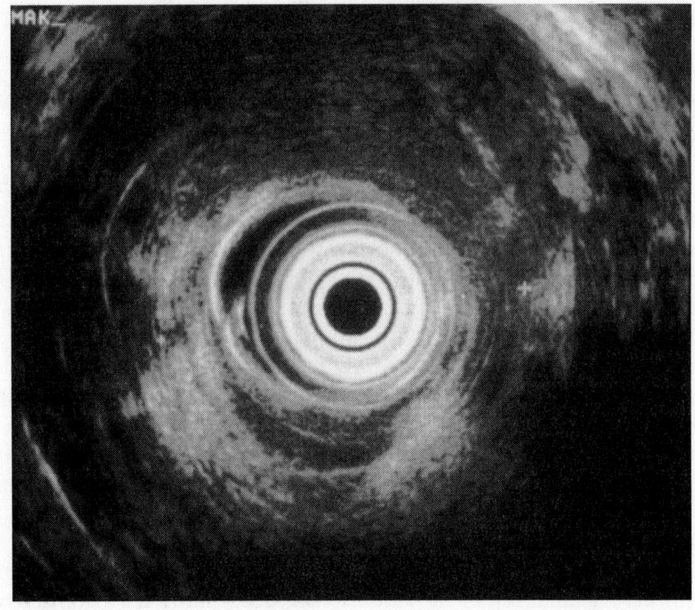

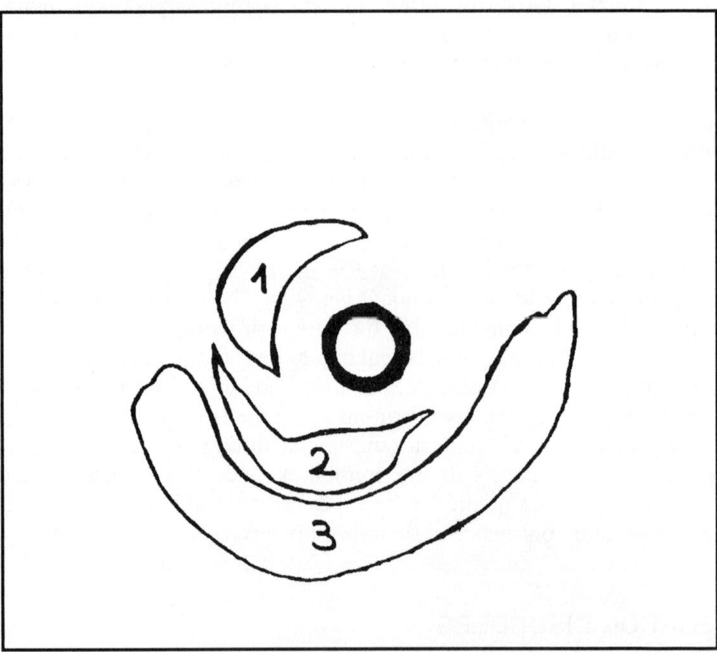

Figure 1a Endosonography of a severely damaged anal sphincter during labour: Middle anal canal: 1, balloon; 2, internal anal sphincter (5–9 o'clock); 3, external anal sphincter (2–8 o'clock)

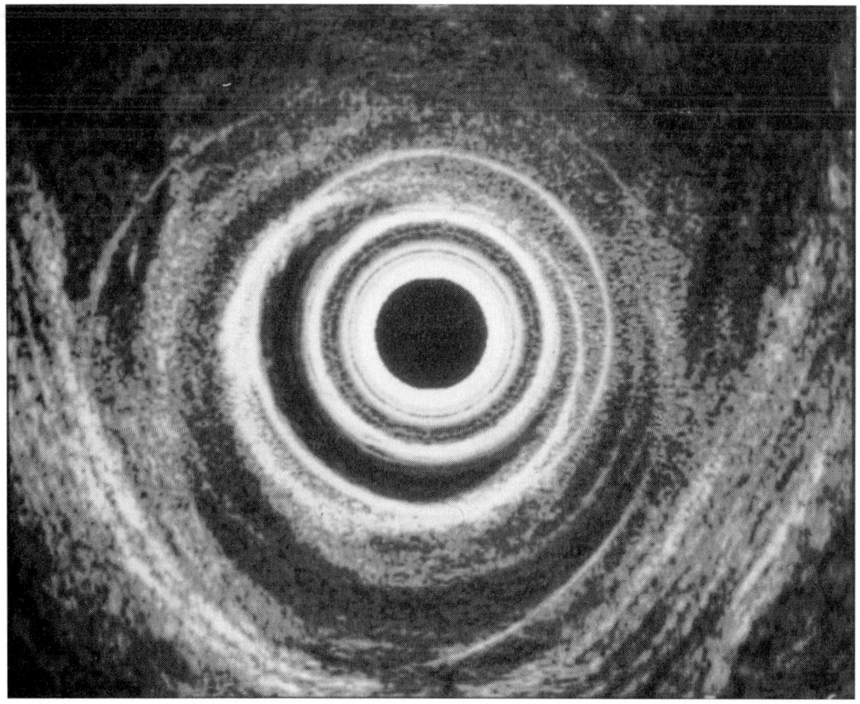

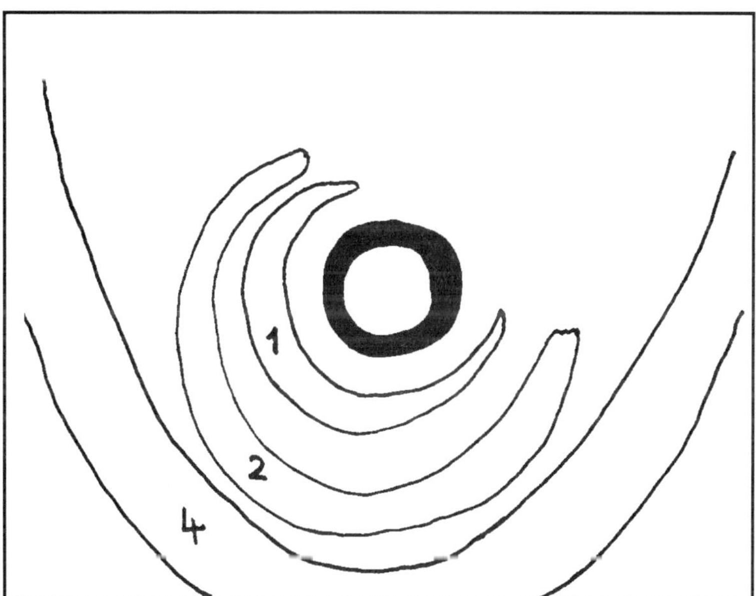

Figure 1b Endosonography of a severely damaged anal sphincter during labour: Upper anal canal: 1, balloon; 2, internal anal sphincter (3–11 o'clock); 4, puborectalis sling

Table 1 Specific questions on the case history with defaecation disorders

Frequency per 24 h:
  Quantity of each evacuation

Consistency: formed   hard
                               soft
               loose
               liquid (watery)
               variable

Intense straining at stool is required when:
  The stool is before the anus and cannot be released
  The whole 'stomach' is full

Feeling of incomplete evacuation

Interrupted evacuation
  A small portion is released after the defaecation
  Repeated evacuation of small portions (staccato)

Urge to defaecate without stool

Urgency of defaecation with or without incontinence

Special manoeuvre needed

Straining needed
  With constipation
  With soft stool

Intake of drugs

This is the job of the doctor. He must, through specific questions (Table 1) be able to deduce the cause (Table 2) and carry out specific examinations in order to make a diagnosis.

Supplementary to the clinical examinations are tests in the anorectal laboratory (measurement of anal pressure, rectal sensation, rectosphincteric reflex, balloon-expulsion test and electrophysiology). Furthermore defaecography, MRI and transit-time measurements are very helpful. In the following sections only the clinical conditions which affect the pelvic floor will be discussed.

Rectocele

A rectocele is a sacculation of the anterior wall of the rectum against the vagina. The formation of rectoceles is controversial. Some gynaecologists see the condition as a hernia in the rectovaginal septum. The rectovaginal septum, however, is judged very differently. DeLancy describes three levels[12]. In the lower level (level III) he found no morphologically discernible septum. Others claim that the Denonvilliers fascia is an adhesive peritoneal duplication of the pouch of Douglas[13]. Studies on plastinated preparations describe a solid connective tissue formation as the rectovaginal fascia[14].

Another reason may be birth trauma or an outlet obstruction. A possible cause of a rectocele is tissue ageing. In an outlet obstruction, forced expulsion puts pressure on the distal anterior rectal wall[15]. This in turn causes a sacculation against the vagina if the anus does not open (anismus, sphincter dysplasia).

Table 2   Differential diagnosis after taking the case history

Case history	Suspected diagnosis/cause
Infrequent small portions	Low-roughage diet
Hard consistency	Low fluid uptake
Loose consistency	Chronic, inflammatory bowel disease (Crohn's disease)
Excessive straining when the stool is felt before the anus	Functional outlet obstruction: sphincter dysplasia, anismus; tumour
Feeling of incomplete evacuation	Rectocele, enterocele, intussusception, proctitis
Small portion a few minutes after evacuation	Rectocele
Frequent secondary evacuation	Enterocele (intussusception)
Urge to defaecate without stool	For example, hypertrophic papilla
Urgency to evacuate	Irritable bowel syndrome, Crohn's disease/ulcerative colitis, sphincter lesion, proctitis (unspecific), acute enteritis

Manipulation
  Pressing up the buttocks
  Pressure against the perineum/vagina
  Traction backwards (anus/vagina)
  Digital evacuation
	
	Pelvic floor hernia,
	Rectocele,
	Sphincter dysplasia,
	Coprostasis (various causes)

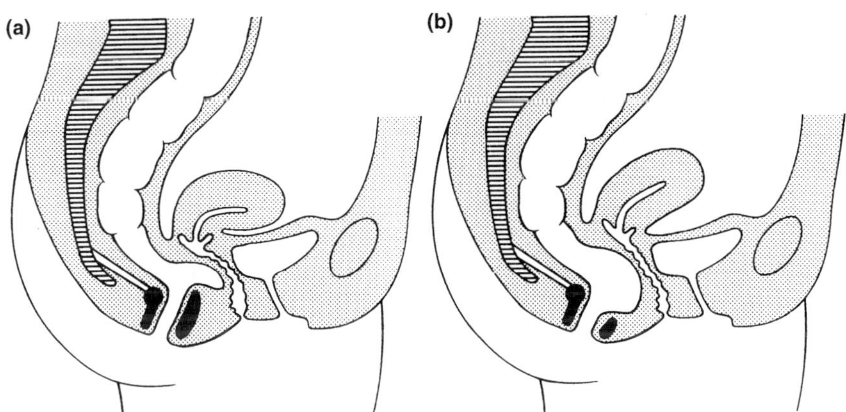

Figure 2   Rectocele: (a) above the anal sphincter, (b) involving the anal sphincter (from ref. 15, with permission from Hans Huber Publishers)

Initially the rectocele is situated cranial of the anal sphincter (Fig. 2a). Among some women the rectocele becomes deeper and extends into the vaginal introitus. With others the rectocele extends distally and evaginates the sphincter ventrally (Fig. 2b).

A rectocele is often found during a rectal examination. The patient does not necessarily have any complaints.

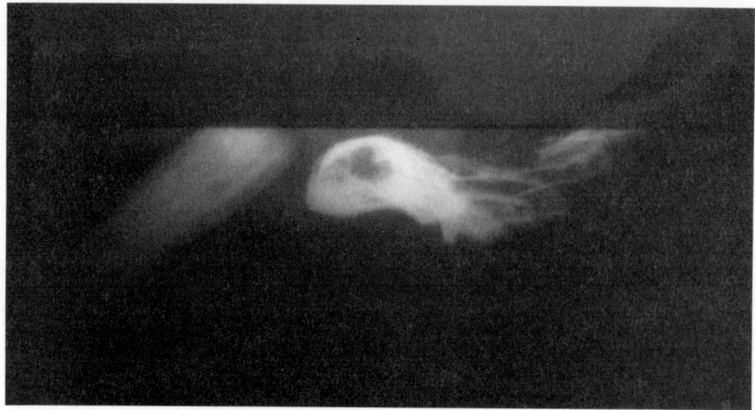

Figure 3 Defaecography of a rectocele above the anal sphincter (barium-soaked tampon in the vagina)

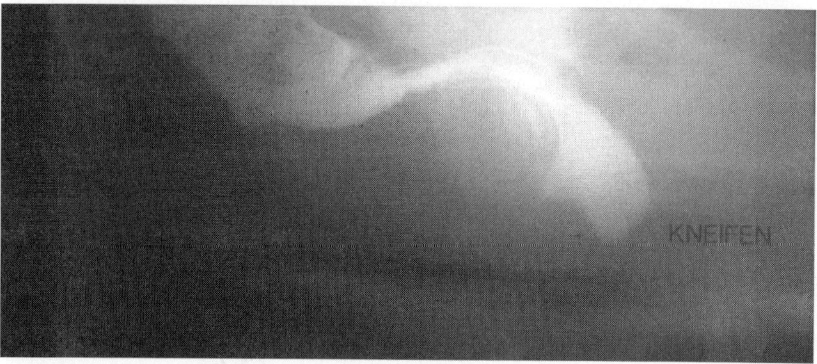

Figure 4 Defaecography of a rectocele involving the anal sphincter

The defaecography can be used to differentiate and display the different types of rectoceles (Figs 3 and 4). The determination of the size of the rectocele is problematic because of disturbed privacy in the radiological unit. Many patients are inhibited whilst being observed, and because of the flatulence. At home, where there is less inhibition, the symptoms may be more severe as patients strain much harder.

Nevertheless, diagnostic imaging is very helpful in planning an operation. Other disorders can thus be discovered which may have been covered up by the main complaints. Female patients with a rectocele above the sphincter typically complain of a need to empty the bowels after defaecation. Faeces which pass into the rectocele while evacuating are released into the upper anal canal, and this in turn causes a defaecation stimulus.

If the sphincter is included in the rectocele (Figs 2b and 4), the puborectalis sling is pulled into the sacculation during squeezing and some bowel contents are pressed outwards. The patient then complains of smearing.

Various operative techniques in treating a rectocele are described. Our therapy of choice is the transanal ampulloplasty, because at the same time the abundant mucosa can be resected[16].

Enterocele

An enterocele (cul-de-sac) is a widened rectovaginal pouch (pouch of Douglas) and extends down to the pelvic floor (Fig. 5). The pouch of Douglas is often filled with the sigma, less often with the caecum or the small intestines. An enterocele generally becomes symptomatic after a hysterectomy. The bowel in the enterocele presses against the rectum during defaecation, which in turn is compressed against the sacrum. This causes a defaecation obstruction which intermittently interrupts or impedes rectal passage. Apart from the defaecation disorders many women describe the feeling of pressing down a large mass into the lower abdomen. This can be illustrated in the defaecography (Fig. 6).

The cause of an enterocele is unclear. One theory is that the rectovaginal pouch extends down to the pelvic floor congenitally and occludes. The Denonvilliers fascia is a result of this occlusion and is described by some as a duplication of the peritoneum[13]. The enterocele can then be regarded as non-occlusion (the same mechanism is seen in a congenital inguinal hernia). A prolapsing uterus may tract the pouch of Douglas caudally and produce an enterocele[17]. Recent studies question the duplication[14].

The fact that the only cause of an enterocele is repeated intense straining at stool over the years is difficult to imagine. One plausible cause is the removal of a large uterus during hysterectomy, creating a gap for the intestine. Another factor is the destabilization of the pelvic floor when the ligaments are insufficiently sutured. During the operation the vaginal stump should be pulled

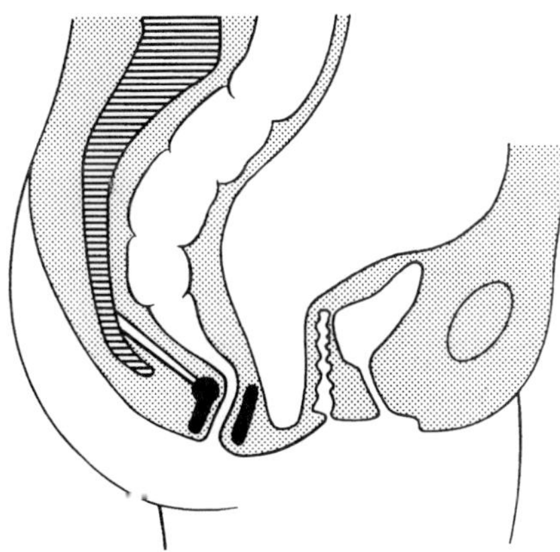

Figure 5 Enterocele (cul-de-sac), after hysterectomy (from ref. 15, with permission from Hans Huber Publishers)

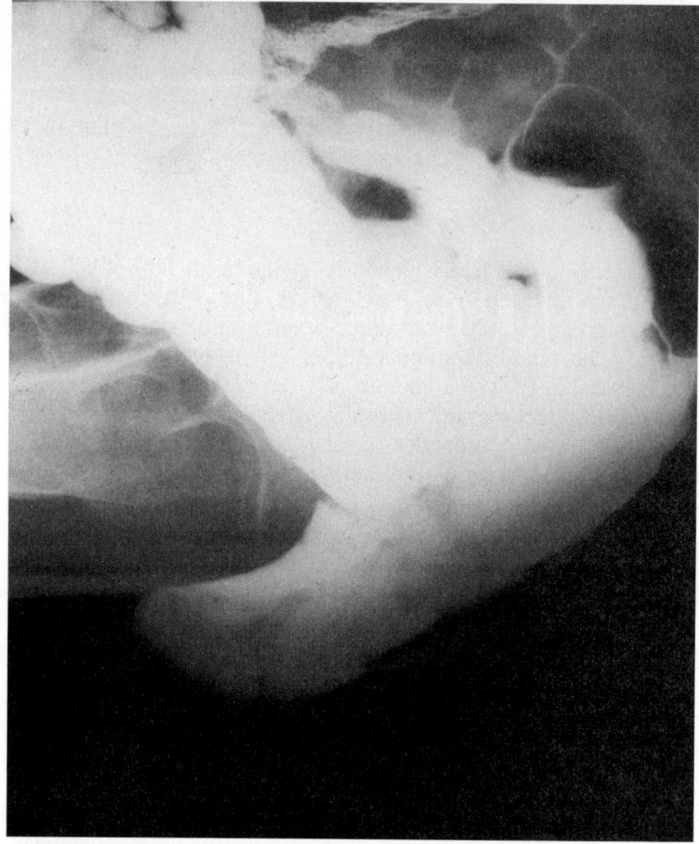

Figure 6 Defaecography of an enterocele with large intestine in the pouch of Douglas obstructing the rectal passage

upwards and sacrally in order to raise the pelvic floor and narrow the recto-vaginal pouch.

Intussusception

The rectum prolapse begins with the invagination of the middle rectal segment in the rectal ampulla. This was first described by Devadhar in 1965, using defaecography[18]. Various theories were developed and discarded: rectovaginal pouch extending down to the pelvic floor, pelvic floor weakness, loose fixation of the rectum in the lower abdomen especially in the peritoneal reflexion[19]. Constipation associated with low-roughage diet could be a possible aetiology. The observation that a change to a high-fibre diet among young patients causes the prolapse to disappear, supports this theory. The same is true for the solitary rectal ulcer. This is a result of anterior rectal wall intussusception.

Laparoscopic rectopexy is our preferred procedure when conservative therapy fails.

Pelvic floor hernia

Pelvic floor hernia is the descent of the posterior wall of the rectum into a gap between the ischiococcygeal muscle and the iliococcygeal muscle. The hernia develops either in the left or the right gap. The gap lies medial of the ischial tuberosity. Defaecography clearly shows the out-pocketing in the ampulla (Fig. 7)[20]. Parks' postanal repair is a possible therapy[9].

If a patient recounts that, during defaecation, one particular spot on the buttock has to be pushed in to evacuate completely, then a pelvic floor hernia has to be assumed.

Sphincter dysplasia or anismus

Anismus, also known as spastic pelvic floor syndrome, is an acquired form of functional outlet obstruction. During normal defaecation the sphincter muscle and the puborectalis sling relax; unlike in anismus, where the sphincter muscle and the puborectalis sling contract. This can be demonstrated by sphincter pressure manometry.

If functional outlet obstruction is not caused by anismus, then the most likely diagnosis is sphincter dysplasia.

This malformation is described in newborns as an anterior displaced anus or an ectopic anus. In young males intense complaints lead to an early diagnosis and an operation is generally performed by the paediatric surgeon. Among girls the diagnosis is most often overlooked, as the symptoms are not so intense. If other family members suffer from the same symptoms then the defaecation disorder is played down.

The autosomal dominant inherited anomaly shows a variable expressivity[21]. Normally the middle portion of the external anal sphincter inserts as connective tissue on the coccyx. These fibres are also known as the anococcygeal ligament, which fixes the dorsal anus to the coccyx. During squeezing the fixation helps the puborectalis sling to stretch passively (Fig. 8a). In sphincter dysplasia these fibres insert in the skin around the natal cleft instead of the coccyx. The inherited disorder can be documented using MRI and shown during the operation (Fig. 9). If the skeletal fixation is lacking the puborectalis (sling) does not open during straining at stool and the posterior circumference moves caudally and ventrally, unlike in healthy individuals where the puborectalis sling moves caudally and dorsally (Figs 8a and 8b). As a result the anus remains shut.

The possibility of an anismus must be excluded before an operation to correct sphincter dysplasia is considered. The balloon expulsion test, together with sphincter pressure manometry, can be used to differentiate between anismus and sphincter dysplasia. In anismus the sphincter remains contracted; in sphincter dysplasia the sphincter becomes lax. The balloon cannot be expelled in both cases.

Biofeedback training in anismus and sphincteropexy in sphincter dysplasia are the therapies of choice. Sphincteropexy is the fixation of the puborectalis sling to the sacrotuberal ligament. With this procedure good long term results are achieved in over 70% of patients[22].

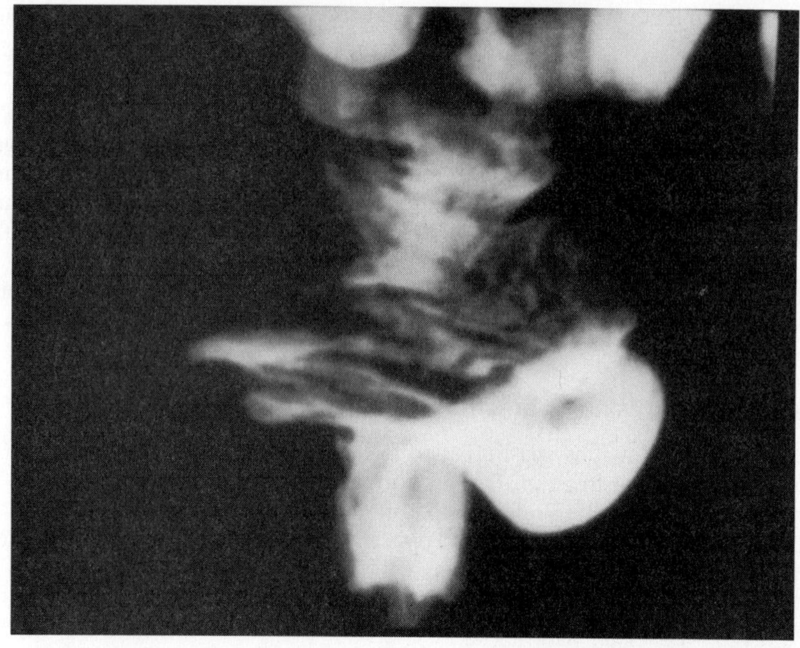

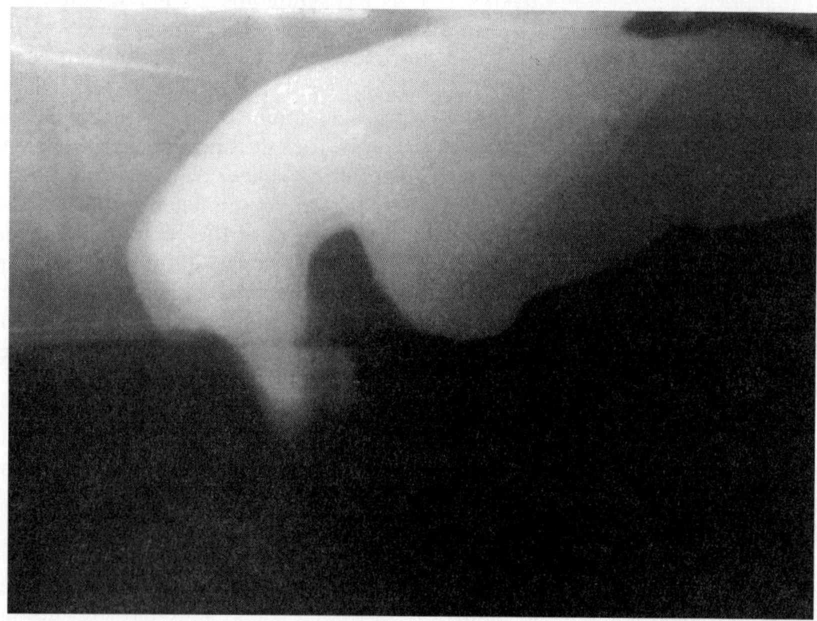

Figure 7 Defaecography of a pelvic floor hernia in the left levator ani muscle

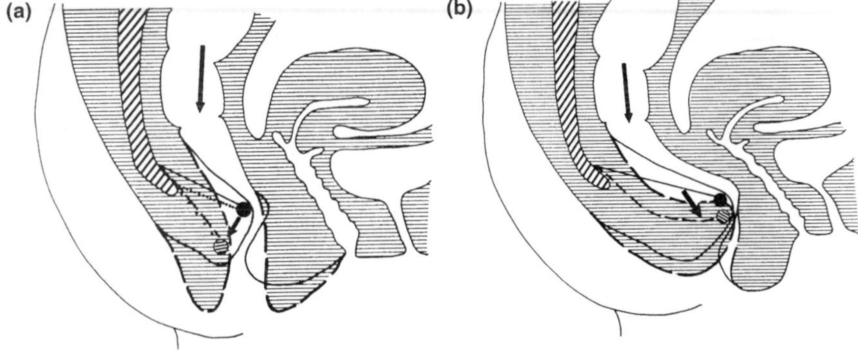

Figure 8 Sphincter dysplasia: (a) Straining for defaecation in healthy persons. Black point = puborectalis sling; dotted line = anococcygeal ligament; interrupted line = position of the levator ani while squeezing. (b) Straining in a patient with sphincter dysplasia (from ref. 22, with permission from S. Karger AG, Basel)

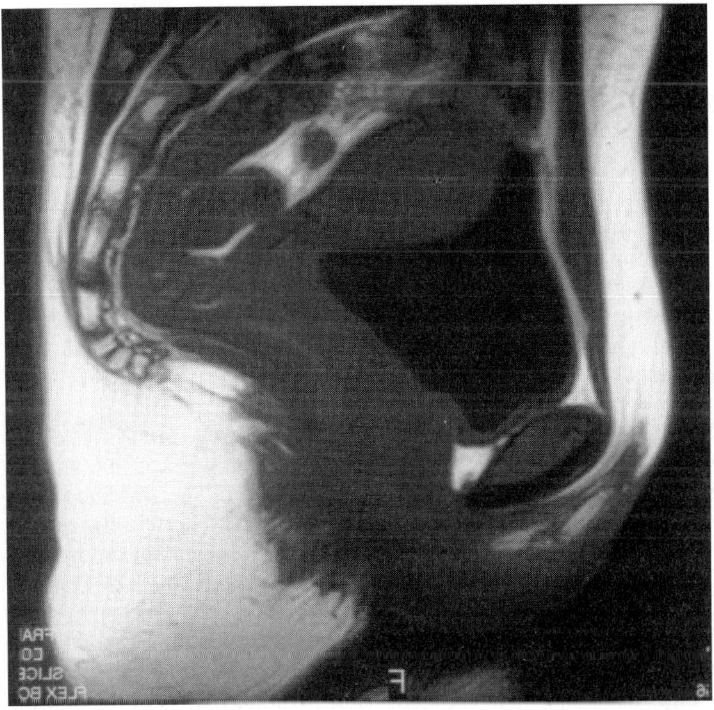

Figure 9 Sphincter dysplasia. (**a**) MRI sagittal cross-section of the middle plane of the pelvis in a normal individual

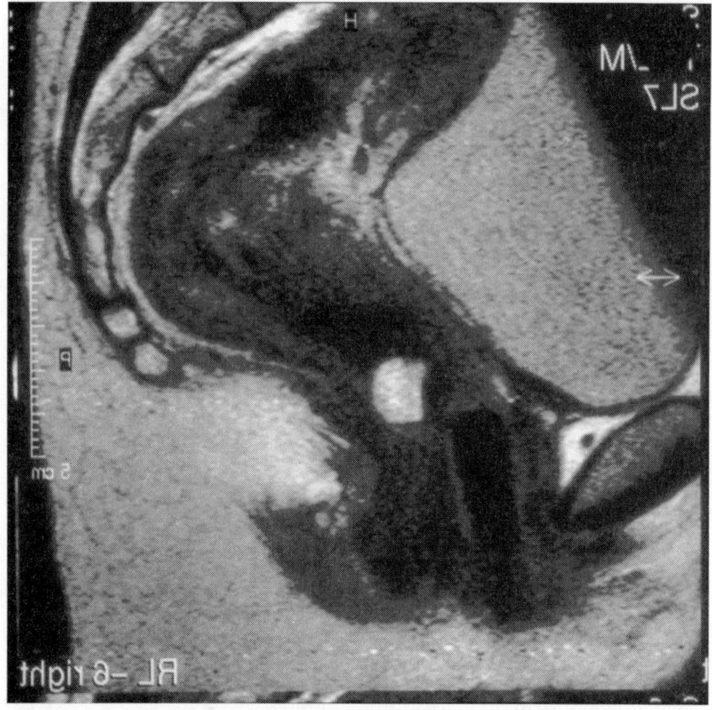

Figure 9(b)   MRI in a female with sphincter dysplasia; note the mass dorsally of the anal canal representing the middle portion of the external anal sphincter, inserting in the skin around the natal cleft

OTHER PELVIC FLOOR DISORDERS

Proctologists, gynaecologists and urologists tend to concentrate on their own compartment of the pelvic floor. It is important to be aware that pelvic floor disorders, although in a common interface, require the involvement of the various specialists.

Apart from an obstruction caused by an enterocele, the passage of stool through the rectum can also be obstructed by a retroversion of the uterus or a leiomyoma. The fundus of a retroverted uterus impinges on the anterior rectal wall, especially during the act of straining at stool. The so-called 'ball-valve' phenomenon interferes with undisturbed propulsion of stool in the rectum[23]. The same phenomenon occurs with leiomyomata when located at the isthmus or the cervix, or when a myoma on a pedicle is trapped in the pouch of Douglas.

The cause of genital prolapse is a matter for speculation, and is associated by some with a relaxation of the pelvic floor[24]. The same applies to the cystouretherocele.

Pudendal nerve damage, together with an impaired function of the sympathetic and parasympathetic nervous system, result in urinary incontinence. This may occur with or without an idiopathic faecal incontinence. The cause of stool incontinence, either ageing or pudendal neuropathy, is controversial and is a matter for discussion.

The pelvic floor must be investigated further, and hopefully research will combine all three compartments in the future.

References

1. Jorge JM, Wexner SD. Anatomy and physiology of the rectum and anus. Eur J Surg. 1997;163: 723–31.
2. Fröhlich B, Hotzinger H, Fritsch H. Tomographical anatomy of the pelvis, pelvic floor, and related structures. Clin Anat. 1997;10:223–30.
3. Wedel T, Roblick U, Gleiss J et al. Organization of the enteric nervous system in the human colon demonstrated by whole-mount immunohistochemistry with special reference to submucous plexus. Ann Anat. 1999;181:327–37.
4. Kamm MA. Diagnostic, pharmacological, surgical and behavioural developments in benign anorectal disease. Eur J Surg. 1998;582:119–23.
5. Buchmann P. Stuhlinkontinenz. In: Buchmann P, editor. Lehrbuch der Proktologie. Bern: Verlag Hans Huber, 1994:122–5.
6. Marti MC. Anal incontinence. In: Marti MC, Givel JC, editors. Surgical Management of Anorectal and Colonic Disease. Berlin: Springer, 1998:191–2.
7. Rasmussen OØ, Christiansen J, Tetzschner T, Sörensen M. Pudendal nerve function in idiopathic fecal incontinence. Dis Col Rectum. 2000;43:633–7.
8. Buchmann P, De Lorenzi D, Müller A. Re-Eingriffe bei sekundärer Inkontinenz. Chirurg. 1996;67:491–7.
9. Parks AG. Anorectal incontinence. Proc R Soc Med. 1975;68:681–90.
10. Pinho M, Ortiz J, Oya M, Panagamuwa B, Asperer J, Keighley MRB. Total pelvic floor repair for the treatment of neuropathic fecal incontinence. Am J Surg. 1992;163:340–3.
11. Marti MC. Descending perineum. In: Buchmann P, Brühlmann W, editors. Investigation of Anorectal Functional Disorders. Berlin: Springer, 1993:87.
12. DeLancy JOL. The analomy of the pelvic floor. Curr Opin Obstet Gynecol. 1994;6:313–16.
13. Huber A, v Hochstetter AHC, Allgöwer M. Transsphinktere Rektumchirurgie. Berlin: Springer, 1983:26.
14. Ludowikowski B, Kovacs P, Fritsch H. Das Rektovaginale Septum – Entwicklung, Verlauf und Funktion. Ann Anat. 1999;181:16.
15. Buchmann P. Defaekationsprobleme. In: Buchmann P, editor. Lehrbuch der Proktologie. Bern: Verlag Hans Huber, 1994:190–208.
16. Sullivan ES, Leaverton GH, Hardwick CE. Transrectal perineal repair: an adjunct to improved function after anorectal surgery. Dis Col Rectum. 1968;11:106–14.
17. Read CD. Hernia of the pouch of Douglas. In: Bourne AW, Nixon WCW, editors. Transactions of the Twelfth British Congress of Obstetricians and Gynaecologists. London: Australia Press, 1950:189–205.
18. Devadhar DSC. A new concept of mechanism and treatment of rectal proctidentia. Dis Col Rectum. 1965;8:75–7.
19. Gemsenjäger E. Rectal prolapse, solitary rectal ulcer syndrome, and descending perineal syndrome. In: Marti MC, Givel JC, editors. Surgical Management of Anorectal and Colonic Disease. Berlin: Springer, 1998:351–3.
20. Hauck R. Rectal outpocketing. In: Buchmann P, Brülmann W, editors. Investigation of Anorectal Functional Disorders. Berlin: Springer, 1993:149–61.
21. Zorzi A, Schinzel A, Hirsig J. Analsphinkterdysplasie als Ursache chronischer Defaekationsstörungen: eine klinische und genetische Studie. Schweiz Med. Wochenschr 1991;121:1567–75.
22. Buchmann P, Bruhin R, Sartoretti Ch, De Lorenzi D. Sphincteropexy: a new operation to cure outlet obstruction in adults. Dig Surg. 1997;14:413–18.
23. Hudson CN. Female genital prolapse and pelvic floor deficiency. Int Colorect Dis 1988;3:181–5
24. Hudson CN. Gynaecological conditions and coloproctology. In: Henry MM, Swash M, editors. Coloproctology and the Pelvic Floor. Oxford: Butterworth–Heinemann, 1992:459–60.

3
Intrinsic innervation and innervational abnormalities of the colorectum – from morphology to molecular genetics

H.-J. KRAMMER, T. WEDEL, K.-H. SCHÄFER,
T. H. K. SCHIEDECK, U. J. ROBLICK and H.-P. BRUCH

INTRODUCTION

About 100 years ago, in 1899, the Danish pediatrician Harald Hirschsprung[1] published a case report entitled 'Constipation of newborns due to dilatation and hypertrophy of the colon'. He described a congenital megacolon caused by intestinal aganglionosis in twin brothers who died of subsequent enterocolitis. However, Hirschsprung was not aware of the underlying pathology. It took two decades to discover that in congenital megacolon the primary morphological defect resides within the enteric nervous system (ENS). These histopathological observations were communicated by Dalla-Valle[2], and illustrated for the first time that structural abnormalities of the ENS are capable of provoking severe disturbances of intestinal motility. The advancing knowledge of the morphology of the ENS has led to the recognition of a wide range of ENS pathologies associated with distinct gastrointestinal motility disorders[3]. As for the colon, motor dysfunctions cause conditions which are clinically characterized by a delayed colonic transit time and, in some instances, by a concomitant development of a megacolon. To assess and classify the underlying histopathological alterations of the ENS, a comprehensive demonstration of the entire nerve plexus components within the human colonic wall is required.

INNERVATION OF THE COLORECTUM

Gastrointestinal functions are controlled by neural, humoral and myogenic mechanisms. The neural control involves intrinsic and extrinsic components. The well-known sympathetic and parasympathetic nervous systems provide the extrinsic innervation. However, the gastrointestinal tract is characterized additionally by an extensive and very differentiated intrinsic nervous system, the ENS. Basic functions such as motility, absorption and secretion are regulated by the ENS virtually independently from the central nervous system. The ENS comprises all nervous elements located within the gastrointestinal tube from the oesophagus to the internal anal sphincter, including the gallbladder, the bile duct system and the pancreas. Only those regions containing striated musculature – the upper part of the oesophagus and the external anal sphincter – are innervated predominantly by extrinsic nerves[4,5].

One of the most characteristic structural features of the ENS is the existence of multiple neuronal networks within the different layers of the intestinal wall (Fig. 1). The arrangement of these intramural plexus has been studied intensively over the past 120 years in various animal species. The number and size of ganglia, the spatial organization of the networks, the neuronal cytoarchitecture as well as the neurotransmitter content vary between the different species and the different intestinal segments. However, in spite of these differences, the general structural patterns of the ENS are basically similar: the majority of nerve cells are localized within the ganglia, the ganglia are connected by nerve fibre strands, both the ganglia and the internodal nerve fibre strands form networks extending throughout the entire intestinal circumference[6,7]. In addition to the ganglionated plexus the intestinal wall also contains aganglionated networks which have no nerve cells and consist of nerve fibre strands.

In contrast to smaller laboratory animals (e.g. rat and guinea-pig), in which only two ganglionated plexus have been described, the human colon exhibits four ganglionated plexus as demonstrated by whole-mount preparations. The *plexus myentericus* (Auerbach)[8] is composed of ganglia and interconnecting

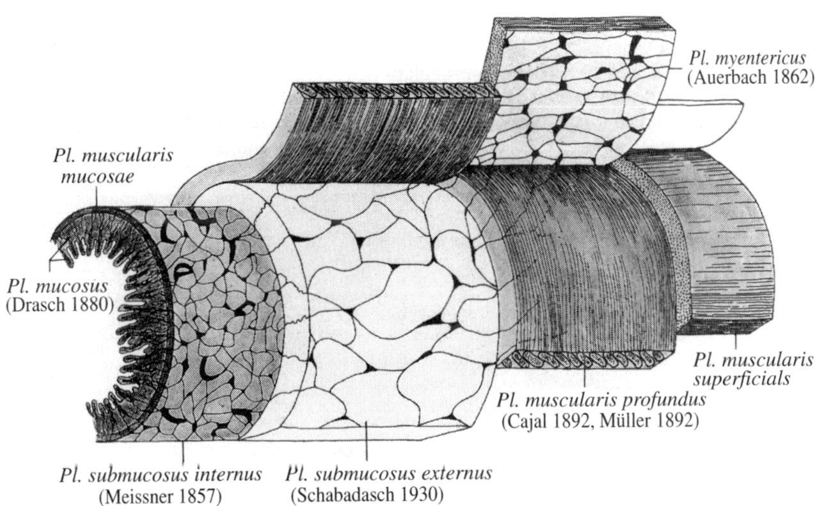

Figure 1 Schematic drawing of the topography, architecture and nomenclature of the ganglionated and aganglionated plexus of the ENS as demonstrated by whole-mount preparations

nerve fibre strands forming a polygonal network within the intermuscular plane delimited by the circular and longitudinal muscle layer. The ganglionated nerve network is arranged more densely in the descending colon than in the ascending colon. Whereas primary and secondary nerve fibre strands establish the connections between the ganglia, tertiary nerve fibre strands ramify into the adjacent muscle layers. Nerve cells are located predominantly within the ganglia, but are also disseminated within all types of nerve fibre strands. The *plexus submucosus extremus* is located at the outermost border of the tela submucosa in close association to the adjacent circular muscle layer. At regular intervals thin nerve fibre strands run almost parallel to the circular muscle layer and form a delicate network which contains single nerve cells as well as small ganglia. Although closely related to the plexus submucosus externus, the plexus submucosus extremus is considered as an independent plexus because of its distinct topography and architecture. The plexus submucosus extremus seems to be involved in the generation of rhythmical slow waves, which originate from the network of intestinal cells of Cajal at the circular muscle–submucosa interface[9,10]. The *plexus submucosus externus* (Schabadasch)[11,12] is located within the outer portion of the tela submucosa and forms a nerve network with relatively wide meshes. Among the three submucosus plexus, the nerve fibre strands and the ganglia of the plexus submucosus externus possess the largest diameters and sizes respectively. The *plexus submucosus internus* (Meissner)[13] is located within the inner portion of the tela submucosa beneath the lamina muscularis mucosae and exhibits an architecture similar to the plexus submucosus externus. However, the meshes of the nerve network are denser and the nerve fibre strands and ganglia show smaller diameters and sizes respectively. The ganglia predominantly have a round shape and exceed the plexus submucosus externus in number. The following plexus compartments are considered to be aganglionated: plexus muscularis superficialis or longitudinalis, plexus muscularis profundus or circularis, plexus muscularis mucosae and plexus mucosus[14–16].

Another important feature of the ENS is the morphological variety of neurons reflecting its functional complexity. The first and most popular classification was inaugurated by Dogiel[17] in 1896, who differentiated between type I and type II neurons. The existence of a type III neuron has been less accepted because of its indistinct description[18]. Whereas Dogiel and other authors classified according to shape only, Stach and colleagues have defined and used further morphological criteria for the differentiation of enteric nerve cells[19]. In addition to the shape of pericarya and of the neuronal processes these criteria include the course of axonal projections, intercellular relationships, topographic arrangement within the ganglia and regional distribution patterns. This more sophisticated classification is based on silver-impregnated whole-mount preparations and has led to a "multi-neuron-theory" comprising up to eight enteric nerve cell types.

INNERVATIONAL ABNORMALITIES OF THE COLORECTUM

The knowledge of the normal structure of the ENS in the human colon is of clinical significance, as several gastrointestinal motility disorders are associated with defects of the ENS residing within the colon[3]. Thus, the above-described morphological characteristics may serve as a baseline for the assessment of structural alterations of the colonic ENS. The crucial role of a morphologically intact ENS for normal intestinal motility is best illustrated if enteric nerve cells are completely lacking within defined segments of the gut. However, decreases, increases or an abnormal topographic distribution of ENS components are also capable of provoking severe disturbances of colonic transit. The following structural abnormalities of ENS have been found in adult patients with chronic colonic motility disorders including the development of a megacolon[20,21].

Aganglionosis

Intestinal aganglionosis is encountered in classic Hirschsprung's disease and defined by the complete absence of nerve cells within caudal regions of the gastrointestinal tract. Aganglionosis is not confined to newborns or children, but is also observed in adults[21]. Instead of a ganglionated network thickened nerve fibre strands pass through the intermuscular zone in a craniocaudal direction and are irregularly distributed within the tela submucosa (Figs 2 and 3). Proximal to the aganglionic segment appears a transitional zone of variable extent with disseminated clusters of nerve cells.

Hypoganglionosis

In comparison to a normally configurated myenteric plexus, hypoganglionosis is characterized by a considerable reduction of the number of ganglia per intestinal length. The ganglia are smaller, contain less neurons and predominantly show round shapes (Fig. 4). Depending on the extent of the quantitative alterations hypoganglionic conditions can be classified into different degrees of severity. In particular moderate forms of hypoganglionosis require a subtle morphometric analysis to be confirmed, as they are not so readily recognized in conventional cross-sections.

Hyperganglionosis

The term hyperganglionosis refers to the submucous plexus and describes hyperplastic changes of both ganglia and nerve fibre strands. The histopathological features include submucous giant ganglia with a two- to three-fold increase in the content of nerve cells and the presence of hypertrophied nerve fibre strands (Fig. 5). These findings have been previously described by Meier-Ruge et al.[22] as intestinal neuronal dysplasia (IND). IND is frequently combined with myenteric aganglionosis and hypoganglionosis, but may also be found as an isolated form.

Heterotopic ganglia

In addition to hypoganglionic changes, ectopically localized ganglia represent another form of non-aganglionic innervation disorder observed in patients with colonic motor dysfunctions. In contrast to normotopic ganglia positioned between the circular and longitudinal muscle layer, heterotopic ganglia are located outside the intermuscular zone within the tunica muscularis (Fig. 6).

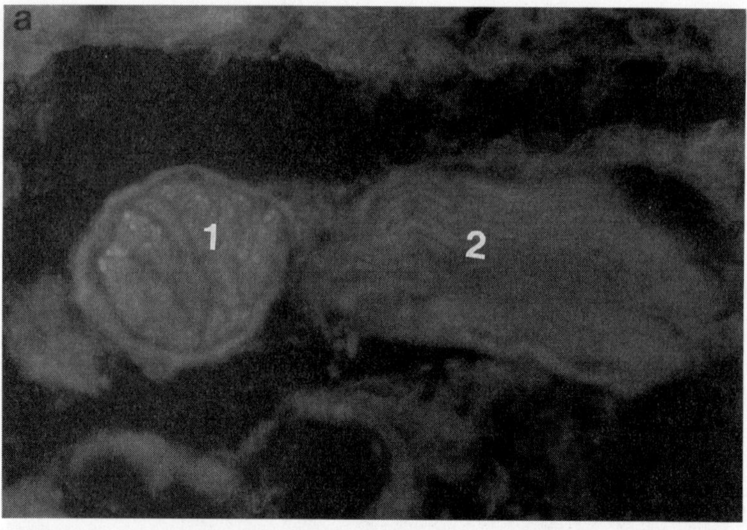

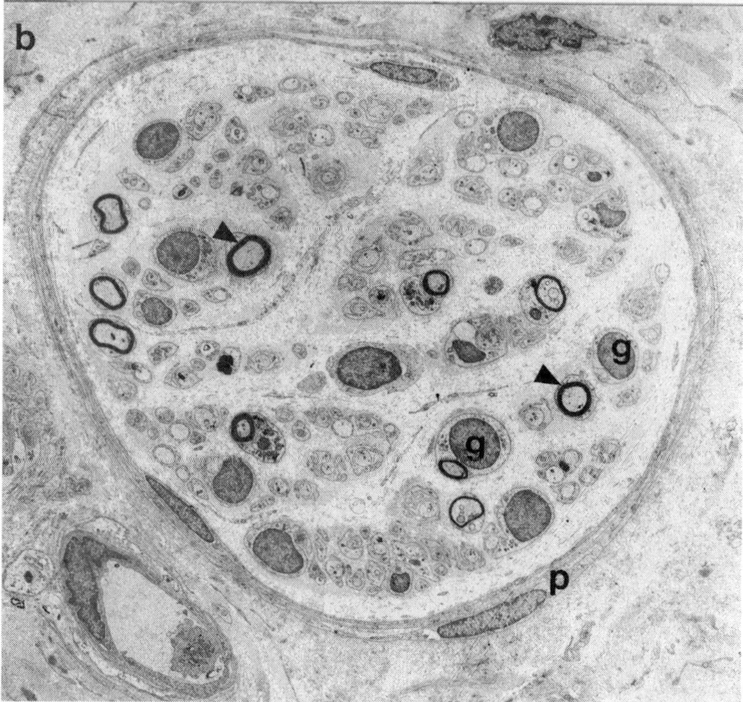

Figure 2 Aganglionosis (Morbus Hirschsprung). (a) Transverse (1) and longitudinal (2) section through hypertrophied nerve fibre bundles running within myenteric plexus plane. (b) Electron micrograph of a hyertrophied nerve fibre bundle showing the perineural sheath (p) and the endoneural space filled with multiple myelinated axons (arrow-heads) and glial cells (g)

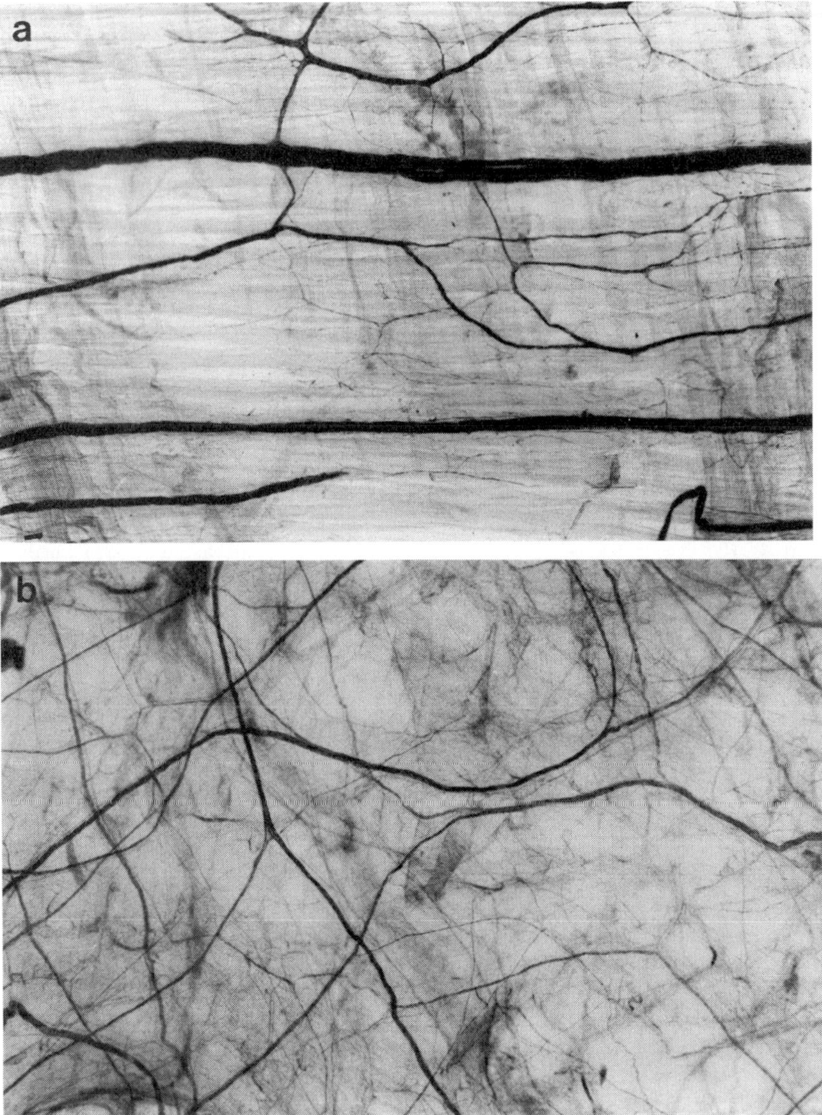

Figure 3 Aganglionosis (Morbus Hirschsprung). (a) Whole-mount preparation of the tunica muscularis showing thickened nerve fibre strands running parallel in craniocaudal direction. (b) Wholemount preparation of the tela submucosa which contains an irregular network of nerve fibre strands devoid of nerve cells and ganglia

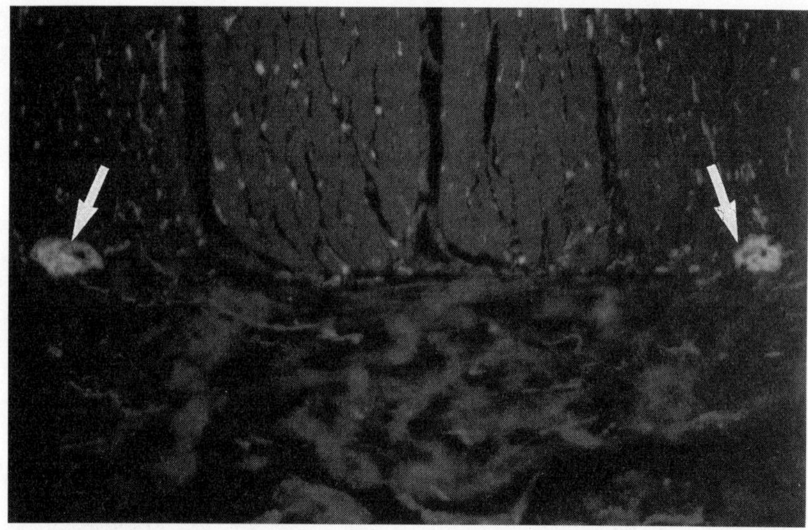

Figure 4 Hypoganglionosis in a section. The myenteric plexus exhibits a decreased ganglionic density, the remaining ganglia (arrows) are smaller, contain less neurons and show round shapes

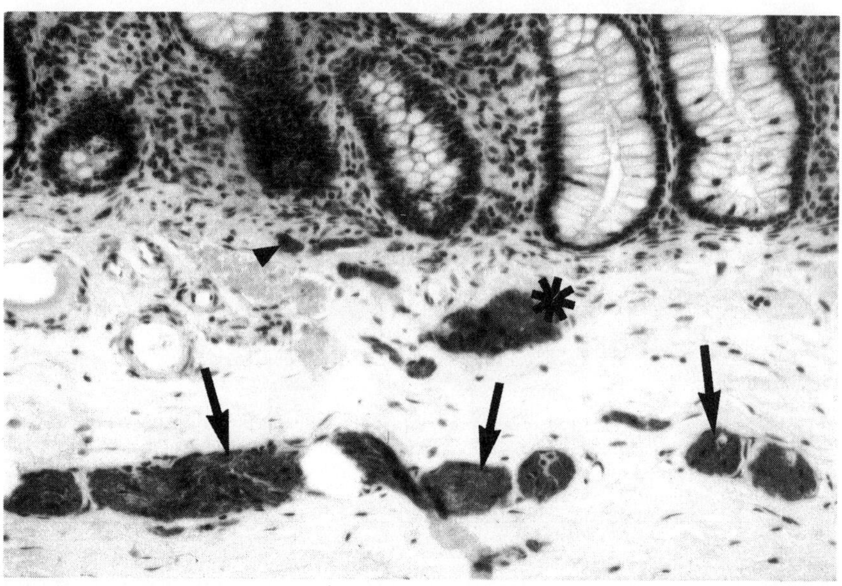

Figure 5 Intestinal neuronal dysplasia (IND) in a section. The submucous plexus is characterized by numerous hypertrophied nerve fibre strands (arrows) and giant ganglia (asterisk) with an increased content of nerve cells

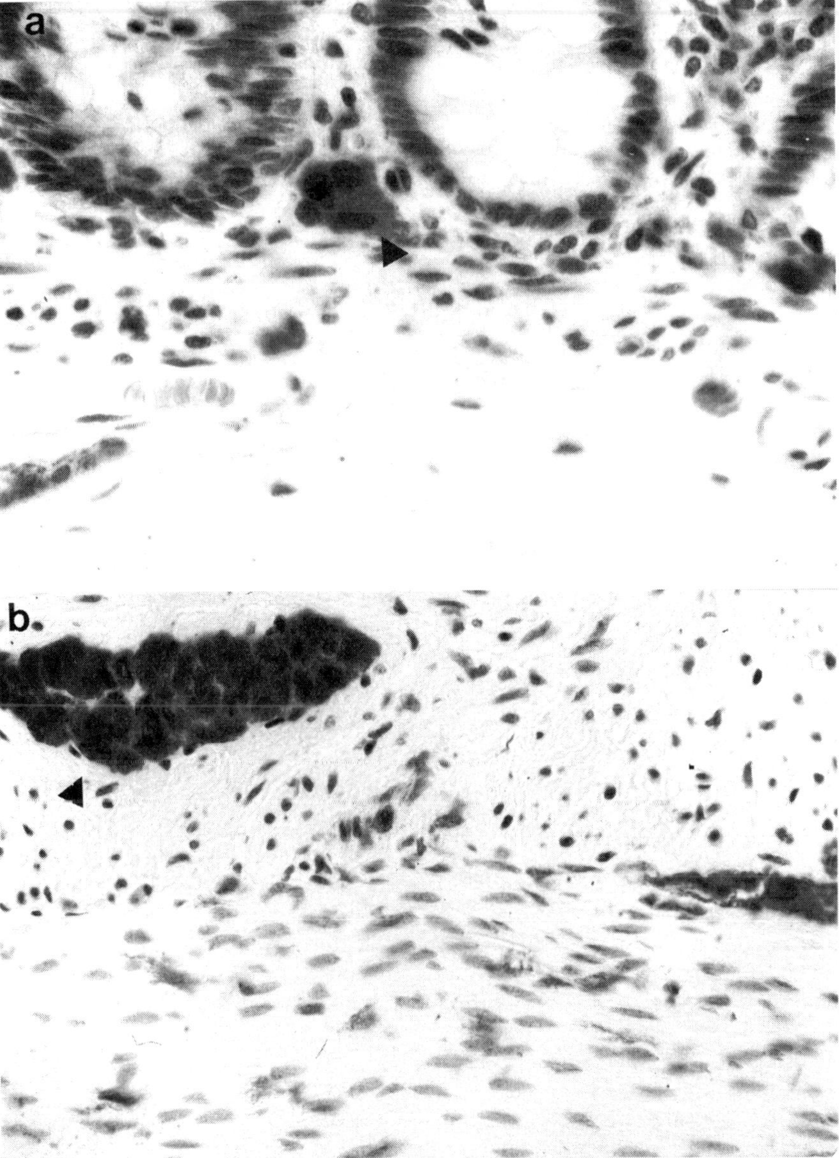

Figure 6 Heterotopic ganglia. (a) Ectopic ganglion (arrow-head) located within the lamina propria mucosae between two adjacent epithelia crypts. (b) Ectopic ganglion (arrow-head) located outside the intermuscular zone (myenteric plexus plane) within the muscle layer

MOLECULAR GENETICS OF ENTERIC INNERVATIONAL ABNORMALITIES

Studies of knockout animal models and mutant strains have provided novel insights into the development of the ENS and the pathogenesis of intestinal motility disorders. To date, mutations at six distinct gene loci involved in the normal development, proliferation and differentiation of cell systems responsible for the generation of intestinal motility have been described. They are discussed briefly below:

1. The ret proto-oncogene, which encodes for a tyrosine kinase receptor, is necessary for the normal development of the mammalian ENS. Mutations of a locus containing the ret oncogene occur in sporadic and familial Hirschsprung's disease – perhaps more frequently in long-segment rather than in short-segment forms[23–26].
2. Mutations of a gene encoding the glial cell-derived neurotrophic factor (GDNF), a ligand for the tyrosine kinase receptor, have been described in a few patients with Hirschsprung's disease[27].
3. Homozygous mutations in the endothelin 3/endothelin B-receptor system result in the autosomal recessive Waardenburg–Shan syndrome characterized by piebaldism, heterochromasia of the iris, sensorineural deafness and congenital megacolon[28–30] (Fig. 7). Heterozygous mutations occur in 5–10% of patients with Hirschsprung's disease.
4. The Sox 10 transcription factor is crucial for the development of the ENS from migrating neural crest cells[31]. Mutations occur in the Waardenburg–Shan syndrome[32].
5. The proto-oncogene c-kit encodes for a tyrosine kinase receptor that facilitates the development of interstitial cells of Cajal, the intestinal pacemaker cells[33,34]. A relative deficiency of c-kit-positive interstitial cells of Cajal has been reported in Hirschsprung's disease and in cases of chronic intestinal pseudo-obstruction[35,36].

The lack or deficiency of receptors or transcription factors lead to failures in the migration of precursor cells of the ENS from the neural crest to the bowel. If the appropriate setting of neurotrophic factors is not supplied at defined developmental stages, various syndromes or diseases may result depending on the factor lacking[37]. Measurements of the amount of neurotrophins in the gut wall of patients with Hirschsprung's disease show considerable differences between the affected and non-affected intestinal segments. Whereas the content of GDNF decreases from the proximal to the aganglionic segment, no significant alterations are observed for the classical nerve growth factor (personal observation). For an undisturbed growth and development of the ENS during organogenesis of the intestine and also beyond birth, the appropriate composition and combination of trophic factors is absolutely essential.

CONCLUSIONS

Conventional cross-sections combined with whole-mount preparations improve the visualization of the ENS and allow a two-dimensional assessment of each of the intramural plexus layers. The diagnosis and classification of structural

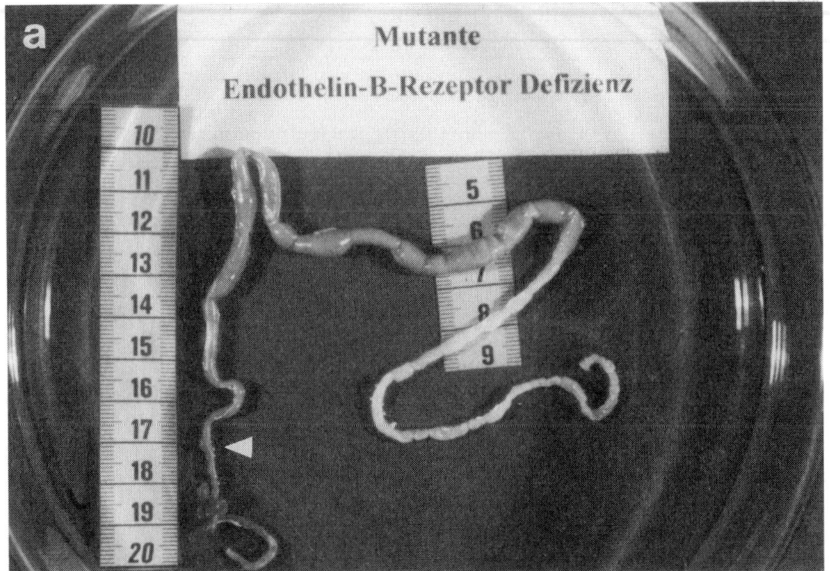

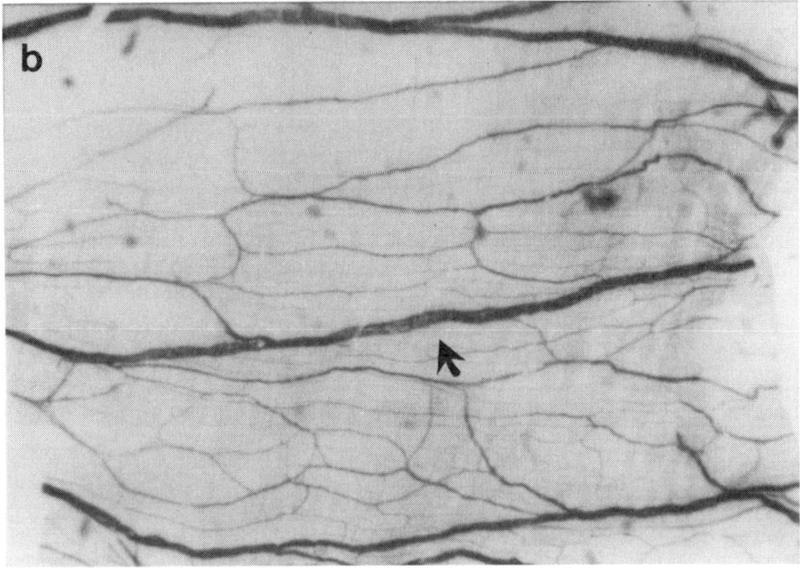

Figure 7 Homocygous endothelin B-receptor-deficient rat. (a) The distal ileum, caecum and colon (arrow-head) are constricted. Orally to the narrowed segments the intestine is dilated. (b) The whole-mount preparation of the constricted colon shows a complete aganglionosis with hypertrophied nerve fibre bundles arranged in a pattern similarly observed in patients with Hirschsprung's disease (compare to Fig. 3a)

innervational disorders affecting the human colon are thereby facilitated. Between aganglionosis encountered in classic Hirschsprung's disease and normoganglionosis exists a range of non-aganglionic structural abnormalities of the ENS. They include hypoganglionosis and heterotopic ganglia of the myenteric plexus as well as hyperplastic changes of the submucous plexus. Obviously, non-aganglionic alterations are also capable of provoking severe disturbances of intestinal motility including the development of a megacolon. In chronically constipated patients without megacolon the neuropathological defects are less frequent and pronounced. However, the assessment of whole-mount preparations frequently reveals structural alterations of the ENS involving both the myenteric plexus (hypoganglionosis) and the submucous plexus (hyperplastic changes).

Severe intestinal innervation disorders are generally diagnosed in early childhood. Minor alterations may remain unrecognized during infancy and adolescence and may not cause aggravated symptoms until adulthood. As a consequence, in adult patients with long-standing intractable constipation in whom secondary causes and upper gastrointestinal tract motility disorders have been previously excluded, a histopathological assessment of the ENS is recommended. Deep submucous biopsies are suitable for the diagnosis of Hirschsprung's disease and for the evaluation of the submucous plexus layers. However, as myenteric hypoganglionosis represents a common histopathological finding in these patients, full-thickness biopsies provide a more comprehensive assessment of the morphology of the ENS. After a careful clinically based preselection, this procedure may serve as an additional tool for the diagnostic and therapeutic approach in patients with chronic motor dysfunction of the colon.

Acknowledgements

The authors thank Mrs S. Tögel, Mrs W. Maaß, Mrs K. Budler and Mrs G. Knebel for their painstaking technical assistance and for their help in the preparation of the manuscript. The work was supported by grants from the Deutsche Forschungsgemeinschaft (DFG Kr 1257/2-2) and the Research Foundation of the Medical Universtiy of Lübeck (1599/J-25).

References

1. Hirschsprung H. Stuhlträgheit Neugeborener in Folge von Dilatation und Hypertrophie des Kolons. Jahrb Kinderh. 1899;27:1–7.
2. Dalla-Valle A. Ricerche istologische su di un caso megacolon congenito. Pediatria. 1920;28:740–52.
3. Goyal RK, Hirano I. Mechanisms of disease. The enteric nervous system. N Engl J Med. 1996; 334:1106–15.
4. Furness JB, Costa M. The Enteric Nervous System. New York: Churchill Livingstone, 1987.
5. Stach W, Brehmer A, Krammer H-J. Übersicht über das Nervensystem. In: Waldeyer A, Mayet A, editors. Anatomie des Menschen 1: Berlin, Walter de Gruyter, 1993, pp. 146–69.
6. Radke R, Krammer H-J. Enteric nervous system (ENS) similarities and differences in the gastrointestinal tract, gallblader, and pancreas. Neurogastroenterologia. 1996;3:93–105.
7. Krammer HJ, Zhang M, Kühnel W. Distribution of NADPH-diaphorase-positive neurons in the enteric nervous system of the human colon. Ann Anat. 1994;176:137–41.
8. Auerbach L. Über einen Plexus myentericus, einen bisher unbekannten ganglionervösen Apparat im Darmkanal der Wirbeltiere. Breslau: E Morgenstern, 1862.
9. Christensen J, Rick GA. Intrinsic nerves in the mammalian colon: confirmation of a plexus at the circular muscle–submucosal interface. J Autonom Nerv Syst. 1987;21:223–31.

10. Stach W. Der Plexus entericus extremus des Dickdarms und seine Beziehungen zu den intestitiellen Zellen (Cajal). Z Mikrosk Anat Rosch. 1972;85:245–72.

11. Schabadasch A. Intramurale Nervengeflechte des Darmrohrs. Z Zellforsch Mikrosk Anat. 1930;10:320–85.

12. Stach W. Der Plexus submucosus externus (Schabadasch) im Dünndarm des Schweines. I. Form, Struktur und Verbindungen der Ganglien und der Nervenzellen. Z Mikrosk Anat Forsch. 1977;91:737–55.

13. Meissner G. Über die Nerven der Darmwand. Z Ration Med NF. 1857;8:364–6.

14. Cajal SR y. Sur les ganglions et plexus nerveux de l'intestin. C R Soc Biol. 1893;9:217–23.

15. Müller E. Zur Kenntnis der Ausbreitung und Endigungsweise der Magen, Darm und Pankreasnerven. Arch Mikroskop Anat. 1892;40:390–408.

16. Drasch O. Beiträge zur Kenntnis des feineren Baues des Dünndarms, insbesondere über die Nerven desselben. Sitz Ber Akad Wiss (Wien), Math-Naturw Kl, Abt III. 1880;82:168–98.

17. Dogiel AS. Zwei Arten sympathischer Nervenzellen. Anat Anz. 1896;11:679–87.

18. Dogiel AS. Über den Bau der Ganglien in den Geflechten des Darmes und der Gallenblase des Menschen und der Säugetiere. Arch Anat Physiol. 1899; Anat Abt.4:130–58.

19. Stach W, Brehmer A, Krammer H-J. Structural organisation of enteric nerve cells in large mammals including man. In: Krammer, H-J. Singer MV, editors. Neurogastroenterology – From the Basics to the Clinics. Lancaster: Kluwer; 2000, pp. 3–21.

20. Holschneider AM, Meier-Ruge W, Ure BM. Hirschsprung's disease and allied disoders – a review. Eur J Pediatr Surg. 1994;4:260–6.

21. Wheatley MJ, Wesley JR, Coran AG, Polley TZ. Hirschsprung's disease in adolescents and adults. Dis Colon Rectum. 1990;33:622–9.

22. Meier-Ruge W, Gambazzi F, Käufeler RE, Schmid P, Schmidt CP. The neuropathological diagnosis of neuronal intestinal dysplasia (NID B). Eur J Pediatr Surg. 1994;4:267–73.

23. Lyonnet S, Bolino A, Pelet A et al. A gene for Hirschsprung's disease maps to the proximal long arm of chromosome 10. Nature Genet. 1993;4:346–50.

24. Edery P, Lyonnet S, Mulligan LM et al. Mutations of the RET proto-oncogene in Hirschsprung's disease. Nature. 1994;367:378–9.

25. Romeo G, Rochetto P, Yin L et al. Point mutations affecting the tyrosine kinase domain for the RET proto-oncogene in Hirschsprung's disease. Nature. 1994;367:377–8.

26. Attie T, Pelet A, Edery P et al. Diversity of RET proto-oncogene mutations in familial and sporadic Hirschsprung disease. Hum Mol Genet. 1995;4:1381–6.

27. Trupp M, Arenas E, Fainzilber M et al. Functional receptor for GDNF encoded by c-ret proto-oncogene. Nature. 1996;38:785–9.

28. Attie T, Till M, Pelet A et al. Mutation of the endothelin-3 gene in Waardenburg–Hirschsprung disease. Hum Mol Genet. 1995;4:2407–9.

29. Edery P, Attie T, Amiel J et al. Mutation of the endothelin-3 gene in Waardenburg–Hirschsprung disease (Shah–Waadenburg syndrome). Nature Genet. 1996;12:442–4.

30. Greenstein-Baynash A, Hosoda K, Giaid A et al. Interaction of endothelin-3 with endothelin B receptor is essential for development of epidermal melanocytes and enteric neurons. Cell. 1994;79:1277–85.

31. Southard-Smith EM, Kos L, Pavan WJ. Sox 10 mutations disrupts neural crest development in Dom Hirschsprung mouse model. Nature Genet. 1998;18:60–4.

32. Pingault V, Bondurand N, Kuhlbrodt K et al. Sox mutations in patients with Waardenburg–Hirschsprung disease. Nature Genet. 1998;18:171–3.

33. Maeda H, Yamagata A, Nishikawa et al. Requirement of c-kit for development of intestinal pacemaker system. Development. 1992;116:369–75.

34. Huizinga JD, Thuneberg L, Klüppel M, Malysz J, Mikkelsen HB, Bernstein A. W/kit gene required for interstitial cells of Cajal and for pacemaker activity. Nature. 1995;373:347–9.

35. Vanderwinden JM, Rumessen JJ, Liu H, Descamps D, De Laet MH, Vanderhaeghen JJ. Interstitial cells of Cajal in human colon and in Hirschsprung's disease. Gastroenterology. 1996;111:901–10.

36. Isozaki K, Hirota S, Miyagawa JI, Taniguchi M, Shinomura Y, Matzuzawa Y. Deficiency of c-kit cells in patients with a myopathic form of chronic idiopathic intestinal pseudo-obstruction. Am J Gastroenterol. 1997;92:332–4.

37. Gershon M. Genes and lineages in the development of congenital defects of the enteric nervous system. In: Krammer H-J, Singer MV, editors. Neurogastroenterology – From the Basics to the Clinics. Lancaster: Kluwer; 2000, pp. 411–23.

Section II
Dysfunction of the pelvic floor

4
Endosonography in benign anorectal disorders

A. FUERST, M. BURGER, H. MESSMANN and L. HUTZEL

INTRODUCTION

Endosonography of the lower gastrointestinal tract was first described in the 1950s by Wild and Reid[1] in studies on the rectal wall. In 1983 it was introduced into the preoperative assessment of rectal carcinomas[2-4]. As the experience of the examiners grew, indications for this method expanded to the field of benign diseases of the anorectum. Simultaneously the equipment improved with regard to resolution and ease of handling.

Endosonographic examination is also suitable for the investigation of extrarectal structures, and allows sonography-guided biopsies of intra- and extramural processes[5]. It became a valuable tool in localizing pathological changes and influenced clinical decision-making concerning operative procedures for anorectal disorders.

PATIENT'S POSITION AND INVESTIGATION TECHNIQUE

Anorectal endosonography is usually performed in the left lateral decubitus position. The lithotomy position is more suitable if sedating drugs are necessary in patients with painful anorectal disorders and if biopsies are necesary. Normally special preparation of the patient is not required. In case of incomplete evacuation an enema should be performed. Following clinical rectal examination the ultrasound probe is passed into the rectum.

We apply a rotating transducer supplied by Kretz (Combison 310+, Zipf, Austria). This probe allows transversal 360° as well as longitudinal imaging. The transducer measures 16 cm in length and 21 mm in diameter. The frequency can be adjusted between 5.0 and 10.0 MHz during the examination. The maximum focal range is about 7 cm. Details of about 1 mm diameter can be depicted. A latex balloon is put over the hard cone and is filled with degassed water. Usually we prefer a 7.5 MHz transducer, and a 5.0 MHz probe is used for distant processes requiring a longer focal length.

ULTRASOUND ANATOMY

Anal canal and anal sphincter

The morphology of the anal canal was assessed in multiple endosonographic studies in healthy volunteers and anatomical specimens[6–15]. In the proximal part of the anal canal the puborectal muscle can usually be visualized. This is a striated muscle, so it appears highly echogenic and is visible as a U-shaped muscle sling around the anorectal flexure inserting ventrally at the pubic bone. It is close to the caudal part of the levator muscle. Between the U-shaped puborectal sling there is the vagina in women, typically seen as a three-layered structure (hyperechoic–hypoechoic–hyperechoic)[5]. Pulling back the probe the echogenic sling encircles the anal canal ventrally and forms the external anal sphincter. The thickness of the external sphincter is 5–10 mm in diameter[8,10,12,14,16,17]. In females the anterior sphincter is usually shorter and thinner and about 7.7 ± 1.1 mm in diameter; in men it is 8.6 ± 1 mm. Besides gender-specific differences the thickness of the sphincter is also correlated to body weight[16]. Age-related changes of the external sphincter could not be shown[14,17–20]. A uniform anatomical description of the external anal sphincter does not exist. Some authors describe a deep and superficial part with further divisions[21], whereas others see it as one circular muscle[22–24]. The hypoechoic internal sphincter lies inside the external anal sphincter; it is in continuity with the muscularis propria layer of the rectal wall. A diameter of 1–3 mm was found[8,10,12,14,16,25,26]. Thickness and echogenicity of the internal sphincter increase with age in affected as well as in healthy people. This is explained by increased sclerosis during ageing[27]. There is no correlation between body weight or height or gender and sphincter diameter[25].

Between the internal and external anal sphincter a small longitudinal muscle can be visualized by endosonography, which is a hyperechoic band in continuity of the longitudinal muscle of the rectum[10,16,28]. The function of this muscle is not precisely known, but it obviously supports eversion of the anus during defaecation[29].

Rectal wall and pararectal region

The layers of the rectal wall can be identified by endosonography corresponding to the histological layers. This is widely accepted and has been proved in numerous studies[4,30,31]. The five basic layers of the gastrointestinal wall form the standard in the interpretation of rectal endosonography:

1. the hyperechoic layer is the interface between the water-balloon and the mucosal surface;
2. the hypoechoic layer is a combined layer of the mucosa and the muscularis mucosae;
3. the hyperechoic layer is the submucosa;
4. the hypoechoic layer is the muscularis propria;
5. the hyperechoic layer is the interface between the muscularis propria and the perirectal fat, or the serosa if present[31].

The perirectal tissue appears to be of varying echogenicity; it is predominantly hypoechoic. In men the bladder, urethra and prostate; and in women the vagina, uterus and adnexal structures, can be visualized. Parts of the small bowel can also be seen around the proximal third of the rectum.

INDICATIONS FOR ANORECTAL ENDOSONOGRAPHY IN BENIGN DISORDERS

Anal incontinence

One of the most important and most frequent indications for anal endosonography is investigation of the anatomy of the anal canal. Before the introduction of anal endosonography it was believed that damage to the pudendal nerve was the main cause of faecal incontinence[32,33]. However, several endosonographic studies have concluded that obstetric trauma is the most common cause of faecal incontinence[34,35]. In one endosonographic study Sultan *et al.* found sphincter defects in 35% of primi parae after vaginal delivery[34]. The percentage of defects increases up to 80% after instrumental delivery[34]. Even in obviously atraumatic deliveries sphincter traumas occur, as shown in several studies[36–39]. Sphincter defects are found mostly in the anterior side, and in many cases both the internal and external sphincter are affected[34].

Sphincter defects are frequently found after surgical procedures. The defects may be located at any part of the sphincter, depending on the operation. An isolated defect of the internal anal sphincter can frequently be found[17]. These findings are described after haemorrhoidectomies, lateral sphincterotomies, surgery for fistulas, and transanal stapling of coloanal or ileoanal anastomoses[40–43]. Since sphincter defects and faecal incontinence have been recorded, manual anal dilatation cannot be recommended[39,44,45].

By using endosonography, further causes of anal incontinence, such as primary internal sphincter degeneration (leading to a passive anal incontinence) or sclerosis of the internal anal sphincter (occurring in mixed connective disease) could be identified[46,47]. Endosonography is, however, used as the method of choice in many institutions for the demonstration of sphincter defects. This method is simple, accurate, painless and causes little discomfort (Figs. 1 and 2).

Pitfalls

Defects of the external anal sphincter can usually be visualized as hypoechoic gaps in the hyperechoic circular external sphincter. Sometimes, however, the assessment of the anterior part of the sphincter can be compromised by atypically located fibres of the external sphincter or by the transversal perineal muscle, or by air in the vagina[48,49]. In women exact visualization of the anterior external sphincter is important. The additional use of vaginal endosonography could be helpful in some cases. A false-positive posterior external sphincter defect may be assumed, if the hypoechoic triangle of the anococcygeal ligament is misinterpreted[15].

Perianal fistulas and abscesses

Precise assessment of perianal fistulas is often not possible with proctological examination alone. The identification of the inter-, trans-, extra-, or suprasphincteric

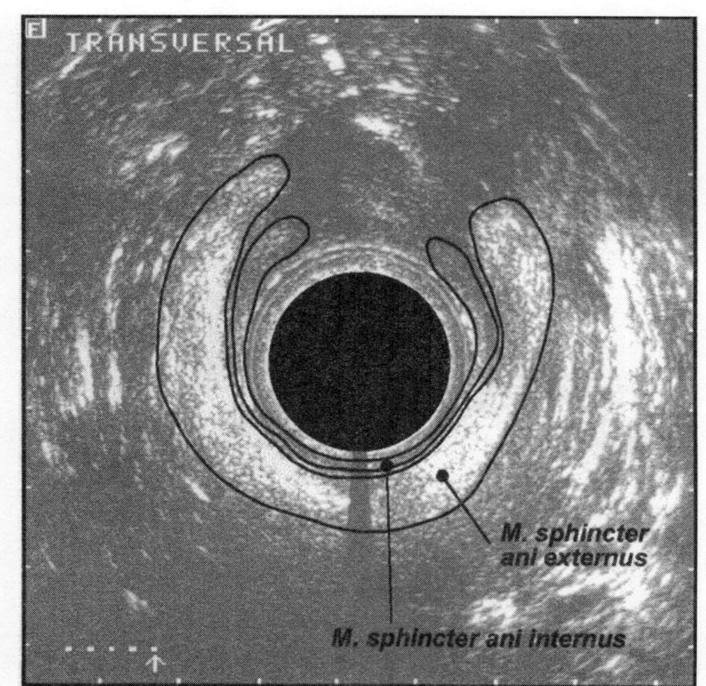

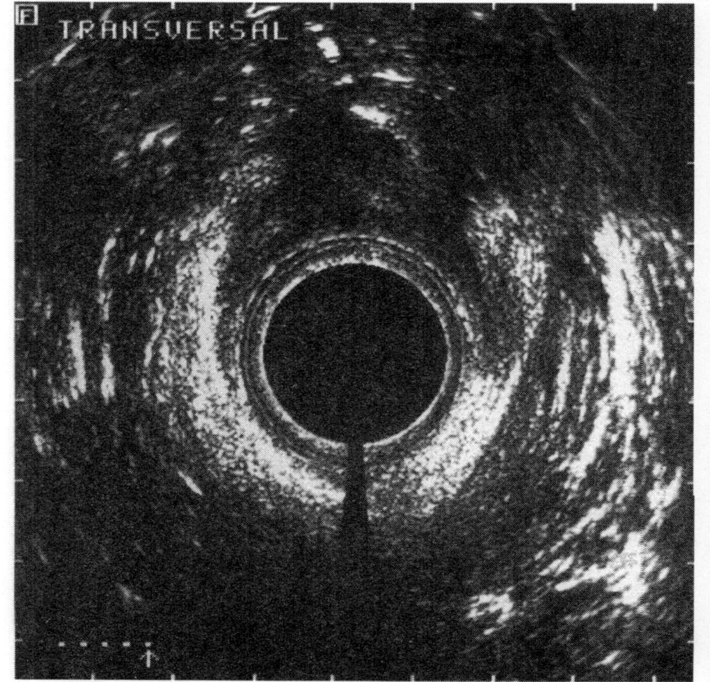

Figure 1   Anal endosonography of a 33-year-old patient suffering from faecal incontinence following obstetric tr divided at the anterior side and retracted laterally. This patient was selected for anal sphincter repair

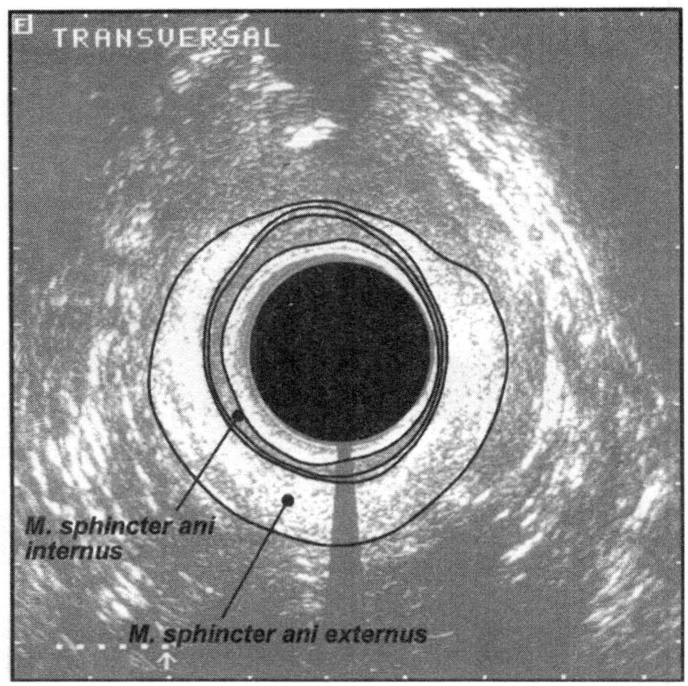

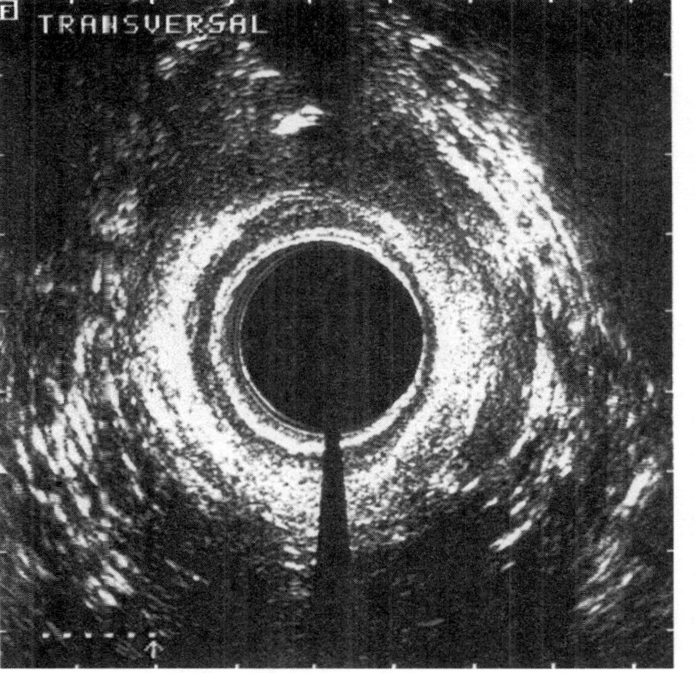

Figure 2 Endosonographic appearance of the anal sphincter in a patient complaining of moderate faecal incontinence sphincter appears thin, but not completely divided. The internal anal sphincter is intact. This patient was selected f

course of a fistula can be very helpful in planning the surgical procedure. The risk of postoperative faecal incontinence can be reduced and preoperative existing defects can be recorded[15]. The risk of recurrence can be reduced if complex fistulas can be detected. The endosonographic differentiation of recent fistulas can be difficult in patients after multiple surgical interventions, because fistulas and scar tissue sometimes appear in a similar echogenicity. The insertion of hydrogen peroxide into the fistula tract increases the accuracy of the fistula tract anatomy[50–52] (Figs 3 and 4). The use of contrast agents has been described in two studies presenting good results, with accuracy rates of 95%[51] and 92%[52]. In these cases transvaginal endosonography can provide additional information[49,53–55]. Perianal abscesses can also be visualized well by endosonography. Differentiation of granulation and scar tissue and abscess membrane is sometimes difficult. MRI is an alternative diagnostic procedure[56,57] and endoanal MRI has some possible advantages in the assessment of perianal fistulas[58]. The accuracy rate in classifying fistulas varies from 64%[56] to 86%[57] compared to surgical exploration. One advantage of endosonography is the possibility of performing diagnostic biopsies or interventional insertion of a drainage. Both diagnostic tools need to be proven in further studies. Endosonographic examinations can be impos-sible due to anal stenosis or in severe painful inflammation. In these cases an additional advantage of endosonography is its use in the operating room[15].

PRE- AND POSTOPERATIVE EVALUATION OF THE ANAL SPHINCTER BY ENDOSONOGRAPHY

Before an excision of a fistula, sphincter defects should be excluded, especially in women. If obstetric sphincter damage is found, a sphincter-preserving procedure such as the musculomucosal advancement flap should be performed instead of a routine fistulotomy[15]. In recurring anal fissures following sphincterotomy the extent of the sphincter defect can be visualized and, depending on the endosonographic assessment, the therapeutic procedure can be considered[59]. In addition to manometry the continuity of the anal sphincter should be assessed by endosonography before intestinal continuity is restored[15]. Faecal incontinence may persist after surgical sphincter repair[60]. The postoperative result should be evaluated by endosonography, since unsatisfactory results can be objectified. The extent of the remaining defect after sphincter repair may affect the degree of continence[17], and repeated surgical operation of the defect can improve continence. In this way patients can be selected for re-operation.

CONSTIPATION

Anorectal endosonography has not been a standard procedure to investigate constipation up to now, but Kamm et al.[61] described a familial myopathy of the internal sphincter with symptoms of constipation and proctalgia. They found a thickening of the internal sphincter exceeding 8 mm in diameter. Histological assessment after partial myotomy showed an autosomal-dominant hereditary defect of the internal sphincter. Non-hereditary dysfunctions of the internal

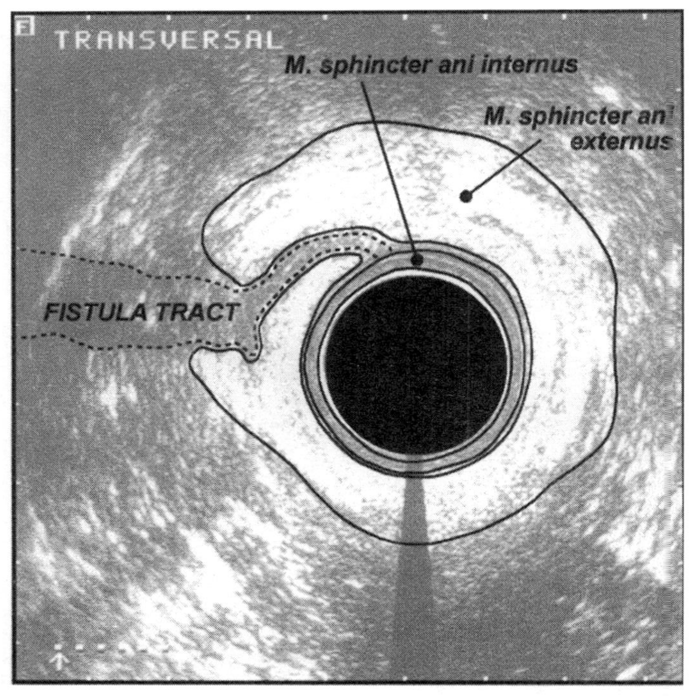

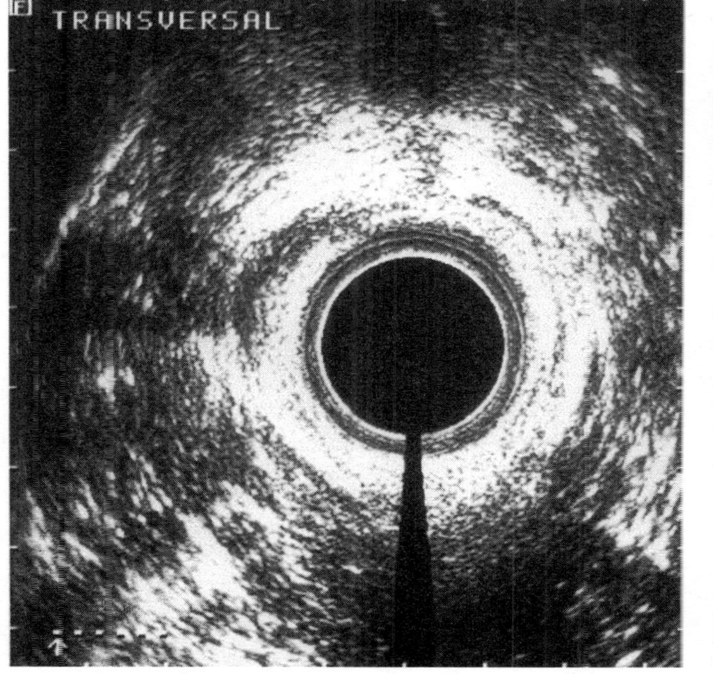

Figure 3 Thirty-one-year-old patient with Crohn's disease and anal fistula. The external opening of the fistula tr internal opening was presumed to be at 11 o'clock. An additional posterior fistula tract could not be excluded

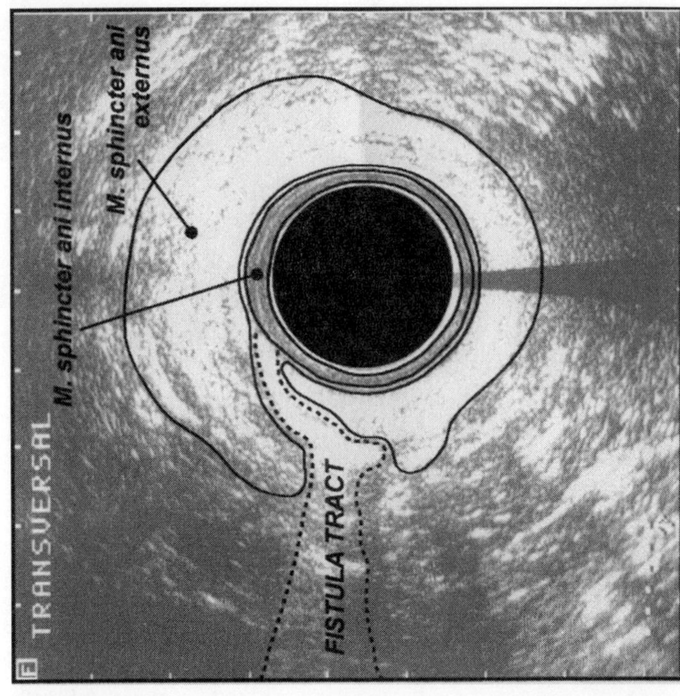

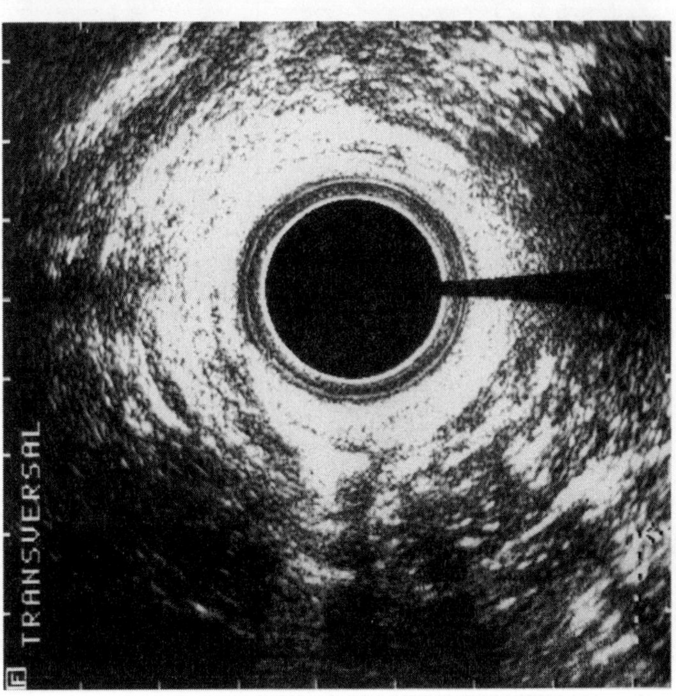

Figure 4 The fistula tract was filled with hydrogen peroxide. The supposed fistula tract was confirmed; additional tr fistula was confirmed in the following operation

sphincter are also described[62]. A hypertrophic internal sphincter is a frequent finding in constipated patients, so endosonography could lead to new perspectives in the therapy of the constipated patient[17].

FURTHER INDICATIONS

Endosonography has been used in other benign anorectal disorders. A thickening of the anal wall was described in acute Crohn's disease[63]. In haemorrhoidal disorders thickened internal and external muscles were found[64]. In proctalgia a specific pathology was not evident[65]. The importance of endosonography in these cases lies in the exclusion of fistulas or occult abscesses or other concomitant disorders.

SUMMARY

Anorectal endosonography has become an important diagnostic tool in benign proctological disorders. Endosonographic examination causes less discomfort than digital palpation. The most important indications are the assessment of faecal incontinence and perianal sepsis. Endosonography should be performed using a standardized procedure. Training and quality management need further evaluation.

Acknowledgement

The authors thank Mr D. Pirner for his support in graphic illustration.

References

1. Wild JJ, Reid JM. Diagnostic use of ultrasound. Br J Phys Med. 1956;19:248.
2. Alzin HH, Kohlberger E, Schwaiger R, Alloussi S. Valeur de l'echographie endorectale dans la chirurgie du rectum. Ann Radiol Paris. 1983;26:334.
3. Dragsted J, Gammelgaard J. Endoluminal ultrasonic scanning in the evaluation of rectal cancer. A preliminary report of 13 cases. Gastrointest Radiol. 1983;8:367.
4. Hildebrandt U, Feifel G, Zimmermann FA, Goebbels R. Significant improvement in clinical staging of rectal carcinoma with a new intrarectal ultrasound scanner. J Exp Clin Cancer Res. 1983;2:53.
5. Sailer M, Leppert R, Fuchs KH, Thiede A. Die endorektale Sonographie. Coloproctology. 1995; 17:149–57.
6. Law PJ, Bartram CI. Anal endosonography: technique and normal anatomy. Gastrointest Radiol. 1989;14:349–53.
7. Eckardt VF, Jung B, Fischer B, Lierse W. Anal endosonography in healthy subjects and patients with idiopathic fecal incontinence. Dis Colon Rectum. 1994;37:235–42.
8. Nielsen MB, Pedersen JF, Hauge C, Rasmussen OO, Christiansen J. Endosonography of the anal sphincter: findings in healthy volunteers. Am J Roentgenol. 1991;157:1199–202.
9. Tjandra JJ, Milsom JW, Stolfi VM et al. Endoluminal ultrasound defines anatomy of the anal canal and pelvic floor. Dis Colon Rectum. 1992;35:465–70.
10. Nielsen MB, Hauge C, Rasmussen OO, Sorensen M, Pedersen JF, Christiansen J. Anal sphincter size measured by endosonography in healthy volunteers. Effect of age, sex and parity. Acta Radiol. 1992;33:453–6.
11. Sultan AH, Nicholls RJ, Kamm MA, Hudson CN, Beynon J, Bartram CI. Anal endosonography and correlation with in vitro and in vivo anatomy. Br J Surg. 1993;80:508–11.

12. Papachrysostomou M, Pye SD, Wild SR, Smith AN. Anal endosonography in asymptomatic subjects. Scand J Gastroenterol. 1993;28:551–6.
13. Gerdes B, Kohler HH, Zielke A, Kisker O, Barth PJ, Stinner B. The anatomical basis of anal endosonography – a study in postmortem specimens. Surg Endosc. 1997;11:986–90.
14. Poen AC, Felt-Bersma RJF, Cuesta MA, Meuwissen SGM. Normal values and reproducibility of anal endosonographic measurements. Eur J Ultrasound. 1997;6:103–10.
15. Poen AC, Felt-Bersma RJF. Endosonography in benign anorectal disease: an overview. Scand J Gastroenterol. 1999;34(Suppl. 230):40–8.
16. Sultan AH, Kamm MA, Hudson CN, Nicholls JR, Bartram CI. Endosonography of the anal sphincters: normal anatomy and comparison with manometry. Clin Radiol. 1994;49:368–74.
17. Nielsen MB. Endosonography of the anal sphincter muscles in healthy volunteers and in patients with defecation disorders. Acta Radiol Suppl. 1998;416:1–21.
18. Papachrysostomou M, Pye SD, Wild SR, Smith AN. Significance of the thickness of the anal sphincter with age and its relevance in faecal incontinence. Scand J Gastroenterol. 1994;29:710–14.
19. Nielsen MB, Pedersen JF. Changes in the anal sphincter with age. An endosonographic study. Acta Radiol. 1996;37:357–61.
20. Schäfer R, Heyer T, Gantke B et al. Anal endosonography and manometry: comparison in patients with defecation problems. Dis Colon Rectum. 1997;40:293–7.
21. Oh C, Kark AE. Anatomy of the external anal sphincter. Br J Surg. 1972;59:717.
22. Ayoub SF. Anatomy of the external anal sphincter in man. Acta Anat. 1979;105:25.
23. Dalley AF. The riddle of the sphincters. The morpho-physiology of the anorectal mechanism reviewed. Am Surg 1987;53:298 (published erratum appears in Am Surg. 1987;53:398).
24. Golligher J. Surgery of the Anus, Rectum and Colon. 5th edn. London:Bailliére Tindall, 1984.
25. Burnett SJ, Bartram CI. Endosonographic variations in the normal internal anal sphincter. Int J Colorectal Dis. 1991;6:2–4.
26. Gantke B, Schäfer A, Enck P, Lübke HJ. Sonographic manometric and myographic evaluation of the anal sphincters morphology and function. Dis Colon Rectum. 1993;36:1037–41.
27. Klosterhalfen B, Offner F, Topf N, Vogel P, Mittermayer C. Sclerosis of the internal anal sphincter – a process of aging. Dis Colon Rectum. 1990;33:606–9.
28. Law PJ, Bartram CI. Anal endosonography: technique and normal anatomy. Gastrointest Radiol. 1989;14:349–53.
29. Lunniss PJ, Phillips R. Anatomy and function of the anal longitudinal muscle. Br J Surg. 1992;79:882–4.
30. Beynon J, Foy DMA, Channer JL. The endosonic appearances of normal colon and rectum. Dis Colon Rectum. 1986;29:810.
31. Kumar A, Scholefield JH. Endosonography of the anal canal and rectum. World J Surg. 2000;24:208–15.
32. Parks AG, Swash M, Urich H. Sphincter denervation in anorectal incontinence and rectal prolapse. Gut. 1977;18:656–65.
33. Snooks SJ, Swash M, Setchell M, Henry MM. Injury to innervation of pelvic floor sphincter musculature in childbirth. Lancet. 1984;2:546–50.
34. Sultan AH, Kamm MA, Hudson CN, Thomas JM, Bartram CI. Anal-sphincter disruption during vaginal delivery. N Engl J Med. 1993;329:1905–11.
35. Kamm MA. Obstetric damage and fecal incontinence. Lancet. 1994;344:730–3.
36. Burnett SJ, Spence-Jones C, Speakman CT, Kamm MA, Hudson CN, Bartram CI. Unsuspected sphincter damage following childbirth revealed by anal endosonography. Br J Radiol. 1991;64:225–7.
37. Law PJ, Kamm MA, Bartram CI. Anal endosonography in the investigation of fecal incontinence. Br J Surg. 1991;78:312–14.
38. Deen KI, Kumar D, Williams JG, Olliff J, Keighley M. The prevalence of anal sphincter defects in fecal incontinence: a prospective endosonic study. Gut. 1993;34:685–8.
39. Farouk R, Bartolo DC. The use of endoluminal ultrasound in the assessment of patients with fecal incontinence. J R Coll Surg Edinb. 1994;39:312–18
40. Felt-Bersma RJ, van Baren R, Koorevaar M, Strijers RL, Cuesta MA. Unsuspected sphincter defects shown by anal endosonography after anorectal surgery. A prospective study. Dis Colon Rectum. 1995;38:249–53.
41. Sultan AH, Kamm MA, Nicholls RJ, Bartram CI. Prospective study of the extent of internal anal sphincter division during lateral sphincterotomy. Dis Colon Rectum. 1994;37:1031–3.

42. Farouk R, Drew P, Duthie G, Lee P, Moson J. Disruption of the internal anal sphincter can occur after transanal stapling. Br J Surg. 1996;83:1400.

43. Silvis R, van Eekelen JW, Delemarre JB, Gooszen HG. Endosonography of the anal sphincter after ileal pouch–anal anastomosis. Relation with anal manometry and fecal continence. Dis Colon Rectum. 1995;38:383–8.

44. Speakman CT, Burnett SJ, Kamm MA, Bartram CI. Sphincter injury after anal dilatation demonstrated by anal endosonography. Br J Surg. 1991;78:1429–30.

45. Nielsen MB, Rasmussen OO, Pedersen JF, Christiansen J. Risk of sphincter damage and anal incontinence after anal dilatation for fissure-in-ano: an endosonographic study. Dis Colon Rectum. 1993;36:677–80.

46. Vaizey CJ, Kamm MA, Bartram CI. Primary degeneration of the anal sphincter as a cause of passive fecal incontinence. Lancet. 1997;349:612–15.

47. Engel AF, Kamm MA, Talbot IC. Progressive systemic sclerosis of the internal anal sphincter leading to passive fecal incontinence. Gut. 1994;35:857–9.

48. Eckardt VF, Jung B, Fischer B, Lierse W. Anal endosonography in healthy subjects and patients with idiopathic fecal incontinence. Dis Colon Rectum. 1994;37:235–42.

49. Poen AC, Felt-Bersma RJF, Cuesta MA, Meuwissen SGM. Vaginal endosonography of the anal sphincter complex is important in the assessment of fecal incontinence and perianal sepsis. Br J Surg. 1998;85:359–63.

50. Cheong D, Nogueras JJ, Wexner SD, Jagelman DG. Anal endosonography for recurrent anal fistulas: image enhancement with hydrogen peroxide. Dis Colon Rectum. 1993;36:1158–60.

51. Poen AC, Felt-Bersma RJF, Eijsbouts QAJ, Cuesta MA, Meuwissen SGM. Hydrogen peroxide enhancement transanal ultrasound in the diagnosis of fistula-in-ano. Dis Colon Rectum. (In press).

52. Iroatulam A, Nogueras J, Chen H. Accuracy of endoanal ultrasonography in evaluating anal fistulas. Gastroenterology. 1997;112(Suppl.A):1450.

53. Wijers O, Tio T, Tygat G. Ultrasonography and endosonography in the diagnosis and management of inflammatory bowel disease. Endoscopy. 1992;24:559–64.

54. Tio TL, Mulder C, Wijers OB, Sars P, Tytgat G. Endosonography of peri-anal and peri-colorectal fistula and/or abscess in Crohn's disease. Gastrointest Endosc. 1990;36:331–6.

55. Schratter SA, Lochs H, Handl ZL, Tscholakoff D, Schratter M. Endosonographic features of the lower pelvic region in Crohn's disease. Am J Gastroenterol. 1993;88:1054–7.

56. Hussain S, Stoker J, Schouten W, Hop W, Lameris J. Fistula in ano: endoanal sonography versus endoanal MR imaging in classification. Radiology. 1996;200:475–81.

57. Lunniss PJ, Barker PG, Sultan AH. Magnetic resonance imaging of fistula in ano. Dis Colon Rectum. 1994;37:708–18.

58. Lunniss PJ, Armstrong P, Barkler PG, Reznek RH, Phillips RK. Magnetic resonance imaging of anal fistulae. Lancet. 1992;340:394.

59. Farouk R, Monson J, Duthie G. Technical failure of lateral sphincterotomy for the treatment of chronic anal fissure: a study using endoanal ultrasonography. Br J Surg. 1997;84:84–5.

60. Nielsen MB, Hauge C, Pedersen JF, Christiansen J. Endosonographic assessment of the anal sphincter after surgical reconstruction. Dis Colon Rectum. 1994;37:434 (paper VII).

61. Kamm MA, Hoyle CH, Burleigh DE. Hereditary internal anal sphincter myopathy causing proctalgia fugax and constipation. A newly identified condition. Gastroenterology. 1991;100:805–10.

62. Nielsen MB, Rasmussen OO, Pedersen JF, Christiansen J. Anal endosonographic findings in patients with obstructed defecation. Acta Radiol. 1993;34:35–8.

63. Solomon MJ, McLeod RS, Cohen EK, Cohen Z. Anal wall thickness under normal and inflammatory conditions of the anorectum as determined by endoluminal ultrasonography. Am J Gastroenterol. 1995;90:547–8.

64. Poen AC, Felt-Bersma RJF, Cuesta MA, Meuwissen SGM. Internal hemorrhoids are associated with endosonographic thickening of the submucosa and hypertrophy of the external anal sphincter. Gastroenterology. 1996;110:A736.

65. Eckardt VF, Dodt O, Kanzler G, Bernhard G. Anorectal function and morphology in patients with sporadic proctalgia fugax. Dis Colon Rectum. 1996;39:755–62.

5
Radiological imaging studies of the pelvic floor

A. LIENEMANN and D. SPRENGER

INTRODUCTION

Clinical investigation of female patients with pelvic floor dysfunction has advanced significantly in recent decades. Although a careful and thorough initial evaluation and physical examination performed to detect all defects remains mandatory, even the most experienced clinicians can sometimes be misled by the findings[1]. Clinicians can refer to a wide range of imaging modalities. These diagnostic adjuncts can confirm clinical suspicion, narrow a differential diagnosis, or reveal unsuspected findings which eventually alter the therapeutic approach[2,3]. This chapter briefly reviews the most commonly used radiological modalities and discusses the clinical applications, strengths, and limitations of the various imaging techniques.

CONTRAST STUDIES OF THE COLON

Enema studies of the colon using positive and/or negative contrast media are well established and provide an excellent overview of the entire large bowel. The technique is easy to perform and widely available. These studies are performed to rule out other concomitant diseases such as colonic cancer or a redundant or displaced sigmoid loop in patients who complain of constipation or anorectal incontinence and obstruction. The enema studies provide only static anatomical information and therefore are not diagnostic in patients with pelvic floor disorders[4].

COLON TRANSIT

The stool frequency reported by patients proved to be inaccurate and only poorly correlated with actual colonic transit time[5]. Using radiopaque markers an objective, clinically applicable and widely available measurement of colonic transit was possible (Fig. 1A). The initial technique was described by Hinton et al.[6].

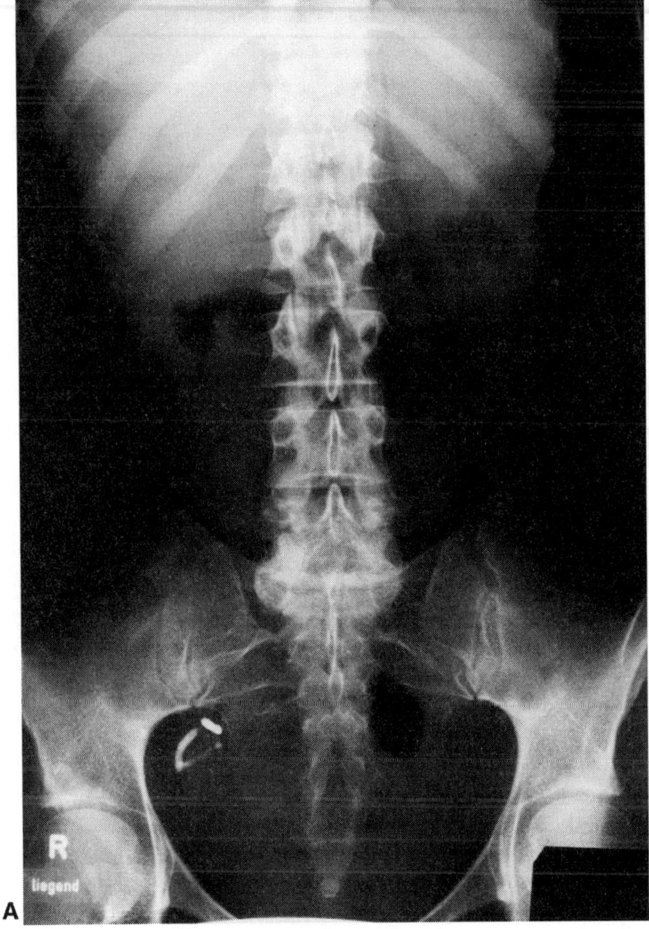

Figure 1   Thirty-two-year-old nulliparous female with chronic pain in the lower abdomen, a sense of something falling down and a feeling of incomplete emptying.
A: The colonic transit time measurement using radiopaque markers revealed no abnormalities. There is still some contrast material from a previous study in the appendix

The premise of this type of study is the fact that the transit of a faecal material, as well as the administered markers through the colon, represents nothing more than the half-life time of such material in the colon.

Prior to the examination all other contrast material from previous studies should be cleared from the small and large bowel. Furthermore patients should continue with their usual diet and daily activities. Laxatives, enemas or any other medication which might alter bowel motility should be avoided.

Radiopaque markers can be obtained commercially or can be prepared. We ask the patient to ingest 20 radiopaque markers, which are packed within a gelatine

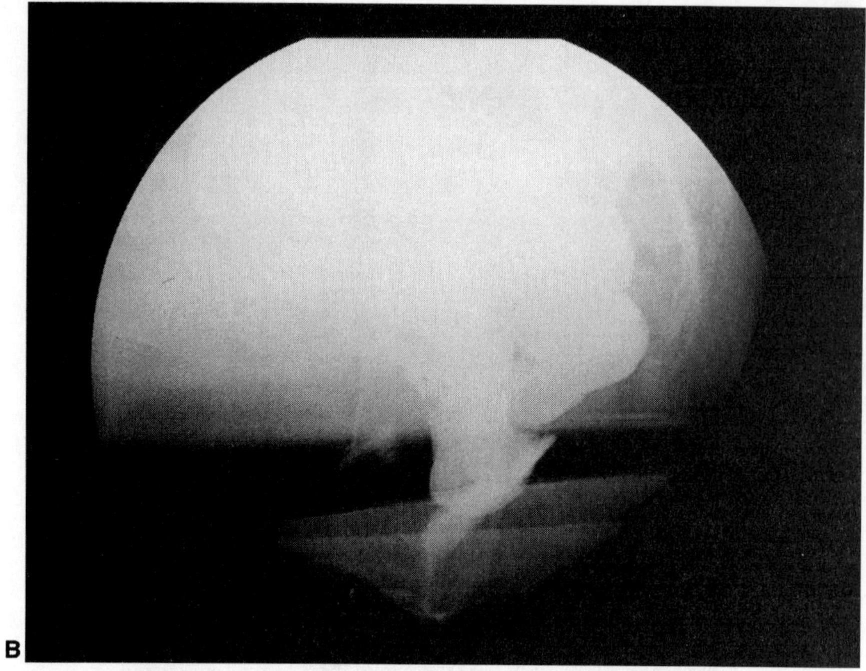

Figure 1 B: On defaecography a rectal intussusception and an enterocele were diagnosed. The vagina was opacified by using a tampon soaked with contrast media

capsule, at the same time of day for 6 successive days. On day 7 an abdominal radiograph is taken with the patient supine. The mean transit time of the colon is calculated by counting the visible markers on the film and multiplying them by a factor of 1.2. A colonic transit time of more than 72 h is considered abnormal[7]. The technique described varies among authors but all are very similar. A good overview is given in ref 7.

Measurement of colonic transit is most appropriate in patients with a long history of constipation which is unexplained by prior routine studies such as endoscopy or barium enema of the colon. It may also monitor surgical therapy and outcome.

The inherent high variability in transit suggests that only major differences from normal should be interpreted as a significant finding[8]. If the markers accumulate in the area of the rectosigmoid, defaecation disorders such as stool outlet obstruction may be present. A delay throughout the entire colon with exclusion of defaecation disorders may represent an abnormal motility of the large bowel.

PELVIC FLUOROSCOPY AND DEFAECOGRAPHY

This technique is still the most commonly used radiological approach to describe pelvic floor dysfunction. During recent decades nearly all experience

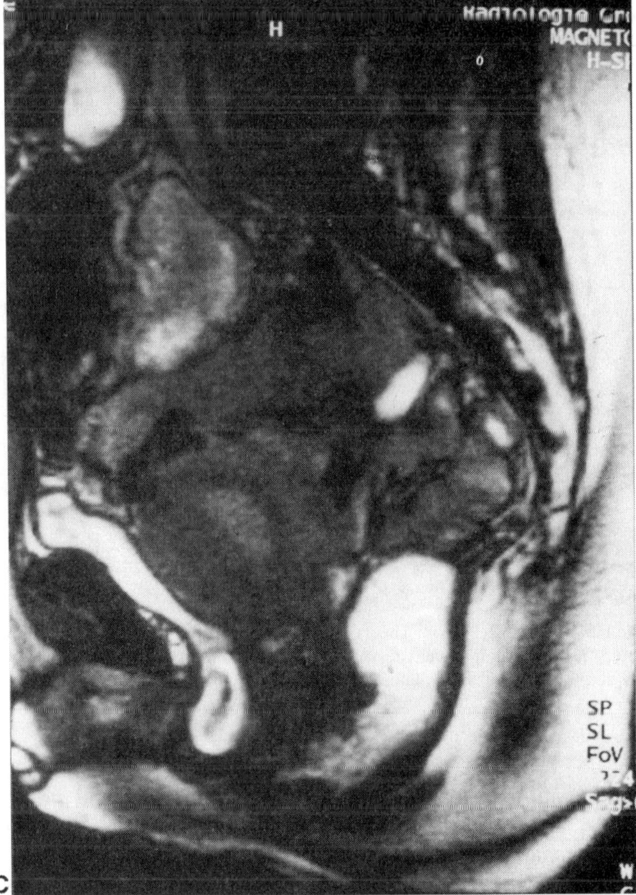

Figure 1 C: Functional MRI (mid-sagittal slice orientation with the patient straining) shows extended findings. The uterovaginal prolapse is accompanied by a cystocele and puts pressure on the ventral wall of the rectum

concerning normal and abnormal pelvic floor anatomy and physiology has been gained using this method. The technique in use today eventually evolved from the myography of the levator ani muscle introduced by Berglas and Rubin[9] and the viscerogram performed by Béthoux and Bory[10].

The technique of radiological visualization of the pelvic floor requires recognition of the midline sagittal anatomy of the pelvis (Fig. 1B). Bony landmarks include the symphysis pubis, the coccyx, the promontory and the ischial tuberosities. Soft-tissue contrast can only be achieved indirectly by opacifying the lumen of relevant organs. To date no commonly accepted scheme has been established. According to Brubaker *et al.*[11] and Kelvin *et al.*[12] a complete

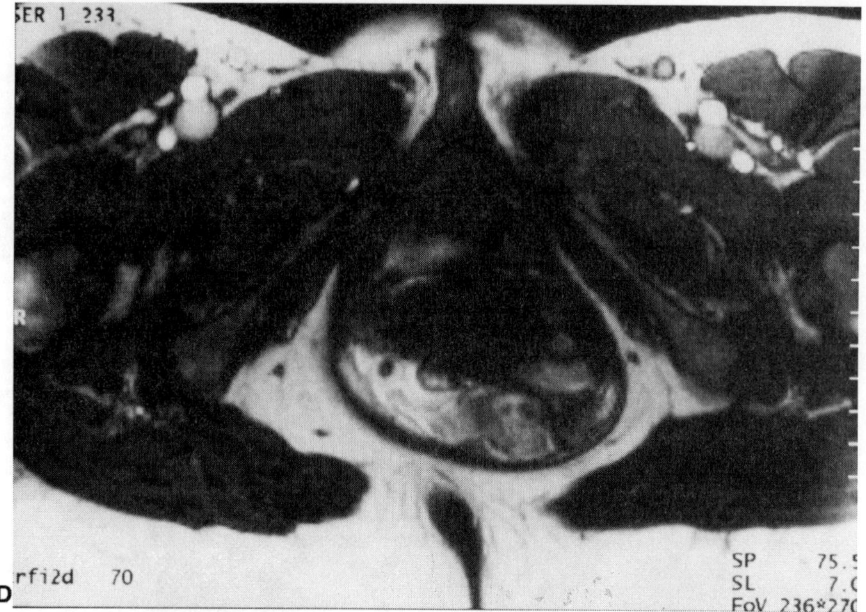

Figure 1 **D**: Functional MRI (axial slice orientation at the level of the ischiatic tubera with the patient straining) reveals a major weakness of the pelvic diaphragm with an eccentric ballooning of the urogenital hiatus to the left and a lateral rectocele

visceral opacification is mandatory. Contrast material should be placed in the urinary bladder, the urethra, the vagina, the rectum and the small bowel to help appreciate their spatial relationship to each other. Our own protocol starts with an opacification of the small bowel with oral barium sulphate suspension 1–2 h prior to the examination. This allows for the identification of enteroceles. Next we empty the bladder and introduce 100 ml of water-soluble iodine contrast media in a sterile fashion via a catheter. The urethra itself is opacified by using a thread soaked with contrast media. Both procedures delineate the bladder, the bladder neck and the position of the urethra with respect to the symphysis pubis. Identification of the vagina is achieved by using barium sulphate paste (approximately 30 ml). The use of a contrast-soaked tampon is not advisable (Fig. 1B); it might splint the prolapse and hinder the assessment of the rectovaginal space[12]. Next, after digital examination, a rectal catheter is put in place and approximately 200–300 ml of a mixture of barium sulphate suspension and starch is introduced. The high viscosity of the mixture is more or less equivalent to normal stool. Liquid contrast media alone is not physiological; as in diarrhoea it stresses the continence mechanism. Although the amount of paste used varies considerably, it should be inserted until the patient reports an urge to relieve the bowel. Due to reflux into the sigmoid colon the volume does not represent the true intrarectal volume. The external anal orifice and perineal surface are best visualized with barium paste. A radiographic ruler is necessary to provide accurate measurements.

The patient then sits on a specially designed commode in an upright position. Fluoroscopic tower and table, as well as radiographic filters, are adjusted accordingly. We use digital fluoroscopy with a filming sequence of one frame per second. Views of the pelvic floor are obtained with the patient at rest, during squeezing and straining with defaecation. The film sequence is mostly taken in the lateral view. This can be combined with an anterior–posterior view. Again a large number of filming protocols are described in the literature.

Measurements and findings in normal subjects and symptomatic patients have shown a considerable overlap of results[13]; therefore measurements by themselves are not reliable. In addition, so far no agreement on standardized measurements and reference lines has been obtained. Some of the most common measurements include the anorectal angle, the width of the anal canal and the position of organs in relation to specific reference lines. A rectocele greater than 4 cm in depth is considered abnormal, especially if it retains contrast material. The various aspects are well summarized by Maglinte *et al.*[3] and Weidner and Low[14].

Fluoroscopic evaluation of the pelvic floor is widely used and available, easy to perform and permits direct visual assessment of the interrelationships. It reflects the physiological position of the patient in everyday life. The exposure to radiation, superimpositions and the visualization only of opacified organs are considered drawbacks of this method. Pelvic fluoroscopy is of value in patients already committed to surgical correction of a clinically known abnormality of the pelvic floor. It can reveal unsuspected findings such as enteroceles. In complex organ prolapse it can clarify the overall anatomical situation and, for example, show a coexisting cystocele and enterocele which were masked by a rectocele.

MAGNETIC RESONANCE IMAGING

Functional MRI of the pelvic floor is currently the most promising tool for the evaluation of patients with pelvic floor dysfunction. In contrast to pelvic fluoroscopy MRI demonstrates the morphology of the pelvic floor with superior soft-tissue differentiation. In addition to the hollow organs of the pelvic floor the pelvic diaphragm (levator ani muscle) itself, as well as the connective tissue, are visualized and muscular defects can be discerned. Unfortunately the in-plane resolution is still limited. Defects of the various parts of the endopelvic fascia cannot be depicted.

This modality also permits multiplanar imaging without superimposition, and avoids ionizing radiation. Therefore static MRI was used in children with anal or rectal atresia, for pelvimetric measurements or to describe the anatomy of the pelvic floor[15].

In 1991 Yang *et al.*[16] and Kruyt *et al.*[17] first introduced functional imaging of the pelvic floor by acquiring only one image taken at rest, during squeezing and straining. They did not use any contrast material for the opacification of organs.

Our own protocol can be divided into seven parts (Figs 1C and 1D); Prior to the examination the patient needs no preparation. No premedication is utilized. The patient should be familiarized with the intention and course of the examination. Next the urinary bladder is emptied.

An adequate opacification of pelvic organs is mandatory. In all cases opacification of the vagina (approx. 50 ml) and the rectosigmoid (approx. 200 ml until the patient expresses an urge to relieve the bowel) using sonography gel is necessary.

MRI is performed with a 1.5 T superconductive magnet unit. The examination requires the patient to be positioned supine, with the request to open the legs slightly. We use a body-array-surface coil. With absorbent pads we prevent running out. We combine static and functional pulse sequences.

The static section includes T2-weighted turbo spin-echo sequences of the pelvis in axial and sagittal orientation. The acquired images are essential for a variety of reasons. The high in-plane resolution allows for a morphological assessment of structures (e.g. pelvic floor muscles). The course of tubular organs such as the rectosigmoid can be traced. Accidental findings (e.g. gartner cysts) may be noticed. Finally, for the functional examination, the urethral complex which is seen on the axial image is used as reference point.

The functional section consists of a T2-weighted True-FISP sequence. Standard single-slice orientation includes a mid-sagittal and an axial (lower rim of the pubic bone) alignment, as well as a coronal stack of slices. The sagittal images visualize all compartments at the same time and allow comparison with standard X-ray procedures (Fig. 1C). The axial images provide information about the urogenital hiatus and its contents (e.g. lateral enterocoeles, rectal descent; Fig. 1D). Muscular defects such as hernias can be best seen on coronal images. Additional slice orientations may be necessary to evaluate unexpected findings on the standard images or to assess complex types of organ prolapse.

During the acquisition of the mid-sagittal or axial images the patient is asked to relax the pelvic floor muscles, contract them slowly, and then relax again. Then the patient is asked to increase the intra-abdominal pressure by straining, and to defaecate. This cycle is repeated twice to a maximum of four times. The coronal images are taken while the patient is straining. The overall time of examination varies between 20 and 30 min.

For evaluation of an organ descent we use two reference lines. The pubococcygeal line (bladder neck or wall, vaginal vault and peritoneal border line) and the ischiopubic line (anorectal junction). These two lines are drawn from the inferior rim of the symphysis to the sacrococcygeal joint and tangent to the inferior rim of the symphysis at the level of the ischiatic tubera. Additional measurements include the width of the urogenital hiatus[18].

In a study population of healthy young nulliparous females we defined the normal range of functional MRI appearances[19].

An increasing number of imaging protocols have been published[20–26]. To date no common accepted method has been established; but most authors agree that functional MRI of the pelvic floor is an alternative to pelvic fluoroscopy, in spite of being performed with the patient in a supine position[23,24].

The main advantage of functional MRI is its modular structure. The individual choice of imaging sequences or different coils produces variable appearances and contrast of the soft-tissue structures. In combination with an endoanal coil high-resolution images of the anal sphincter can be produced[14]. A large field of view, together with a scanning of the abdomen during repeated straining, allows the detection of intra-abdominal adhesions. Even large bowel motility can be recorded using functional MRI.

At present indications for functional MRI of the pelvic floor include any combined forms of organ descent, whenever a dominant type of prolapse, an enterocele or a stool outlet obstruction/defaecation block is suspected or the first-line examinations are inconclusive. Moreover this technique inaugurates a new combined look at the morphology and function of the pelvic floor.

References

1. Kelvin FM, Maglinte DDT, Hornback JA, Benson JT. Pelvic prolapse: assessment with evacuation proctography (defecography). Radiology. 1992;184:547–51.
2. Brubaker L, Retzky S, Smith C, Saclarides T. Pelvic floor evaluation with dynamic fluoroscopy. Obstet Gynecol. 1993;82:863–8.
3. Maglinte DDT, Kelvin FM, Hale DS, Benson JT. Dynamic cystoproctography: a unifying diagnostic approach to pelvic floor and anorectal dysfunction. Am J Radiol. 1997;169:759–67.
4. Karasick S. Does barium enema predict defecographic abnormalities? In: Programs and Abstracts of the 96th Annual Meeting of the American Roentgen Ray Society, San Diego, 1996:83.
5. Manning A, Wyman K, Heaton K. How trustworthy are bowel histories? Comparison of recalled and recorded information. Br Med J. 1976;2:213.
6. Hinton JM, Lennard-Jones JE, Young AC. A new method for studying gut transit times using radiopaque markers. Gut. 1969;10:842–7.
7. Schindlbeck NE, Klauser AG, Müller-Lissner SA. Messung der Kolontransitzeit. Z Gastroenterol. 1990;28:399–404.
8. Metcalf AM, Phillips SF, Zinsmeister AR, MacCarty RL, Beart RW, Wolff BG. Simplified assessment of segmental colonic transit. Gastroenterology. 1987;92:40–7.
9. Berglas B, Rubin IC. Study of the supportive structures of the uterus by levator myography. Surg Gynecol Obstet. 1953;97;677–92.
10. Béthoux A, Bory S. Les mécanismes staiques viscéraux pelviens chez la femme a la lumière de l'exploration fonctionelle du dispositif en position debout. Ann Chir. 1962;16:887–917.
11. Brubaker L, Retzky S, Smith C, Saclarides T. Pelvic floor evaluation with dynamic fluoroscopy. Obstet Gynecol. 1993;82:863–8.
12. Kelvin FM, Maglinte DDT, Hornback JA, Benson JT. Pelvic prolapse: assessment with evacuation proctography (defecography). Radiology. 1992;184:547–51.
13. Shorvon PJ, McHugh S, Diamant NE, Somers S, Stevenson W. Defecography in normal volunteers: results and implications. Gut. 1989;30:1737–49.
14. Weidner AC, Low VHS. Imaging studies of the pelvic floor. Obstet Gynecol N Am. 1998;25: 825–78.
15. DeLancey JOL. Correlative study of paraurethral anatomy. Obstet Gynecol. 1986;68:91–7.
16. Yang A, Mostwin JL, Rosenshein NB, Zerhouni EA. Pelvic floor descent in women: dynamic evaluation with fast MR imaging and cinematic display. Radiology. 1991;179:25–33.
17. Kruyt RH, Delemarre JBVM, Doornbos J, Vogel HJ. Normal anorectum: dynamic MR imaging anatomy. Radiology. 1991;179:159–63.
18. Lienemann A. An easy approach to functional magnetic resonance imaging of pelvic floor disorders. Techn Coloproctol. 1998;2:131–4.
19. Lienemann A, Anthuber C, Baron A, Reiser M. Dynamic MR colpocystorectography assessing pelvic floor descent. Eur Radiol. 1997;7:1309–17.
20. Lienemann A, Sprenger D, Janßen U, Anthuber C, Reiser M. [Functional MRI of the pelvic floor. Method and reference values]. Radiologe. 2000;40:458–64.
21. Healy JC, Halligan S, Reznek RH, Watson S, Bartram C, Phillips R, Armstrong P. Dynamic MR imaging compared with evacuation proctography when evaluating anorectal configuration and pelvic floor movement. Am J Radiol. 1997;169:775–9.
22. Hilfiker PR, Debatin J, Schwizer W, Schoenenberger AW, Fried M, Marincek D. MR defecography: depiction of anorectal anatomy and pathology. J Comput Axial Tomogr. 1998;22:749–55.
23. Fielding JR, Griffiths DJ, Versi E, Mulkern RV, Lee MLT, Jolesz FA. MR imaging of pelvic floor continence mechanisms in the supine and sitting positions. Am J Radiol. 1998;171: 1607–10.

24. Gufler H, Laubenberger J, DeGregorio G, Dohnicht S, Langer M. Pelvic floor descent: dynamic MR imaging using a half-fourier RARE sequence. J Magnet Reson Imag. 1999;9:378–83.
25. Vanbeckevoort D, Van Hoe L, Oyen R, Ponette E, De Ridder D, Deprest J. Pelvic floor descent in females: comparative study of colpocystodefecography and dynamic fast MR imaging. J Magnet Reson Imag. 1999;9:373–7.
26. Comiter CV, Vasavada SP, Barbaric Z, Raz S. Dynamic MRI: a new grading system for pelvic prolapse and pelvic floor relaxation. Neurourol Urodyn. 1999;18:302–3.

6
Dysfunction of the pelvic floor – neurological and neurophysiological diagnostics

W. H. JOST

INTRODUCTION

Technological diagnostics of anorectal continence dysfunctions has become increasingly important for diagnosis and therapy in the past few years. In this respect electrophysiological examinations also play an important role. Unfortunately, at the present time only a few clinics carry out the complete diagnostics of anorectal dysfunctions to a great extent. Interdisciplinary cooperation is rare. In numerous clinics surgeons independently carry out electrophysiological diagnostics such as electromyography (EMG). However, this should be done only if such surgeons have had sufficient experience with the EMG. Interpretation of the findings in the EMG often poses problems even to neurologists with broad EMG experience. Cooperation between surgeon and neurologist is desirable. An optimum result can be reached only through cooperation between diagnostician and therapist.

NEUROLOGICAL DIAGNOSTICS IN ANAL INCONTINENCE

Patients with dysfunctions of the anorectum are usually referred to the neurologist only for 'pelvic floor EMG'. As a rule there is usually a deficit of information, since often the internist or surgeon is not acquainted with the diagnostic possibilities of the neurophysiologist; on the contrary, the neurologist may be unaware of the therapeutic consequences of his examination.

The surgeon and/or internist should have a clear question and be able to hand over the information at his disposal (e.g. anamnesis, complaints, clinical and laboratory findings, findings from other examinations such as defaecography, endosonography, and anal manometry). The neurologist should also ask for an anamnesis (anal operation, trauma, other complaints) and examine the patient (inspection, motoric or sensitive deficits, reflexes, digital examination).

The optimum situation would comprise a neurophysiological examination in the presence of the physician in charge. This would prevent a deficit of information and allow further examinations on the basis of the results obtained.

PUDENDAL LATENCY (PNTML)

An elegant method to determine the latency period – not the nerve conduction velocity – of the pudendal nerve (PNTML = pudendal nerve terminal motor latency) has been described by Kiff and Swash[1,2]. Two stimulating electrodes are placed onto the tip of a fingerstall. The finger is then inserted into the anal canal, and this stimulates the terminal branch of the pudendal nerve next to the origin of the pudendal nerve (the complete equipment is available as 'St Mark's pudendal electrode' from Dantec, Skovlunde, Denmark). A stimulation of the pudendal nerve, by inserting the examining finger into the vagina, is also possible. The recording electrode is glued onto the distal part of the base at the finger. The normal value[2] as indicated is 2.0 ± 0.5 ms.

DETERMINATION OF REFLEX LATENCIES

The determination of reflex latencies in the anal reflex (perianal electric stimulus and derivation by a concentric needle electrode from the external anal sphincter)[3–8], as well as in the bulbocavernosus[9] and the pudendoanal reflex (the latter two are triggered by a stimulus on the penis or the clitoris) has proven to be helpful. Prolonged latencies should be regarded as pathological, and indicate a lesion of the nerve fibres (afference and efference). It is not possible, however, to distinguish between a lesion of the cauda equina and a lesion of the pudendal nerve by this method alone.

EMG WITH SURFACE ELECTRODES

The electromyogram with surface electrodes is very popular[10]. The procedure is easy on the patient, quickly realized and does not require broad neurophysiological knowledge; yet it covers only the gobal activity of the anorectal musculature. This method does not allow diagnosis of either an acute or a chronic denervation. It turns out to be an advantage that the EMG can be derived over a longer period of time and parallel to manometry[5]. Surface electrodes are also used for the determination of reflex latencies and stimulus responses.

EMG WITH THE CONCENTRIC NEEDLE ELECTRODE

In anorectal dysfunctions pelvic floor EMG with the concentric needle electrode is the most important neurophysiological tool[6,11]. The first examinations made in this connection date from the year 1929[12]. With the electromyogram it is possible to judge the functioning of the striated muscle and to estimate the position and extent of a muscular defect or a neurogenic lesion. The existence of a normal EMG apparatus with a derivation canal, and optic as well as acoustic presentation of the signals, are necessary prerequisites. The only contraindications are florid inflammations in the area of the designated registration position and coagulation disorders (treatment with Marcumar™ also).

The examination is carried out with the patient in the left lateral position with the hips and knees in flexion, or in the so-called lithotomy position (dorsosacral position). Prior to the examination the neurologist should inspect the anal region and palpate the anal canal. During the digital examination the patient is asked to squeeze and to press. The sensitivity of the anal canal is clinically tested with a wooden stick and then the anal reflex is triggered[13]. Only then, after disinfection of the skin and eventual removal of extensive hairiness, is the EMG derivation from the external anal sphincter made. This records the activity of the motor units that reflect the anatomical and functional condition of the muscle.

Prior to the insertion of the needle electrode the index finger is inserted into the anal canal. Insertion is made under digital control with a 20–60 mm long concentric (coaxial) needle ($\leqslant 0.6$ mm in diameter) at the left and/or right side of the anal circumference distal of the anocutaneous line. According to the clinical question, any other point of the circumference can be examined, e.g. in muscular defects after perineal tear or fistula operation. On the basis of the derived action potentials the correct position of the needle can be checked. First the derivation is made at rest, then the patient is asked to squeeze, press and finally cough (reflex mechanism)[5,14]. It may be sensible to carry out an additional derivation while the anal reflex is triggered, and during digital dilatation of the sphincter muscles (reflex mechanism).

The pelvic floor muscles are supplied mainly by the pudendal nerve and by the roots (S2) S3 and S4 (their course is above the pelvic floor)[15], the puborectal muscle and the external anal sphincter are supplied by different nerves[16]. In electromyographic examinations of the puborectal sling longer needles (about 60 mm) should be used. In this process the needle is pushed forward on the side of the posterior commissure, laterally or dorsally of the external sphincter. During manometry an EMG can also be derived with a concentric needle electrode, which gives more precise information than do surface electrodes[5].

Electromyography of the internal anal sphincter (smooth muscle) requires a great deal of effort[17]. Its value for the diagnostics of anorectal dysfunctions is controversial. To date there are no standardized values.

Interpretation of the EMG

The musculature of the anorectal continence organ mostly shows a resting activity[6,11]. This is probably due to the examination itself and to digital pre-dilatation. If the patient is sufficiently relaxed this leads to a state of relative stillness[14]. Continuous derivation during relaxation may even produce an 'electric silence'[18]. Normal findings show motor unit potentials (quantitative EMG in at least 20 MUP) with a duration of about 4 ms (3–8 ms, rarely longer than 10 ms). The amplitudes total 0.3 to maximal 2 mV (mean 0.6 mV). Less than 15% of all potentials should be polyphasic potentials (Table 1).

The patient is asked to press (relaxation of the pelvic floor) and this inhibits the resting activity to varying degrees[11,14]. A relative silence can also be observed

Table 1 Pathological EMG – finings of the external anal sphincter

Localization of the lesion	Spontaneous activity	Motor unit potentials	Voluntary activity	Reflex activity
Central	–	Normal	Rarefied	Increased
Acute peripheral	+ (Fi, PSW)	Usually normal	Rarefied	Normal or rarefied
Chronic peripheral	–/+ (Fi, PSW, pm)	Neurogenic change, reinnervation potentials	Rarefied	Normal or rarefied

Fi: fibrillations; PSW: positive sharp waves; pm: pseudomyotonic discharges = high frequent bizarre discharges

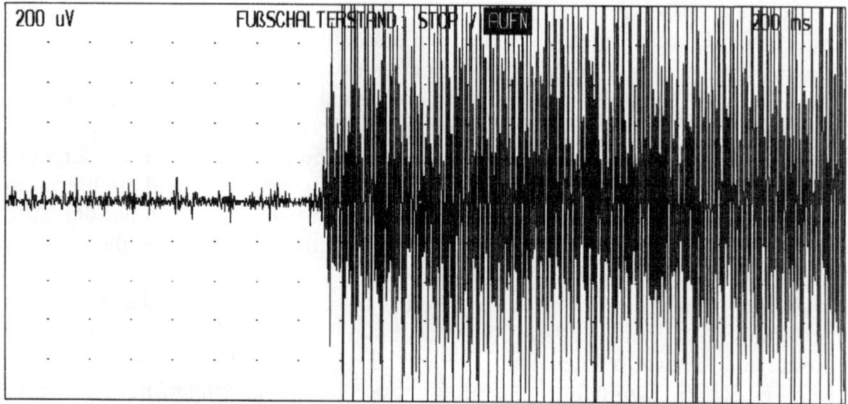

Figure 1 Voluntary contraction through squeezing with interference pattern, in the beginning on the left resting activity

during defaecation. Voluntary contraction through squeezing, but also through reflex activation (e.g. coughing and digital dilatation), produces larger and longer potentials of motor units. A more dense discharging pattern (interference pattern) with partial overlapping of potentials is found during fast registration of particularly vigorous activation (Fig. 1).

Areas of muscular defects or scars show no evidence of muscular actions in the EMG. At rest a spontaneous activity (fibrillations and positive sharp waves, in rare cases also high frequent bizarre discharges) can be observed in neurogenic lesions; during voluntary innervation a prolongation of the motor unit potentials (widened potentials) with higher amplitudes occurs. At the same time polyphasic potentials are frequent. During maximum voluntary innervation the pattern of activity is reduced. With respect to duration, amplitude and shape, central lesions do not cause changes of the single potentials, but lead to a reduced voluntary activity and increased uninhibited reflectory activity. It is doubtful whether solitary myogenic diseases of the external anal sphincter do exist. Myopathies are diagnosed through an EMG of the limb muscles.

EMG WITH THE SINGLE-FIBRE ELECTRODE

In single-fibre electromyography (single-fibre EMG, SFEMG) the electrical activity of single muscle fibres is recorded through extracellular derivation[19,20]. With this method it is possible to determine fibre density. Increased fibre density is a sign for reinnervation processes (sprouting of nerve fibres from preserved motor units). This examination is far more difficult to carry out than is EMG with the concentric needle electrode. It requires a specially equipped EMG amplifier (trigger, high-input impedance and high resolution of time) and special single-fibre electrodes (low profile and small active surface). Moreover, it takes more time and requires an examiner who is familiar with the SFEMG. This method allows quantification of the extent of a neurogenic lesion or an eventual reinnervation. Patients with neurogenic incontinence have an increased fibre density (also in defects in the area of the cauda equina)[19]. A fibre density between 1.3 and 1.8 is considered normal[19]. At the moment this is not a routine method.

EVOKED POTENTIALS AND CENTRAL MOTORIC STIMULATION

Evoked potentials and central motoric stimulation (stimulus is set above the cortex or on the level of the conus medullaris and derivation occurs from the external anal sphincter) are used especially for diagnostics of central disorders and for the localization of medullary lesions[1,21–27]. A total motor conduction time (TMCT) of 19.4 ± 2 ms and a CMCT (central motor conduction time) to L1 of 13.8 ± 1.2 ms[25] are considered normal values for motorically evoked potentials.

By modification of the above-mentioned pudendal electrode it is possible to stimulate via nerve root S3 and subsequently determine pudendal latency[24]. The MEPuL (magnetically evoked pudendal latency) covers a longer distance of the nerve and is therefore less dependent on the examiner than is the PNTML. The normal values are around 2.5 ± 0.4 ms[24] and allow calculation of a CMCT to S3 of 16.9 ± 1.7 ms[25]. The latencies after sacral magnetic stimulation may vary from 2.5 to 11 ms, depending on the distance from the skin[26]. The SNS–PNE latencies (sacral nerve stimulation–percutaneous nerve evaluation) are between 4.5 and 6 ms.

The common somatosensory evoked potentials (SSEP) can also be helpful for diagnosis. Lesions of sensitive fibres are detected through sensitively evoked potentials after stimulus on the penis, the clitoris or the perineum[28]. At the moment only the P40 latency is of diagnostic importance.

DISCUSSION

Anal incontinence can be the result of various neurological disorders. Some of these are traumas or expanding processes of the spinal cord and the caudal nerve roots. However, lesions of the peripheral motoric and sensory nerves are far more frequent, especially lesions of the pudendal nerve or its main branches (the pudendal nerve also contains sensory nerve fibres; mixed nerve)[29,30]. Damage to the pudendal nerve is in most cases caused by overstretching (traction neuropathy) of the nerve[2,29], e.g. in descensus of the pelvic floor or in prolapse of the rectum (e.g. steady pressing during defaecation, overweight, several pregnancies). This causes damage to the afferent and efferent fibres[30]. Often it is a summation of various partial defects. A muscular lesion, for instance (e.g. perineal tear during delivery, sphincterotomy in anal fissure) can exist at the same time as a neurogenic lesion. Incomplete defects of a part of the anorectal continence organ are usually compensated for over a long period of time. However, if an additional disorder of another partial function occurs, then the insufficiency becomes symptomatic. Usually a slow deterioration of continence is of neurogenic origin.

If no muscular lesions can be found as the cause of an incontinence, then the reason is usually denervation of the muscular apparatus, especially of the external anal sphincter and the puborectal muscle. This was proven by histological examinations[29,31] and several EMG studies[5,19]. At the same time there is a group of continence disorders without any muscular defect and without any sign of a neurogenic lesion. Often no cause is found in these cases. Psychogenic disorders are seldom the cause of incontinence in adults and should be suspected only when organic causes have been definitely excluded. The best information for differential diagnosis of incontinence is obtained by EMG of the external anal sphincter with a concentric needle electrode. In muscular defects, conventional EMG is sufficient. With EMG it is possible to locate simple defects and their degree in the striated muscle. In this respect EMG competes with endosonography, which produces comparable evidence but without pain.

Most of the questions in the diagnostics of a neurogenic lesion can be sufficiently answered with the conventional EMG[32]. Together with this, the PNTML, or as an alternative the MEPuL, should always be determined in order to exclude a neuropathy of the pudendal nerve. With the SFEMG it is possible to obtain a more precise quantification of the extent of the neurogenic lesion. If the electrophysiological examinations show increased fibre density in the SFEMG, and a prolonged latency of the anal reflex, then this is proof of damage to the nerve roots and/or peripheral nerves that supply the pelvic floor[5]. However, the realization of a SFEMG is far more difficult than conventional EMG. For routine diagnostics SFEMG appears unnecessary[33] and should be reserved for special indications.

Myogenic changes are certainly very seldom the cause of incontinence. The fact that some authors found myogenic changes in more than 20%[34], and myogenic or neuromyogenic lesions in more than a third of the incontinent patients, is most likely due to false interpretation of the motor unit potentials. On the one hand the motor units of the external anal sphincter are smaller than those of the striated limb muscles; on the other hand reinnervation potentials have probably been taken as a sign of myogenic transformation of motor units. In hundreds of examinations during recent years we never saw a myogenically changed external anal sphincter in patients without a general muscular disease.

Since it is rare that incontinence is caused by only one disorder, other possible deficits must also be taken into consideration. An additional neurogenic lesion in muscular defects, that had existed preoperatively, can worsen the result of a sphincter reconstruction. In the case of an unknown anterior muscle defect (e.g. episiotomy scar), postanal repair (PAR) surgery for neurogenic incontinence may worsen the continence function, since the defect can be worsened through the gathering of the musculature. Another indication for pelvic floor EMG is for the estimation of anal incontinence (e.g. post-traumatic). The problem here is to discover which partial functions of the continence organ are damaged and/or had been damaged before.

Extensive neurophysiological examinations should be reserved for special indications, and carried out only by experienced examiners.

A further important dysfunction of the pelvic floor is functional outlet obstruction. In some cases such obstructions are related to central or peripheral nervous disorders. We object to the non-critical use of the term 'anismus' for any type of functional outlet obstruction, as the blurring of distinct pathophysiological entities into a single diagnostic term obscures not only the proper differential diagnosis but also differential treatment options appropriate for each type of defaecatory dysfunction. We strongly suggest that the term 'anismus' should be reserved for the extremely rare form of focal dystonia of the external anal sphincter and/or puborectal muscle which is a form of extrapyramidal movement disorder, as discussed above. The term 'spastic pelvic floor syndrome' should never be used as a synonym for outlet obstruction. Spastic pelvic floor syndrome is defined as a specific form of reflex hypercontraction of the musculature supplied by the pudendal nerve following lesions of the upper motoneurons. The definition 'contraction of the voluntary sphincters instead of relaxation' or 'paradoxical puborectalis contraction' is incorrect.

Both patients with anismus and patients with spastic pelvic floor syndrome should undergo a primary neurological examination in order to identify accompanying clinical signs and the underlying aetiology of the disorder. By far the most frequent cause of functional outlet obstruction is dyscoordination of the anal sphincter apparatus. In addition to a concise history, thorough clinical examination and manometry the diagnostic process for evacuation disorders necessitates concentric needle EMG carried out by an experienced examiner in order to make the correct diagnosis as a prerequisite for an appropriate therapeutic decision. With the surface electrode it is not possible to differentiate definitely between external anal sphincter and puborectal muscle.

References

1. Kiff ES, Swash M. Normal proximal and delayed distal conduction in the pudendal nerves of patients with idiopathic (neurogenic) faecal incontinence. J Neurol Neurosurg Psychiatry. 1984;47:820–3.
2. Kiff ES, Swash M. Slowed conduction in the pudendal nerves in idiopathic (neurogenic) faecal incontinence. Br J Surg. 1984;71:614–16.
3. Henry MM, Swash M. Assessment of pelvic-floor disorders and incontinence by elektrophysiological recording of the anal reflex. Lancet. 1978;1:1290–1.
4. Henry MM, Parks AG, Swash M. The anal reflex in idiopathic faecal incontinence; an electrophysiological study. Br J Surg. 1980;67:781–3.
5. Neill ME, Parks AG, Swash M. Physiological studies of the anal sphincter musculature in faecal incontinence and rectal prolapse. Br J Surg. 1981;68:531–6.
6. Pedersen E. Electromyography of the sphincter muscles. Contemp Clin Neurophysiol (EEG Suppl.) 1978;34:405–16.
7. Pedersen E, Harving H, Klemar B, Tørring J. Human anal relexes. J Neurol Neurosurg Psychiatry. 1978;41:813–18.
8. Pedersen E, Klemar B, Schrøder HD, Tørring J. Anal sphincter responses after perianal electrical stimulation. J Neurol Neurosurg Psychiatry. 1982;45:770–3.

9. Bors E, Blinn KA. Bulbocavernosus reflex. J Urol. 1959;82:128–30.

10. O'Donnell P, Beck C, Doyle R, Eubanks C. Surface electrodes in perineal electromyography. Urology. 1988;32:375–9.

11. Floyd WF, Wallis EW. Electromyography of the sphincter ani externus in man. J Physiol. 1953; 122:599–609.

12. Beck A. Elektromyographische Untersuchungen am Sphincter ani. Pflüg Arch Ges Physiol. 1930;224:278–92.

13. Rossolimo G. Der Analreflex, seine Physiologie und Pathologie. Neurologisches Centralblatt. 1891;10:257–9.

14. Parks AG, Porter NH, Melzak J. Experimental study of the reflex mechanism controlling the muscles of the pelvic floor. Dis Colon Rectum. 1962;5:407–14.

15. Percy JP, Neill ME, Swash M, Parks AG. Electrophysiological study of motor nerve supply of pelvic floor. Lancet. 1981;1:16–17.

16. Juenemann KP, Lue TF, Schmidt RA, Tanagho EA. Clinical significance of sacral and pudendal nerve anatomy. J Urol. 1988;139:74–80.

17. Braun J, Silny J, Schumpelick V. Methodische und analytische Probleme elektromyographischer Untersuchungen des inneren Analschließmuskels im Rahmen der anorektalen Funktionsdiagnostik. Colo-Proctology. 1987;9:199–209.

18. Allert ML, Jelasic F. Das Ruhe-EMG des gesunden Blasen- und Analschließmuskels. Dtsch Ztschr Nervenheilk. 1968;194:252–60.

19. Neill ME, Swash M. Increased motor unit fibre density in the external anal sphincter muscle in ano-rectal incontinence: a single fibre EMG study. J Neurol Neurosurg Psychiatry. 1980;43: 343–7.

20. Snooks SJ, Barnes PRH, Swash M. Damage to the innervation of the voluntary anal and periurethral sphincter musculature in incontinence: an electrophysiological study. J Neurol Neurosurg Psychiatry. 1984;47:1269–73.

21. Ertekin C, Hansen MV, Larsson LE, Sjödahl R. Examination of the descending pathway to the external anal sphincter and pelvic floor muscles by transcranial cortical stimulation. Electroenceph Clin Neurophysiol. 1990;75:500–10.

22. Ghezzi A, Callea L, Zaffaroni M, Monatanini R, Tessera G. Motor potentials of bulbocavernosus muscle after transcranial and lumbar magnetic stimulation: comparative study with bulbocavernosus reflex and pudendal evoked potentials. J Neurol Neurosurg Psychiatry. 1991;54: 524–6.

23. Haldemann S, Bradley WE, Bhatia NN, Johnson BK. Pudendal evoked responses. Arch Neurol. 1982;39:280–3.

24. Jost WH, Schimrigk K. Magnetic stimulation of the pudendal nerve. Dis Colon Rectum. 1993; 37:687–9.

25. Jost WH, Schimrigk K. A new method to determine pudendal nerve motor latency and central motor conduction time to the external anal sphincter. Electroenceph Clin Neurophysiol. 1994; 93:237–9.

26. Sato T, Konishi F, Kanazawa K. Variations in motor evoked potential latencies in the anal sphincter system with sacral magnetic stimulation. Dis Colon Rectum. 2000;43:966–70.

27. Snooks SJ, Swash M, Henry MM. Abnormalities in central and peripheral nerve conduction in patients with anorectal incontinence. J Roy Soc Med. 1985;78:294–300.

28. Osterhage J, Ludolph AC, Mazur H. Evozierte Potentiale in der Diagnostik der erektilen Dysfunktion. Kontinenz. 1993;2:175–81.

29. Parks AG, Swash M, Urich H. Sphincter denervation in anorectal incontinence and rectal prolapse. Gut. 1977;18:656–65.

30. Roe AM, Bartolo DCC, McC. Mortensen NJ. New method for assessment of anal sensation in various anorectal disorders. Br J Surg.1986;73:310–12.

31. Beersiek F, Parks AG, Swash M. Pathogenesis of ano-rectal incontinence. J Neurol Sci. 1979;42:111–27.

32. Bartolo DCC, Jarratt JA, Read NW. The use of conventional electromyography to assess external sphincter neuropathy in man. J Neurol Neurosurg Psychiatry 1983;46:1115–18.

33. Vodusek DB, Janko M, Lokar J. EMG, single fibre EMG and sacral reflexes in assessment of sacral nervous system lesions. J Neurol Neurosurg Psychiatry. 1982;45:1064–6.

34. Athanasiadis S. Elektromyographische und funktionsanalytische Befunde bei obstruktiven Defäkationsstörungen. Langenbecks Arch Chir. 1992;377:244–52.

7
Pelvic floor dysfunction – conservative management

H. HINNINGHOFEN and P. ENCK

HISTORY OF BIOFEEDBACK IN PELVIC FLOOR DISORDERS

The term 'biofeedback' describes a therapeutic instrument, which derives from the psychological 'theory of learning'. Its basis is 'learning through reinforcement' in the tradition of I. P. Pawlow and B. F. Skinner: the principle is that any reinforced behaviour is likely to be repeated[1].

While Skinner and others restricted such 'operant conditioning' to observable behaviour, it was subsequently shown that even functions of the autonomic nervous system can be influenced by operant conditioning. A body function, which cannot be perceived by the subject under normal conditions, is measured by a technical device and demonstrated to the subject. Biofeedback is based on the fact that electrical impulses, generated by an active muscle, can be fed back in the form of audible and visible signals, so that patients can be taught to recognize and consciously influence normally unconscious body functions. The reinforcer in adult humans is usually 'the result'; for patients the symptomatic improvement.

The first use of biofeedback in gastroenterology was reported by Haskell and Rovner in 1967[2]; they taught their patients, by means of a needle EMG, to contract the external anal sphincter. Patients were instructed to synchronize voluntary contractions with electrically applied stimuli to the muscle, and to perform home exercises. Patients with only partial denervation showed good improvement of incontinence symptoms. Due to the painfulness of this procedure this technique did not gain a clinical future.

The stage for biofeedback training in pelvic floor disorders was set by a case report by Kohlenberg[3] in 1973: The author treated a 13-year-old boy showing faecal incontinence (encopresis and soiling) after colorectal surgery for (questionable) Hirschsprung's disease 2 years previously. At the time of the study the boy was supposed to undergo colectomy. A balloon system was used to provide visual feedback of the anal sphincter function. However, it remains unclear from the publication whether the authors provided feedback from the internal anal sphincter (resting pressure) only, or also from the external anal sphincter and rectum. The treatment resulted in a resting pressure increase from 35 mmHg baseline to 50 mmHg post-treatment – very low anyway to reliably maintain continence. Consequently, clinical improvement is poorly documented and reported.

In these days, balloon systems are widely replaced by transcutaneous EMG recording, first reported by MacLeod in 1979[4]. The EMG biofeedback system consists of surface electrodes mounted on an anal plug, and a monitor or LED display to visualize the signals. After placing the plug in the anal canal these electrodes record EMG signals from the external anal sphincter. These are then displayed on a monitor to provide instant visual feedback to the patient regarding performance. Over time several devices and methods have become available to perform this training.

Today the historical roots of biofeedback training have mostly been lost by most investigators using this technique; it very often occurs as, and is attributed to, physical therapy and rehabilitation. Consequently, its specific application in the treatment of constipation – from 1980 onwards[5] – was predominantly proposed and performed by paediatric and adult surgeons. Another case report in 1979 may also landmark this conversion of a psychology-generated and theory-driven therapeutic strategy into clinical medical routine: Schiller et al.[61] successfully used the rectal infusion of saline as a training mode to improve sphincter functions in a patient with incontinence and chronic diarrhoea.

BIOFEEDBACK THERAPY IN PELVIC FLOOR DISORDERS IN THE LITERATURE

To date there have been 27 papers published concerning biofeedback application in adults with faecal incontinence, and a total of 25 papers reporting treatment of chronic constipation in adults by means of biofeedback. After a basic description of the principles of biofeedback training the currently published literature will be reviewed. This review extends and updates a previous survey paper on the same subject[7]. Since then, another four papers have evaluated the use of biofeedback training in patients with chronic pelvic (anal or rectal) pain which were included in this survey.

Biofeedback treatment of faecal incontinence

The definition proposed by the Rome criteria is: continuous or recurrent uncontrolled passage of faecal material (>10 ml) for at least 1 month in an individual older than 3 years of age[29]. Faecal incontinence can be caused by neurological or muscular damage. It is a serious problem that affects men and women of all ages. Continence is the result of a complex cooperation of neuromuscular and anatomical mechanisms. There are three components in anorectal function that can be the aim for biofeedback therapy in incontinent patients. The aim may be to improve the strength of the anal sphincter, or the coordination of the rectum and the sphincter, or to improve the sensory awareness of stool in the rectum. The treatment protocol for every patient will depend on the underlying dysfunction.

External anal sphincter improvement

After a manometric probe is placed in the anorectum the patient is instructed to squeeze the anus and to maintain the squeeze for at least 10 s. During this exercise the patient receives visual feedback generated by the EMG activity of the anal sphincter. The instruction for this manoeuvre is to selectively squeeze the anal muscles, not the abdominal, gluteal or thigh muscles[9,10]. To explain the correct manoeuvre, a normal pressure recording can be shown[11].

Coordination of rectum and anal sphincter

The aim of this training is to squeeze the anal sphincter with a maximum contraction in a minimum time after a balloon distention in the rectum[12]. By means of visual feedback the patients are taught to squeeze their anal sphincter without increasing the intra-abdominal pressure, because many patients with incontinence show an inappropriately high intra-abdominal pressure during squeezing.

Sensory perception training

The aim is to teach the patient to perceive a smaller distention of the rectum with the same intensity as they had previously perceived a larger distention[13]. After inflating a balloon in the rectum until an urge to defaecate, the balloon volume is decreased stepwise. The subject is instructed to note the pressure changes in the rectum and to use the biofeedback signal as a cue for volumes that are not perceived. Through a process of trial and error, lower thresholds for rectal perception will be established.

Biofeedback training and the evaluation of outcome require the use of anorectal testing techniques. It is necessary to have: a measure of sphincter contraction, a measure of abdominal wall pressure (pressure in a rectal balloon), and graded distention of the rectum with an airfilled balloon.

Several types of biofeedback systems are available. An anal plug with electrodes and a recording system is used in many studies. This device is suitable for strengthening the anal sphincter; it is not useful for coordination or sensory perception training. For these goals a system with an additional rectal balloon is necessary.

The number of training sessions required to reach clinical improvement is variable. It depends not only on the severity of the symptoms but also on the patient's motivation and ability to learn. The number of training sessions should be based on the patient's needs. To improve the long-term outcome of biofeedback training, follow-up assessments and training lessons should be performed at intervals.

The 27 data-based studies reported in peer-reviewed international journals (see Tables 1 and 4) derive from almost as many centres around the world. All institutions belong to gastroenterological or surgical clinics or were closely associated with them. Although biofeedback training is of psychological origin, none of the studies has been undertaken in a psychological setting. This indicates that the application in (lower) intestinal functions is restricted to medical settings in which invasive diagnostic and therapeutic approaches are available, feasible and ethical.

Table 1 Biofeedback studies in faecal incontinence (1)

First author	Year	Ref.	No.	Age	Range	Sex (F:M)	Origin[a]
Engel	1974	12	7	40.7	6–54	5:2	5:2
Cerulli	1979	10	50	46.0	5–97	36:12	35:14
Goldenberg	1980	62	12	n.r.	12–78	6:6	6:6
Wald	1981	9	17	46.9	10–79	11:6	4:13
Latimer	1984	19	8	30.1	8–72	4:4	5:3
Whitehead	1985	14	18	72.7	65–92	15:3	3: 15
Buser	1986	63	13	53.6	13–66	7:6	9:4
McLeod	1987	4	113	56.0	25–88	67:46	79:34
Berti Riboli	1988	64	21	61.0	14–84	15:6	15:6
Loening-Baucke	1990	24	8	63.0	35–78	8:0	n.r.
Miner	1990	20	25	54.6	17–76	17:8	16:9
Chiarioni	1993	65	14	48.1	24–76	10:4	3:11
Keck	1994	48	15	39.0	29–65	13:2	6:9
Guillemot	1995	23	24	60.7	39–78	19:5	3:19
Sangwan	1995	66	28	52.9	30–74	22:6	13:25
Rao	1996	11	19	50.0	17–78	20:2	14:5
Ko	1997	41	25	63.0	31–82	21:4	25:3
Rieger	1997	67	30	68.0	29–85	28:2	27:3
Patankar	1997	22	25	66.0	34–85	13:12	8:17
Patankar[b]	1997	21	72	70.0	34–87	43:29	30:42
Glia	1998	75	26	61	32–82	22:4	19:7
All			570		5–97	401:169	

[a] Surgical/obstetric vs. medical patients.
[b] Multicentre trial.
n.r. = Not reported.

A total of almost 650 patients of all ages have been treated over the years; most of them were women. Although anal incontinence is found more frequently in people older than 65, only one study[14] included geriatric patients only. Except for the five studies discussed in the following section, the patients entered into these studies usually had quite different underlying causes of incontinence. Patient selection depended on whether the setting was surgical or medical. While the initial studies had relatively small sample sizes, these have increased over the years, as has the duration of patients' follow-up after treatment: A recent multicentre trial across three different laboratories in the USA[15] included 72 patients, and long-term follow-up studies of 2 years and more were reported[16,17] (Table 3).

While the initial studies from the Baltimore group focused on internal and external sphincter muscle *coordination* as the major goal of biofeedback training, subsequently both sensory components, as well as voluntary muscle control,

Table 2 Biofeedback studies in faecal incontinence (2)

First author	Year	Ref.	Init.[a]	End[b]	Treatment goals			No. of sessions	Add.[c]
					Coordination	Sensitivity	Voluntary contraction		
Engel	1974	12	yes	yes	yes	no	no	1 – 4	no
Cerulli	1979	10	yes	yes	yes	yes	no	1	no
Goldenberg	1980	62	yes	no	no	yes	no	> 1	no
Wald	1981	9	yes	no	yes	yes	yes	1 + 1	home
Latimer	1984	19	yes	yes	yes	yes	yes	8 (2/week)	home
Whitehead	1985	14	yes	yes	no	no	yes	8 (2/week)	home
Buser	1986	63	yes	yes	no	yes	yes	1 – 3	home
McLeod	1987	4	no	yes	no	no	yes	3.3	no
Berti Riboli	1988	64	yes	yes	yes	yes	yes	12 (2/week)	no
Loening-Baucke	1990	24	yes	yes	yes	yes	yes	3	home
Miner	1990	20	yes	yes	yes	yes	yes	3	no
Chiarioni	1993	65	yes	yes	no	no	yes	2 + 1	home
Keck	1994	48	yes	yes	no	yes	yes	3 (1–7)	home
Guillemot	1995	23	yes	yes	no	no	yes	4/week	home
Sangwan	1995	66	no	yes	no	yes	yes	33.75 (1–7)	home
Rao	1996	11	yes	yes	yes	yes	yes	7 (4–13)	home
Ko	1997	41	yes	no	no	no	yes	5 (2–13)	home
Rieger	1997	67	(yes)	no	no	no	yes	6	home
Patankar	1997	22	no	no	no	no	yes	7 (5–11)	home
Patankar[d]	1997	21	no	no	no	no	yes	7 (2–11)	home
Glia	1998	75	yes	yes	no	yes	yes	max. 10	no

[a] Initial evaluation (manometry, EMG).
[b] End evaluation (manometry, EMG).
[c] Additional treatment (home training).
[d] Multicentre-studies.
Data in parentheses indicate that only some of the patients were evaluated.

were entered into the treatment programmes (see Table 2). After biofeedback training becomes more common some of the investigators involved had shown that sensory perception from the rectum is necessary for treatment[13] and determines the outcome[18]. Two studies[19,20] have shown that sensory retraining is probably the most important factor in biofeedback training in incontinence.

The availability of non-invasive transcutaneous EMG biofeedback devices for clinical and for home training has led to an increase in the training of voluntary anal sphincter muscle contraction as the major goal in recent years, while the other goals tend to diminish (Table 2). A change in outcome evaluation can also be noted in the published literature. While earlier studies have incorporated initial and end evaluation of physiological functions of the pelvic floor by means of

Table 3 Biofeedback studies in faecal incontinence (3)

First author	Year	Ref.	Criteria[a]	Evaluation type	Follow-up	Efficacy[b]	Control[c]
Engel	1974	12	n.r.	interv.	6–16 months	57	no
Cerulli	1979	10	>90%	n.r.	4–108 weeks	72	no
Goldenberg	1980	62	n.r.	n.r.	10–96 weeks	83	no
Wald	1981	9	>75%	interv.	2–38 months	71	no
Latimer	1984	19	n.r.	diary	6 months	88	within subjects
Whitehead	1985	14	>75%	diary	6 months	77	waiting list
Buser	1986	63	n.r.	n.r.	16–30 months	92	no
McLeod	1987	4	>90%	subj.	6–60 months	63	no
Berti Riboli	1988	64	>90%	n.r.	3 months	86	no
Loening-Baucke	1990	24	>75%	diary	12 months	50	conventional treatment
Miner	1990	20	subj.	diary	<2 years	76	three-arm crossover
Chiarioni	1993	65	>75%	interv.	14.5 months	85	no
Keck	1994	48	subj.	interv.	8 months (1–23)	73	no
Guillemot	1995	23	subj.	diary	30 months (24–36)	56	no treatment
Sangwan	1995	66	subj.	interv.	20 months (4–47)	75	no
Rao	1996	11	>67%	diary	1 year	53	no
Ko	1997	41	n.r.	diary	not done	87.5	no
Rieger	1997	67	>80%	interv.	6–12 months	67	no
Patankar	1997	22	>75%	subj.	not done	70	no
Patankar[d]	1997	21	>75%	subj.	not done	83.3	no
Glia	1998	75	>50%	interv.	21 months (12–46)	53.7	no

[a] Efficacy criteria: percentage decrease in incontinence symptoms.
[b] Percentage patients improved.
[c] Control group employed.
[d] Multicentre study. n.r. = not reported; interv. = interview; subj. = subjective rating.

manometry, EMG, and other diagnostic tools, this also has become neglected, with increased usage of biofeedback treatment into routine clinical management of patients[21,22].

Despite a broad agreement that biofeedback is the treatment of choice in patients with faecal incontinence, the training modalities are far less consistent: neither the total number of training sessions necessary, nor their frequency, the duration of treatment, or the supplementation of therapy by home training with or without technical devices are standardized at present (Table 3). Most recent studies incorporate home exercises, but these are usually not controlled for compliance and efficacy.

Symptom evaluation was mostly done with the help of diary cards, monitoring progress during the course of treatment. Others have used interview techniques and questionnaires, which may bear the risk of false or incomplete memory, if the period to recall is too long. Control of the efficacy of an incontinence therapy by means of diary cards allows an estimate of the progress when the events are frequent and the recording period sufficiently long (at least 2 weeks or longer), since the percentage of decrease of such events can easily be calculated; this is much more difficult with infrequent events, as is the case in chronic constipation (see below).

All but one of the published studies reported a success rate greater than 50%, with efficacy criteria ranging between 75% and 90% reduction in the frequency of incontinence events. The overall success (percentage of improved patients) is approximately 70%, supporting the view that, even if there are only a few studies which incorporated control groups, the effects cannot be attributed to placebo alone.

Biofeedback training in faecal incontinence in homogeneous patient groups

In addition to the studies above, in which patients with different underlying causes of incontinence have been treated by the same biofeedback training, five studies with homogeneous patient groups have been published: in one study patients with diabetes mellitus[25], in three studies[26–28] patients with various surgical conditions (prolapse, sphincter surgery, low anterior resection and colectomy), and in one case patients with 'idiopathic (neurogenic) faecal incontinence'[6]. It is surprising and noteworthy to find only the latter with a rather poor outcome – no treatment effect at all – while the others claim response rates which are well within the range of studies cited above. A surprising outcome, because the other study groups (e.g. refs 26 and 28) most certainly had also included some patients with idiopathic (neurogenic) faecal incontinence. Unfortunately, documentation is rather poor in this study: no EMG data prior to treatment are reported, except the statement of 'severe denervation', or incontinence symptom recordings by dairy pretreatment, during or post-treatment which would allow differentiation between individuals. The mean increase in squeeze pressure was small, but at least some patients showed marked improvement of anal sphincter performance. Training was home training only, with four outpatient visits, but again, compliance of the patient to the programme is not reported.

The only controlled study is the one by Hämäläinen *et al.*[26], who used a 'no treatment by biofeedback' control group in patients undergoing surgery for rectal prolapse. Biofeedback was performed presurgery for 4–6 weeks to reduce postsurgery incontinence. It is questionable whether such a prospective study would still show significant improvement after operation in comparison to controls if an unspecific treatment option – to control for attention and other psychological effects – and/or if a specific treatment option – e.g. pelvic floor exercises without biofeedback support – had been chosen as control.

Table 4 Biofeedback studies in faecal incontinence in homogeneous patient groups

First author	Year	Ref.	No.	Pathology	Age	F:M	Evaluation	Dur
Wald	1984	25	11	diabetes	52.2	8:3	Manometry	n.r
van Tets	1996	6	12	neurogenic	48.0	n.r.	Manometry, EMG	12 w
Ho	1996	28	13	LAR, Col	62.1	3:10	Manometry	4 w
Hämäläinen	1996	26	11	prolapse	61.2	9:2	Manometry	4–6 w
Jensen	1997	27	28	sphinc surg	34.0	n.r.	diary	3–4 sessions/w

[a] Percentage patients improved.
n.r. = Not recorded.
LAR = Low anterior resection.
Col = Colectomy.

Biofeedback treatment of chronic constipation

Constipation can be defined by three parameters: symptoms, frequency of defaecation, and physiological measurements[30]. According to the Rome criteria constipation is defined as the presence of two or more of the following symptoms for at least 3 months: (1) straining at defaecation at least one-fourth of the time, (2) lumpy and/or hard stools at least one-fourth of the time, (3) sensation of incomplete evacuation at least one-fourth of the time, and (4) two or fewer bowel movements per week. Constipation can be divided into two categories with regard to its pathophysiological mechanism: slow colonic transit and anorectal dysfunction (outlet obstruction); the two may coexist. Symptoms compatible with constipation are found in 3–20% of the population; the prevalence increases to 20–25% in the elderly[31]. Up to 50% of patients with constipation suffer from 'outlet obstruction'[32]. This disorder is characterized by a failure of rectoanal coordination with paradoxical anal sphincter contraction, inadequate anal sphincter relaxation during defaecation, and/or impaired rectal sensation[33,34]. In such patients the goals of retraining are to correct each of these pathophysiological disturbances. The patient has to learn to evacuate stool without using laxatives, suppositories, or digital manipulations.

Rectoanal coordination

The goal of this exercise is to lead to a useful coordination between intra-abdominal pressure and anal sphincter relaxation during defaecation. After placing an EMG plug with a rectum balloon in the anorectum, the patient sits down in front of a monitor and is asked to bear down as if to defaecate. On the monitor the pressure tracings from the abdominal pressure and the anal sphincter are shown. The patient is asked to vary the abdominal and anal effort. The goal is to achieve simultaneously an increase in intra-abdominal pressure and a decrease in anal sphincter pressure. It may be helpful to show first a normal pattern of rectoanal coordination.

Rectal sensory perception

The goal is to diminish the thresholds for rectal sensory perception as descibed above for faecal incontinence. By a process of trial and error the patient is taught to perceive increasingly smaller volumes of balloon distention.

To perform an appropriate training for constipated patients a biofeedback system is necessary that records both anal and rectal pressures. The distended balloon can also be pulled through the anus to simulate the act of defaecation, and to give the patient an example of the correct feeling of this procedure[35].

The number of biofeedback training sessions should be customized for each patient, as discussed previously. Normally, three to six 45-min training sessions may be required.

The application of biofeedback training in chronically constipated patients has a much shorter tradition, but is obviously gaining more attention today since a total of 25 papers have been published in the past 12 years. More than 700 patients were treated in many different centres, with all except one[36] being surgical departments, presumably indicating that surgeons more often than internists are confronted with therapy-refractory chronic constipation and are asked for surgical therapy of dubious efficacy such as colectomy[37] (Table 5). It was, consequently, surgery and surgery-associated physiology laboratory testing which revealed two types of constipation that may be distinguished: slow colonic

Table 5 Biofeedback studies in chronic constipation (1)

First author	Year	Ref.	No.	Age	Range	Sex (F:M)	Duration
Bleijenberg	1987	39	10	32.0	10–48	n.r.	>6 years
Weber	1987	69	22	n.r.	18–35	22:0	n.r.
Lestar	1991	44	16	42.5	n.r.	10:6	n.r.
Kawimbe	1991	40	15	45.0	22–76	12:3	8.8 years
Dahl	1991	70	9	41.0	20–60	15:0	18 years (4–40)
Wexner	1992	71	18	67.7	10–84	13:5	26.9 years
Fleshman	1992	45	9	49.4	35–62	8:1	n.r.
Turnbull	1992	72	7	35.7	29–42	7:0	12 years (1–30)
Keck	1994	48	12	62.0	17–82	10:2	n.r.
Papachrysostymou	1994	47	22	42.0	32–50	17:5	3–25 years
Bleijenberg	1994	49	20	37.0	20–50	15.5	7 years (2–15)
Koutsomanis	1994	46	20	34.0	18–53	18:2	n.r.
Koutsomanis	1995	52	60	40.5	20–64	53:7	13 years
Siproudhis	1995	42	27	46.0	21–77	20:7	35 months (6–192)
Leroi[a]	1996	43	15	41.2	n.r.	15:0	n.r.
Ho	1996	28	62	48.0	n.r.	28:24	4.8 years
Park	1996	38	68	65.9	15–90	44:24	20 years
Ko	1997	41	17	50.0	22–82	12:5	8.1 years
Rao	1997	36	25	50.0	21–87	16:10	n.r.
Glia	1997	50	26	55.0	28–78	23:3	11 years
Karlbohm	1997	73	28	46.0	22–72	23:5	9 years (1–30)
Rieger	1997	74	19	63.0	16–78	18:1	n.r.
Patankar	1997	22	30	65.3	33–86	24:6	n.r.
Patankar[b]	1997	21	116	73.0	33–85	88:28	n.r.
Chiotakakou[c]	1998	16	100	40.0	10–79	87:13	n.r.
All			773		10–90	601:162	

[a] Sexually abused women.
[b] Multicentre study.
[c] Long-term follow-up.
n.r. = Not recorded.

transit and so-called 'outlet obstruction'-type ('spastic pelvic floor syndrome', anismus, pelvic floor dyssynergia), and only the latter one being subject to biofeedback treatment in most studies (see below).

Patients with chronic constipation are on average younger than their incontinent counterparts, but female predominance persists. If reported in the studies, constipation history may date back to childhood in some, or back a few months only in other patients. The pathomechanism by which functional outlet obstruction occurs is still unknown, and it is questionable whether all patients resemble one clinical entity only. At least one study[37] claims to have identified different types of 'animus', and another has found at least one cause of anismus to be sexual abuse in childhood or adulthood[37].

Since the diagnosis of functional outlet obstruction is based only in part on clinical symptoms (laxative use, necessity to excessive straining, digital assistance with defaecation), all studies have used elaborate laboratory testing to confirm the diagnosis: this usually included manometry, defaecography or related imaging techniques, anal sphincter EMG, and the balloon expulsion test. Most centres have also used large-bowel transit studies to *exclude* slow-transit constipation. Others[39] have ignored this, or have challenged its necessity by consecutive inclusion of patients with constipation of both types[40,41]. While one can assume that colonic transit measurement may be comparable across centres, neither manometry nor defaecography is a standardized clinical procedure so far, and the same holds true for balloon expulsion. No agreement is currently available as to how many and which tests need to be pathological to confirm the diagnosis.

Probably the most surprising finding is that most centres have *not* included psychological evaluation of the patients included (Table 6), although it has been known for many years that many patients with chronic constipation suffer from overt psychopathology. In some studies treatment failure has been attributed to psychopathology (e.g. refs 39, 42 and 43), and psychological counselling was offered.

While the initial paper[39] and a second group[5] suggested the necessity for hospital admission and inpatient treatment of 4 weeks and longer, subsequent research has shown that outpatient management is feasible without losing efficacy. From an economic standpoint this modification was necessary to allow biofeedback treatment to become widely accepted. Whether or not a single treatment session[44] will become the preferred and most effective mode in most cases is, however, questionable.

Treatment efficacy is usually assessed by comparing clinical symptoms prior to and after treatment, but some studies[45–47] have evaluated sphincter perfomance in physiological tests instead. Outcome is assessed sometimes by diary card, but often by reviews, interviews, and questionnaires. It should be kept in mind that these evaluation techniques are even more unreliable if the event to be recorded – e.g. defaecation – is infrequent in nature. However, stool diaries would have to be used for longer periods than in faecal incontinence to gain the same sensitivity.

Different from incontinence training, re-education of paradoxical pelvic floor behaviour is achieved in a shorter period of time – within a few sessions – and maintained for longer after the training. Only one study called the results disappointing[48], but does admit efficacy in selected cases. This indicates that patient

Table 6 Biofeedback studies in chronic constipation (2)

First author	Year	Ref.	Diagnostic evalua		
			Manometry	Defaecography	Colonic transit
Bleijenberg	1987	39	no	yes	yes
Weber	1987	69	yes	no	no
Lestar	1991	44	yes	no	no
Kawimbe	1991	40	yes	yes	no
Dahl	1991	70	yes	yes	yes
Wexner	1992	71	yes	yes	yes
Fleshman	1992	45	yes	yes	yes
Turnbull	1992	72	yes	yes	yes
Keck	1994	48	yes	(yes)	(yes)
Papachrysostymou	1994	47	yes	yes	yes
Bleijenberg	1994	49	yes	no	no
Koutsomanis	1994	46	yes	yes	yes
Koutsomanis	1995	52	no	no	yes
Siproudhis	1995	42	yes	yes	no
Leroi	1996	43	(yes)	no	no
Ho	1996	28	yes	yes	yes
Park	1996	38	yes	yes	yes
Ko	1997	41	yes	(yes)	yes
Rao	1997	36	yes	yes	yes
Glia	1997	50	yes	yes	yes
Karlbohm	1997	73	yes	yes	yes
Rieger	1997	74	yes	yes	(yes)
Patankar	1997	22	no	no	no
Patankar[a]	1997	21	no	no	no
Chiotakakou	1998	16	no	no	(yes)

[a] Multicentre trial.

selection – and the appropriate diagnostic tools to differentiate between slow transit and outlet obstruction – may still be a matter of controversy. The sensitivity and specificity of these diagnostic tests (manometry, EMG, defaecography, transit studies) may also vary significantly.

While all studies compared treatment outcome with the initial complaints of patients, no comparison to non-biofeedback treatment (e.g. through conventional medical or dietary management) was attempted (or achieved). Only a few studies state that failure to a standardized conventional procedure, e.g. dietary management, was a prerequisite for entering the study. It is, however, tempting to speculate whether a similar response may also be gained by other strategies, and may be due to unspecific placebo effects.

Two studies[49,50] compared different modes of the biofeedback signal on therapy outcome: EMG recording from the anal sphincter muscle – recorded transcutaneously through anal plug devices – versus a feedback signal from a pressure signal (balloon, manometry catheter) – neither was superior. However, pressure sensors in the anal canal carry a risk: the signal may be disturbed through confounding pressure events (increases) in the rectum. A further study[51] compared the efficacy of biofeedback therapy between two groups of patients with different types of anismus, and showed that only those patients with 'classical' anismus, i.e. with a shortening of the anorectal angle with attempts to strain – would profit from biofeedback therapy.

In a more recently published study[52] the investigators compared a group which received verbal feedback from an instructor with a group receiving feedback using a visual display of pelvic floor EMG during straining. It was shown that the reponse rate was similar in both groups, and resulted in symptom improvement of approximately 50%. The authors concluded[52] that 'training in abdominal muscle contraction with pelvic floor relaxation is equally effective with or without a measuring device', but admit that constant encouragement and praise from an instructor is necessary, as is a 'good rapport between patient and instructor' (p. 99).

From a psychological standpoint it is not surprising to learn that verbal instruction and reinforcement can be as effective a feedback mode as a visual- or auditory-mediated technical feedback display – it may only be surprising for physicians not used to sitting beside their patients for much longer than a few minutes. The more important question, generated by this chapter, is whether constant verbal instruction is the more practical (and affordable) way of biofeedback mode than through simple designed technical measurement devices (and not a physiological laboratory, as implied) which may be taken home with the patient, and which would allow more training, in more privacy, and with lower total costs than this study suggests and others have speculated. Interestingly, about half of the studies – and not those claiming biofeedback to be helpful in *all* cases of chronic constipation – have incorporated home training procedures into the treatment programme, but, as with faecal inontinence, patient compliance to such training advices has never been controlled.

Biofeedback therapy in chronic anal or rectal pain

Anorectal pain compatible with the levator ani syndrome and proctalgia fugax occur in 5–8% of the population[53]. The levator ani syndrome is defined as a

Table 7 Biofeedback training in chronic constipation (3)

First author	Year	Ref.	Follow-up	Sessions	Additional home training
Bleijenberg	1987	39	7 months (1–18)	daily	yes
Weber	1987	69	no	2–4	
Lestar	1991	44	no	1	yes
Kawimbe	1991	40	6.2 months	2/day	yes
Dahl	1991	70	6 months	5	yes
Wexner	1992	71	9 months (1–17)	9	no
Fleshman	1992	45	>6 months	2×6	no
Turnbull	1992	72	2–4 years	15	yes
Keck	1994	48	1–8 months	3	yes
Papachrysostymou	1994	47	no	>3	yes
Bleijenberg	1994	49	no	8	yes
Koutsomanis	1994	46	6–12 months	2–6	yes
Koutsomanis	1995	52	2–3 months	1–7	no
Siproudhis	1995	42	1–36 months	1–7	no
Leroi	1996	43	6–10 months	16	no
Ho	1996	28	no	4	yes
Park	1996	38	no	11	no
Ko	1997	41	no	4	yes
Rao	1997	36	<2 months	2/week, 2–4 weeks	yes
Glia	1997	50	no	1–2/week, <10 week	yes

Karlbohm	1997	73	>1 year	8	no
Rieger	1997	74	>6 months	6 (1/week)	yes
Patankar	1997	22	no	7 (5–11), 1/week	no
Patankar	1997	21	no	8 (2–14), 1/week	no
Chictakakou	1998	16	12–44 months	4 (1–4)	no

[a] Efficacy as percentage patients reporting improvement.
[b] Depending on the type of anismus.
n.r = Not recorded; tel. interv. = telephone interview; quest. = questionnaire.

Table 8 Biofeedback studies in pain syndromes

First author	Year	Ref.	No.	Diagnosis	Age	Sex (F:M)	Evaluation
Grimaud	1991	54	12	anal pain	54.0	8:4	interview
Ger	1993	58	14	rectal pain	71.0	8:6	questionnair
Gilliland	1997	59	86	rectal pain	68.0	55:31	interview
Heah	1997	60	16	levator ani syndrome	50.1	7:9	interview

[a] Efficacy as percentage patients reporting improvement.
[b] Change into other therapy arm but not randomized.
n.r. = Not recorded.

chronic or intermittent dull, aching pain or discomfort in the rectum that is worse when sitting than when standing[29]. The symptoms include a chronic sensation of rectal fullness and urge to defaecate. The levator ani syndrome often occurs with pelvic floor dyssynergia[54]. Proctalgia fugax involves infrequent episodes of sharp, fleeting pains from the anal canal or rectum. The physiological reason for the pain is unknown in most patients. The diagnosis is based on excluding other diseases. Some authors discussed excessive anal canal pressure as a cause[55], or ultra-slow wave activity. In some patients with severe proctalgia a myopathy of the internal anal spincter was found[56].

Application of biofeedback training has been reported for both disorders: treatment for chronic anal[58] or rectal pain[59] or levator ani syndrome[60]. These papers do not demonstrate how training of striated pelvic floor muscle contractions and relaxations would allow the pain to influence if it originates from smooth muscle tone of the anus – as in proctalgia fugax – or from the rectum – as in IBS – or from the external anal sphincter, as for the levator ani syndrome. The patients description is poor in these studies.

SUMMARY

Biofeedback therapy of pelvic floor disorders has gained wide acceptance in the past 25 years, and has become the major approach in patients with faecal incontinence and constipation. Biofeedback is safe, inexpensive, easy to administer, and has been shown to improve symptoms and objective parameters of anorectal function. Despite broad agreement concerning its efficacy, the modes of treatment have not yet been standardized, and the major components of their success have not yet been identified. New applications such as in patients with anal or anorectal pain syndromes have been tested preliminarily, and introductions into routine clinical management have been approached. It is tempting to speculate whether, in another few years, behavioural medicine approaches such as biofeedback training will become a reimbursable part of clinical management in most countries.

References

1. Skinner BF. Science and Human Behavior. New York: Macmillan, 1953.
2. Haskell B, Rovner H. Electromyography in the management of the incompetent anal sphincter. Dis Colon Rectum. 1976;10:81–4.
3. Kohlenberg RJ. Operant conditioning of human anal sphincter pressure. J Appl Behav Anal. 1973;6:201–8.
4. MacLeod JH. Management of anal continence by biofeedback. Gastroenterology. 1987;93:291–4.
5. Denis P, Crayon G, Galmiche JP. Biofeedback: the light at the end of the tunnel? Maybe for constipation. Gastroenterology. 1980;80:23–4.
6. van Tets WF, Kuipers JHC, Bleijenberg G. Biofeedback treatment is ineffective in neurogenic faecal incontinence. Dis Colon Rectum. 1996;39:992–4.
7. Enck P. Biofeedback training in disordered defaecation. A critical review. Dig Dis Sci. 1993;38: 1953–60.
8. Giebel GD, Lefering R, Troidl H, Blöchl H. Prevalence of faecal incontinence: what can be expected? Int J Colorect Dis. 1998:13;73–7.
9. Wald A. Biofeedback therapy for faecal incontinence. Ann Intern Med 1981;95:146–9.
10. Cerulli MA, Nikoomanesh P, Schuster MM. Progress in biofeedback conditioning for faecal incontinence. Gastroenterology. 1979;76:742–6.

11. Rao SSC, Welcher KD, Happel J. Can biofeedback therapy improve anorectal function in faecal incontinence? Am J Gastroenterol. 1996;91:2360–6.
12. Engel BT, Nikoomanesh P, Schuster MM. Operant conditioning of rectosphincteric responses in the treatment of faecal incontinence. N Engl J Med. 1974;290:646–9.
13. Wald A. Biofeedback for neurogenic faecal incontinence: rectal sensation is a determinant of outcome. J Pediator Gastroenterol Nutr. 1983;2:302–6.
14. Whitehead WE, Burgio KL, Engel BT. Biofeedback treatment of faecal incontinence in geriatric patients. J Am Geriatr. Soc. 1985;33:320–4.
15. Rao SSC, Welcher KD, Happel J. Can biofeedback therapy improve anorectal function in faecal incontinence? Am J Gastroenterol. 1996;91:2360–6.
16. Chiotakakou-Faliakou E, Kamm MA, Roy AJ, Storrie JB, Turner IC. Biofeedback provides long term benefit for patients with intractable, slow and normal transit constipation. Gut. 1998;42:517–21.
17. Enck P, Däubling G, Lübke HJ, Strohmeyer G. Long-term efficacy of biofeedback training for faecal incontinence. Dis Colon Rectum. 1994;37:997–1001.
18. Whitehead WE, Engel BT, Schuster MM. Perception of rectal distension is necessary to prevent faecal incontinence. In: Adam G, Meszaros I, Banyai EI, editors. Advances in Physiological Sciences, vol. 17: Brain and Behavior. Pergamon Press, Oxford. 1981:203–9.
19. Latimer PR, Campbell D, Kasperski J. A component analysis of biofeedback in the management of faecal incontinence. Biofeedback Self-Regul. 1984;9:311–24.
20. Miner PB, Donelly TC, Read NW. Investigation of the mode of action of biofeedback in treatment of faecal incontinence. Dig Dis Sci. 1990;35:1291–8.
21. Patankar SK, Ferrera A, Levy JR, Larach SW, Williamson PR, Perozo SE. Biofeedback in colorectal practice. A multicenter, statewide, three-year experience. Dis Colon Rectum. 1997;40:827–31.
22. Patankar SK, Ferrera A, Larach SW, Williamson PR, Perozo SE. Levy JR, Mills YES; Electromyographic assessment of biofeedback training for fecal incontinence and chronic constipation. Dis Colon Rectum. 1997;40:907–11.
23. Guillemot F, Bouche B, Gower-Rousseau C et al. Biofeedback for the treatment of faecal incontinence. Dis Colon Rectum. 1995;38:393–7.
24. Loening-Baucke V. Efficacy of biofeedback training in improving faecal incontinence and anorectal physiologic function. Gut. 1990;31:1395–1402.
25. Wald A, Tunuguntla AK. Anorectal sensorimotor dysfunction in faecal incontinence and diabetes mellitus. N Engl J Med. 1984;310:1282–7.
26. Hämäläinen KPJ, Raivio P, Natila S, Palmu A, Mecklin JP. Biofeedback therapy in rectal prolapse patients. Dis Colon Rectum. 1996;39:262–5.
27. Jensen LL, Lowry AC. Biofeedback improves functional outcome after sphincteroplasty. Dis Colon Rectum. 1997;40:197–200.
28. Ho YH, Chiang JM, Tan M, Low JY. Biofeedback therapy for excessive stool frequency and incontinence following anterior resection or total colectomy. Dis Colon Rectum. 1996;39:1289–92.
29. Drossman DA, Funch-Jensen P, Janssens J, Talley NJ, Thompson WG, Whitehead WE. Identification of subgroups of functional gastrointestinal disorders. Gastroenterol Int. 1990;3:159–72.
30. The Functional Gastrointestinal Disorders: diagnosis, pathophysiology and treatment. New York: Little, Brown, 1994.
31. Drossman DA, Li Z, Andruzzi E, Temple RD, Talley NJ, and Thompso WG. U.S. householder survey of functional gastrointestinal disorders. Prevalence, sociodemography, and health impact. Dig Dis Sci. 1993;38:1569–80.
32. Surrenti E, Rath DM, Pemberton JH, Camilleri M. Audit of constipation in a tertiary referral gastroenterology practice. Am J Gastroenterol. 1995;90:1471–5.
33. Preston DM, Lennard-Jones JE. Anismus in chronic constipation. Dig Dis Sci. 1985;30:413–18.
34. Rao SSC, Welcher KD, Leístikow JS. Obstructed defaecation: a failure of rectoanal coordination. Am J Gastroenterol. 1998;93:1042–50.
35. Rao SS. The technical aspects of biofeedback therapy for defaecation disorders. Gastroenterologist. 1998;6:96–103.
36. Rao SSC, Welcher KD, Pelsang RE. Effects of biofeedback therapy on anorectal function in obstructed defaecation. Dig Dis Sci. 1997;42:2197–205.
37. Camilleri M, Phillips SF, Loening-Baucke V, Anuras S, Schuffler MD, Krishnamurthy S. Colectomy for severe constipation. Dig Dis Sci. 1988;33:1196–8.
38. Park UC, Choi SK, Piccirillo MF, Verzaro R, Wexner SD. Patterns of anismus and the relation to biofeedback therapy. Dis Colon Rectum. 1996;39:768–73.

39. Bleijenberg G, Kuijpers HC. Treatment of the spastic pelvic floor syndrome with biofeedback. Dis Colon Rectum. 1987;30:108–11.

40. Kawimbe BM, Papachrysostomou M, Clare N, Smith AN. Outlet obstruction constipation (anismus) managed by biofeedback. Gut. 1991;32:1175–9.

41. Ko CY, Tong J, Lehman RE, Shelton A, Schrock TR, Welton M. Biofeedback is effective therapy for faecal incontinence and constipation. Arch Surg. 1997:829–34.

42. Siproudhis L, Dautreme S, Ropert A *et al*. Anismus and biofeedback: who benefits? Eur J Gastroenterol Hepatol. 1995;7:547–52.

43. Leroi AM, Duval V, Roussignol C, Berkelmans I, Reninque P, Denis P. Biofeedback for anismus in 15 sexually abused women. Int J Colorect Dis. 1996;11:187–90.

44. Lestar B, Penninckx F, Kerremans R. Biofeedback defaecation training for anismus. Int J Colorect Dis. 1991;6:202–7.

45. Fleshman JW, Dreznik Z, Meyer K, Fry RD, Carney R, Kodner IJ. Outpatient protocol for biofeedback therapy of pelvic floor outlet obstruction. Dis Colon Rectum. 1992;35:1–7.

46. Koutsomanis D, Lennard-Jones JE, Kamm MA. Prospective study of biofeedback treatment for patients with slow and normal transit constipation. Eur J Gastroenterol Hepatol. 1994;6:131–7.

47. Papachrysostomou M, Smith AN. Effects of biofeedback on obstructed defaecation – reconditioning of the defaecation reflex. Gut. 1994;35:252–6.

48. Keck JO, Staniunas RJ, Coller YES *et al*. Biofeedback training is useful in faecal incontinence but disappointing in constipation. Dis Colon Rectum. 1995;37:1271–6.

49. Bleijenberg G, Kuijpers HC. Biofeedback treatment of constipation: comparison of two methods. Am J Gastroenterol. 1994;89:1021–6.

50. Glia A, Gylin M, Gullberg K, Lindberg G. Biofeedback retraining in patients with functional constipation and paradoxical puborectais contraction. Dis Colon Rectum. 1997;40:889–95.

51. Park UC, Choi SK, Piccirillo MF, Verzaro R, Wexner SD. Patterns of anismus and the relation to biofeedback therapy. Dis Colon Rectum. 1996;39:768–73.

52. Koutsomanis D, Lennard-Jones JE, Roy AJ, Kamm MA. Controlled randomised trial of visual biofeedback versus muscle training without a visual display for intractable constipation. Gut. 1995;37:95–9.

53. Thompson WG. Proctalgia fugax. J R Coll Phys Lond. 1980;14:247–8.

54. Grimaud JC, Bouvier M, Naudy B, Guien C, Salducci J. Manometric and radiologic investigations and biofeedback treatment of chronic idiopathic anal pain. Dis Colon Rectum. 1991;34:690–5.

55. Rao SSC, Hatfield RA. Paroxysmal anal hyperkinesis: a characteristic feature of proctalgia fugax. Gut. 1996;39:609–612.

56. Kamm MA, Hoyle CHV, Burleigh D *et al*. Hereditary internal anal sphincter myopathy causing proctalgia fugax and constipation. A newly identified condition. Gastroenterology. 1991;100:805–10.

57. Diamant NE, Kamm MA, Wald A, Whitehead WE. American Gastroenterological Association Medical Position. Anorectal Testing Techniques. Gastroenterology. 1999;116:732–60.

58. Ger GC, Wexner SD, Jorge JMN *et al*. Evaluation and treatment of chronic intractable rectal pain – a frustrating endeavor. Dis Colon Rectum. 1993;36:139–45.

59. Gilliland R, Heymen JS, Altomare DF, Vickers D, Wexner SD. Biofeedback for intractable rectal pain. Dis Colon Rectum. 1997;40:190–6.

60. Heah SM, Ho YH, Tan M, Leong AFP. Biofeedback is effective treatment for levator ani syndrome. Dis Colon Rectum. 1997;40:187–9.

61. Schiller LR, Santa Ana C, Davis GR, Fordtran JS. Fecal incontinence in chronic diarrhea. Report of case with improvement after training with rectally infused saline. Gastroenterology. 1979;77:751–3.

62. Goldenberg DA, Hodges K, Hersh T, Jinich H. Biofeedback therapy for fecal incontinence. Am J Gastroenterol. 1980;74:352–5.

63. Buser WD, Miner PB. Delayed rectal sensation with fecal incontinence. Successful treatment using anorectal manometry. Gastroenterology. 1986;91:1186–91.

64. Berti Riboli F, Frascio M, Pitto G, Reboa G, Zanolla R. Biofeedback conditioning for fecal incontinence. Arch Phys Med Rehabil. 1988;69:29–31.

65. Chiarioni G, Scattlini C, Bonfante F, Vantini I. Liquid stool incontinence with severe urgency: anorectal function and effective biofeedback treatment. Gut 1993;34:1576–80.

66. Sangwan YP, Coller JA, Barrett RC, Roberts PL, Murray JJ, Schoetz DJ. Can manometric parameters predict response to biofeedback therapy in fecal incontinence. Dis Colon Rectum. 1995;38:1021–5.

67. Rieger NA, Wattchow Da, Sarre RG, *et al*. Prospective trial of pelvic floor retraining in patients with fecal incontinence. Dis Colon Rectum. 1997;40:821–6.

68. Glia A, Gylin M, Akerlund JE, Lindfors U, Lindberg G. Biofeedback training in patients with fecal incontinence. Dis Colon Rectum. 1998;41:359–64.

69. Weber J, Ducrotte P, Touchais JY, Roussignol C, Denis P. Biofeedback training for constipation in adults and children. Dis Colon Rectum. 1987;30:844–6.

70. Dahl J, Lindquist BL, Tysk C, Leissner P, Philipson L, Järnerot G. Behavioral medicine treatment in chronic constipation with paradoxical anal sphincter contraction. Dis Colon Rectum. 1991;34:769–76.

71. Wexner SD, Cheape JD, Jorge JMN, Heyman SR, S.N., Yesgelman DG. Prospective assessment of biofeedback for the treatment of paradoxical puborectalis contraction. Dis Colon Rectum. 1992;35:145–50.

72. Turnbull GK, Ritvo PG. Anal sphincter biofeedback relaxation treatment for women with intractable constipation symptoms. Dis Colon Rectum. 1992;35:530–6.

73. Karlbohm U, Hallden M, Eeg-Olofsson, Pahlman L, Graf W. Result of biofeedback in constipated patients. A prospective study. Dis Colon Rectum. 1997;40:1149–55.

74. Rieger NA, Wattchow DA, Sarre RG, *et al*. Prospective study of biofeedback for treatment of constipation. Dis Colon Rectum. 1997;40:1143–8.

75. Glia A, Gylin M, Akerlund JE, Lindfors U, Lindberg G. Biofeedback training in patients with fecal incontinence. Dis Colon Rectum. 1998;41:359–64.

8
Surgical therapy of pelvic floor disorders

T. H. K. SCHIEDECK, U. J. ROBLICK,
H. J. DÜPREE and H. P. BRUCH

INTRODUCTION

Pelvic floor disorders usually comprise multiple factors and can be on different levels. The symptoms vary considerably. For the treatment of such disorders it is crucial to distinguish between primary causes and secondary changes. In this context we can distinguish between conditions originating from intra-abdominal changes and those having their origin in the pelvic floor. A sigmoidocele III° with pronounced cul-de-sac syndrome, for example, forces the patient to intensively press for defaecation. Years of doing so can lead to rectal prolapse combined with masked incontinence. The characteristic symptoms of pelvic floor disorders are rectal or genital prolapse, faecal or urine incontinence, constipation or outlet obstruction and pain. Descensus perinei is a syndrome that unites pelvic floor disorders of various forms and degrees. In this scenario it must be particularly borne in mind that a muscular deficiency of the pelvic floor can often be accompanied by impaired innervation (overstretching of the n. pudendus) or can cause this[1-3].

The various lesions and symptoms must be established during an extensive diagnosis and should be evaluated with regard to their pathophysiological significance. An initial conservative treatment is often justified. If it fails to be successful, surgical intervention is indicated. The procedures shown in Table 1 are available. In principle, causal treatment should be distinguished from purely symptomatic treatment.

Whereas, for example, the cause for the outlet obstruction is eliminated by the resection of a sigmoidocele in the case of cul-de-sac syndrome, reconstructive pelvic floor measures (e.g. pelvic floor repair and rectocele repair) are restricted to a sole therapy of the local findings.

It goes without saying that age and general condition of the patient must be considered when indicating the various procedures.

Table 1 Operative procedures available

Pelvic floor	Abdominal
Muscle plasty (preanal, postanal, total pelvic floor)	Rectopexy with or without resection
Rectocele repair	Abdominoperineal (Zacharin)
Rehn–Delorme	Sacrocolpopexy
Thiersch ring, silastic band, etc.	Reconstruction of the Douglas

SURGICAL PROCEDURES

Rectocele repair

Rectocele is characterized by a defect in the rectovaginal septum. In this context a trauma during delivery is suspected. Rectocele is frequently accompanied by other changes, such as descensus perinei or sigmoidocele III° in outlet obstruction. Surgical therapy is indicated only for symptomatic patients. Major symptoms are first-degree partial incontinence, the feeling of incomplete evacuation and chronic constipation. This is occasionally accompanied by an ulcus recti simplex. The necessity of patients to manually support defaecation is always an indication for surgical intervention.

Several procedures are available (Table 2). The transvaginal technique has the advantage that the operation can be combined with a levatorplasty. The disadvantage of this approach is the fact that excess rectal mucosa cannot be resected. The transanal approach is considerably more effective in this case.

The success rate largely depends on the question of whether the rectocele is the primary cause or the secondary consequence of another condition. Whenever there are additional changes that are not being treated (e.g. sigmoidocele, slow-transit constipation, anism) the relapse rate is high.

Muscular reconstruction of the pelvic floor

A muscular reconstruction is indicated in cases of incontinence II–III°, possibly accompanied by a sphincter defect. Unfortunately, long-term observation reveals that the widespread plication procedure is often not a lasting success. Nerve degeneration often plays a crucial role. On a long-term basis an impaired n. pudendus leads to a fatty degeneration of the muscles and consequently an insufficient function[12,13].

Postanal repair (posterior levatorplasty)

Sir Alan Parks originally introduced postanal repair to treat incontinence. The aim was to reduce the anorectal angle and extend the anal canal by a posterior levatorplasty in connection with the repair of m. sphincter ani externus, thus improving continence. The literature reports success rates of 15–87% (Table 3). In the majority of cases direct postoperative results may be good, but long-term figures are not encouraging (cf. Table 4). According to Setti-Carraro et al.[26] the result of postanal repair is significantly less favourable if n. pudendus is impaired.

Table 2 Rectocele repair, operative technique and success rate

Reference	Year	No.	Procedure	Success rate (%)
Arnold et al.[4]	1990	35	Transvaginal	46
		29	Transanal	46
Janssen and van Dijke[5]	1994	76	Transanal	92
Infantino et al.[6]	1995	8	Transvaginal	75
		13	Transanal	81
Mellgren et al.[7]	1995	25	Transvaginal	88
Karlbom et al.[8]	1996	34	Transanal	79
Murthy et al.[9]	1996	31	Transanal	92
Khubchandani et al.[10]	1997	123	Transanal	82
Ommer et al.[11]	1998	41	Transperineal	75

Table 3 Improvement of continence immediately post-operation following postanal repair

Reference	Year	No.	Continence (%)
Browning (UK)[45]	1984	140	74
Keighley (UK)[14]	1984	89	63
Henry and Simson (UK)[15]	1985	129	56
Womack et al. (UK)[16]	1988	16	87
Miller et al. (UK)[17]	1988	17	59
Yoshioka and Keighley (UK)[18]	1989	116	34
Scheuer et al. (NL)[19]	1989	39	15
Orrom et al. (UK)[20]	1991	17	59
Deen et al. (UK)[21]	1993	12	40

Table 4 Long-term improvement following postanal repair

Reference	No.	Postoperative (%)	1st year (%)	3rd year (%)	5th year (%)	After 5 years (%)
Keighley (UK)[14]	105	63			24	
Jameson et al. (UK)[22]	36	83		53		27
Briel and Schouten (NL)[23]	37		65	46		
Athananasiadis et al. (D)[24]	31				32	
Setti-Carraro and Nicholls (UK)[25]	9	58	45			22
Setti-Carraro et al. (UK)[26]	34					26

Preanal repair

Preanal repair aims at improving sphincter and pelvic floor function by an anterior repair of m. puborectalis and m. sphincter ani externus. The success rate ranges from 33% to 62%[20,21,27].

Total pelvic floor repair

With the help of total pelvic floor repair (TPFR), the reconstruction of the entire posterior and mesial compartment of the pelvic floor is attempted. According to the literature a success rate 40–70% with regard to incontinence is achieved. Various comparative studies indicate that TPFR is superior to both sole postanal repairs and to preanal repairs[21,28]. It must be taken into account, however, that TPFR is the latest plication procedure. With longer follow-up periods unfavourable results must also be anticipated for this procedure. Unfavourable results are described in cases of obesity, neurogenic impair (n. pudendus) or descensus perinei[29,30].

ABDOMINAL PROCEDURES

Procedure in cases of rectal prolapse

A number of different procedures have been developed for the treatment of rectal prolapse. It is now generally acknowledged that abdominal techniques are superior to perineal surgery with regard to the relapse rate. Therapeutic concepts that are solely based on restricting the anus (e.g. Thiersch wire, silastic banding) are obsolete. Perineal procedures, such as perineal resection of the prolapse according to Altemeier[31] or Rehn–Delorme plication[32] must be considered only for very old patients or those with a poor general condition.

The rectum can be fixed via an abdominal access by various methods. However, it is important, at any rate, to extend the preparation to the pelvic floor. The Wells or Ripstein techniques use artificial material for the pexy, whereas Sudeck is restricted to suture–rectopexy. As an alternative, Frykman–Goldberg introduced a combination of pexy and sigmoid resection (with respect to high anterior rectal resection). Relapse rates of either procedure (with or without resection) are basically identical. However, following sole pexy a higher rate of evacuation disorders (constipation) must be anticipated postoperatively. According to Novell and colleagues[33] with regard to relapse rates there is no difference between pexy procedures using artificial material and those that do not. However, the functional results of patients with net implants are less favourable[34]. Stelzner has pointed out that it is important to remove the rectosigmoidal junction (high-pressure zone)[35]. In our own case material ($n = 72$), no new prolapses developed following laparoscopy in a follow-up of 3 years (Frykman–Goldberg and Sudeck rectopexy). Preoperative tendency to constipation was improved in 76% of cases.

It has now been confirmed by several authors that the therapy of rectal prolapse is ideally implemented by using laparoscopy[36–41]. In specialist clinics this technique is considered the treatment of choice.

Outlet obstruction due to sigmoidocele

Jorge and Wexner[42] have suggested a classification of sigmoidocele. As a consequence, surgery is indicated in cases of sigmoidocele II to III°. However, the patient's symptoms, rather than radiological findings, are the major criterion. The 'feeling of incomplete evacuation' in these cases is an indication to use surgical therapy. In particular this applies to the mechanical outlet obstruction, such as the cul-de-sac syndrome which is characterized by the fact that a sigma loop falling deeply into the small pelvis presses on the rectum, thereby representing a mechanical obstacle to evacuation. More often than not one is also faced with a more or less pronounced rectal prolapse, so that not only a sigma resection, but also a reconstruction of the Douglas and a rectopexy must be carried out. Usually, elderly or old patients are affected, and the extent of the resection is also determined by the often-limited sphincter function[43].

A pronounced descensus perinei represents particular problems. The primary therapy is almost always conservative. However, whenever abdominal problems, such as a cul-de-sac syndrome, are present, surgical therapy will be chosen at an early stage to avoid an aggravation of the symptoms. The circulus vitiosus between pelvic floor prolapse–overstretching of the pudendal nerves–myatrophy–pelvic floor prolapse must be interrupted. More often than not it is not only that the posterior compartment is impaired, but the patient also suffers a prolapse of the vaginal stump (vaginal vault) and/or cystoptosis. Therefore, an interdisciplinary approach is advisable. In these cases the resection rectopexy must often be combined with an anterior levatorplasty (abdominoperineal procedure according to Zacharin and Hamilton[44]). Other advisable surgical therapies can be sacrocolpopexy or a Burch-plasty. To what extent such an intervention will be a lasting success depends not least upon the question to which degree the affected nerves and muscles can recover. Postoperative biofeedback could be a good approach.

CONCLUSIONS

The term pelvic floor disorder describes various clinical pictures. The characteristic symptoms are basically rectal prolapse, anal incontinence and constipation or outlet obstruction. It should be borne in mind that the pelvic floor often represents only the 'endpoint' of pathological changes that derive from 'upper floors'.

The therapeutic strategies must consider such aspects. More often than not, conservative therapies are primarily justified; surgical procedures must be based on an extensive physical examination and diagnostic evaluation.

The major objective of any therapeutic intervention must, on the one hand, focus on reducing the pressure onto the pelvic floor, and on the other hand on reconstructing morphologically destroyed areas. Given the difference in symptoms and severity of conditions, a wide range of surgical options can be applied, such as local procedures (e.g. rectocele repair, levatorplasty, postanal or total pelvic floor repair), intra-abdominal procedures (rectopexy, generally combined with sigmoid resection, sacropelvic fixation) and simultaneously combined procedures (e.g. the Zacharin procedure).

Any plication procedures solely repairing muscles have recently been increasingly criticized since it has emerged that long-term results are relatively poor, so that such techniques should be restricted to very old and multi-morbid patients. It must be borne in mind, however, that the alternative therapy for many patients would be a stoma, unless sphincter replacement techniques (dyn. graciloplasty or artificial bowel sphincter) can be applied. If it is also considered that all anal repair techniques are more or less without complications, they represent a reasonable alternative for the elderly.

Patients suffering rectal prolapse show excellent long-term results following surgical intervention. Patients who are able to undergo abdominal surgery should be treated by a transabdominal procedure, rather than a transperineal or transanal procedure.

Any patients with a pronounced obstructing component or a so-called cul-de-sac syndrome should also undergo resecting surgery.

Establishing the correct indication is crucial for the success rate. The result for a rectocele repair in cases of slow-transit constipation, for example, is very poor.

A restitutio ad integrum is practically impossible; however, a considerable improvement of the condition, especially when combined with conservative therapies (e.g. biofeedback, electrostimulation), is quite realistic.

References

1. Girona J. [Diagnosis and therapeutic possibilities of descending perineum syndrome]. Leber Magen Darm. 1992;22:44–6.
2. Girona J. [Diagnosis of the descending perineum syndrome]. Dtsch Med Wochenschr. 1989; 114:301–2.
3. Pinho M, Yoshioka K, Ortiz J, Oya M, Keighley MR. The effect of age on pelvic floor dynamics. Int J Colorectal Dis. 1990;5:207–8.
4. Arnold MW, Stewart WR, Aguilar PS. Rectocele repair. Four years' experience. Dis Colon Rectum. 1990;33:684–7.
5. Janssen LW, van Dijke CF. Selection criteria for anterior rectal wall repair in symptomatic rectocele and anterior rectal wall prolapse. Dis Colon Rectum. 1994;37:1100–7.
6. Infantino A, Masin A, Melega E, Dodi G, Lise M. Does surgery resolve outlet obstruction from rectocele? Int J Colorectal Dis. 1995;10:97–100.
7. Mellgren A, Anzen B, Nilsson BY et al. Results of rectocele repair. A prospective study. Dis Colon Rectum. 1995;38:7–13.
8. Karlbom U, Graf W, Nilsson S, Pahlman L. Does surgical repair of a rectocele improve rectal emptying? Dis Colon Rectum. 1996;39:1296–302.
9. Murthy VK, Orkin BA, Smith LE, Glassman LM. Excellent outcome using selective criteria for rectocele repair. Dis Colon Rectum. 1996;39:374–8.
10. Khubchandani IT, Clancy JP 3rd, Rosen L, Riether RD, Stasik JJ Jr. Endorectal repair of rectocele revisited [See comments]. Br J Surg. 1997;84:89–91.
11. Ommer A, Kohler A, Athanasiadis S. [Results of transperineal levator-plasty in treatment of symptomatic rectocele]. Chirurg. 1998;69:966–72.
12. Dimpfl T, Jaeger C, Mueller-Felber W et al. Myogenic changes of the levator ani muscle in premenopausal women: the impact of vaginal delivery and age. Neurourol Urodyn. 1998;17:197–205.
13. Stelzner F. [Anorectal incontinence–cause and treatment]. Chirurg. 1991;62:17–24.
14. Keighley MR. Postanal repair for faecal incontinence. J R Soc Med. 1984;77:285–8.
15. Henry MM, Simson JN. Results of postanal repair: a retrospective study. Br J Surg. 1985;72 (Suppl.)S17–19.
16. Womack NR, Morrison JF, Williams NS. Prospective study of the effects of postanal repair in neurogenic faecal incontinence. Br J Surg. 1988;75:48–52.
17. Miller R, Bartolo DC, Locke-Edmunds JC, Mortensen NJ. Prospective study of conservative and operative treatment for faecal incontinence. Br J Surg. 1988;75:101–5.
18. Yoshioka K, Keighley MR. Critical assessment of the quality of continence after postanal repair for faecal incontinence [published erratum appears in Br J Surg. 1990;77:356]. Br J Surg. 1989;76:1054–7.

19. Scheuer M, Kuijpers HC, Jacobs PP. Postanal repair restores anatomy rather than function. Dis Colon Rectum. 1989;32:960–3.
20. Orrom WJ, Miller R, Cornes H, Duthie G, Mortensen NJ, Bartolo DC. Comparison of anterior sphincteroplasty and postanal repair in the treatment of idiopathic fecal incontinence. Dis Colon Rectum. 1991;34:305–10.
21. Deen KI, Oya M, Ortiz J, Keighley MR. Randomized trial comparing three forms of pelvic floor repair for neuropathic faecal incontinence [See comments]. Br J Surg. 1993;80:794–8.
22. Jameson JS, Speakman CT, Darzi A, Chia YW, Henry MM. Audit of postanal repair in the treatment of fecal incontinence. Dis Colon Rectum. 1994;37:369–72.
23. Briel JW, Schouten WR. [Disappointing results of postanal repair in the treatment of fecal incontinence]. Ned Tijdschr Geneeskd. 1995;139:23–6.
24. Athanasiadis S, Sanchez M, Kuprian A. [Long-term follow-up of Parks posterior repair. An electromyographic, manometric and radiologic study of 31 patients]. Langenbecks Arch Chir. 1995;380:22–30.
25. Setti-Carraro P, Nicholls RJ. Postanal repair for faecal incontinence persisting after rectopexy. Br J Surg. 1994;81:305–7.
26. Setti-Carraro P, Kamm MA, Nicholls RJ. Long-term results of postanal repair for neurogenic faecal incontinence. Br J Surg. 1994;81:140–4.
27. Miller R, Orrom WJ, Cornes H, Duthie G, Bartolo DC. Anterior sphincter plication and levatorplasty in the treatment of faecal incontinence. Br J Surg. 1989;76:1058–60.
28. Lehur PA, Bruley des Varannes S, Dutre J, Guiberteau-Canfrere V, Galmiche JP, Le Borgne J. [Pre- and retro-anal myorrhaphy in the treatment of severe anal incontinence. Clinical and manometric results]. Ann Chir. 1995;49:621–7.
29. Korsgen S, Deen KI, Keighley MR. Long-term results of total pelvic floor repair for postobstetric fecal incontinence. Dis Colon Rectum. 1997;40:835–9.
30. van Tets WF, Kuijpers JH. Pelvic floor procedures produce no consistent changes in anatomy or physiology. Dis Colon Rectum. 1998;41:365–9.
31. Takesue Y, Yokoyama T, Murakami Y et al. The effectiveness of perineal rectosigmoidectomy for the treatment of rectal prolapse in elderly and high-risk patients. Surg Today. 1999;29:290–3.
32. Muller-Lobeck H, Duschka L, Schleifer P, Henne T. [Rehn–Delorme operation in pelvic floor insufficiency]. Zentralbl Chir. 1996;121:692–7.
33. Novell JR, Osborne MJ, Winslet MC, Lewis AA. Prospective randomized trial of Ivalon sponge versus sutured rectopexy for full-thickness rectal prolapse. Br J Surg. 1994;81:904–6.
34. Duthie GS, Bartolo DC. Abdominal rectopexy for rectal prolapse: a comparison of techniques. Br J Surg. 1992;79:107–13.
35. Stelzner F. [Etiology and therapy of rectal prolapse. Experiences with 308 cases 1956-1991]. Chirurg. 1994;65:533–45.
36. Berman IR. Sutureless laparoscopic rectopexy for procidentia. Technique and implications. Dis Colon Rectum. 1992;35:689–93.
37. Bruch HP, Herold A, Schiedeck T, Schwandner O. Laparoscopic surgery for rectal prolapse and outlet obstruction. Dis Colon Rectum. 1999;42:1189–94; discussion 1194–5.
38. Cuesta MA, Borgstein PJ, de Jong D, Meijer S. Laparoscopic rectopexy. Surg Laparosc Endosc. 1993;3:456–8.
39. Cuschieri A, Shimi SM, Vander Velpen G, Banting S, Wood RA. Laparoscopic prosthesis fixation rectopexy for complete rectal prolapse. Br J Surg. 1994;81:138–9.
40. Darzi A, Henry MM, Guillou PJ, Shorvon P, Monson JR. Stapled laparoscopic rectopexy for rectal prolapse. Surg Endosc. 1995;9:301–3.
41. Stevenson AR, Stitz RW, Lumley JW. Laparoscopic-assisted resection–rectopexy for rectal prolapse: early and medium follow-up. Dis Colon Rectum. 1998;41:46–54.
42. Jorge JM, Yang YK, Wexner SD. Incidence and clinical significance of sigmoidoceles as determined by a new classification system. Dis Colon Rectum. 1994;37:1112–17.
43. Schiedeck T, Schwandner O, Bruch H. Laparoskopische Therapie der chronischen Obstipation. Zentralbl Chirurg. 1999;124:818–24.
44. Zacharin RF, Hamilton NT. Pulsion enterocele: long-term results of an abdominoperineal technique. Obstet Gynecol. 1980;55:141–8.
45. Browing GG, Motson RW. Results of Parks operation for faecal incontinence after anal sphincter injury. Br Med J. 1984;286:1873–5.

Section III
Radiation damage in proctology

9
Radiation sequelae in proctology: a radiotherapist's statement

M. NIEWALD, K. SCHNABEL[†] and CH. RÜBE

INTRODUCTION

Walsh[1] was the first to report on radiation side-effects to the bowel. In 1897, only 2 years after detection of X-rays, he published a paper entitled 'Deep tissue traumatism after Roentgen ray exposure'. He reported quickly occurring and fully reversible symptoms caused by radiation exposure to the bowel mucosa. Füth and Ebeler[2] described chronic radiation injuries to the bowel (stenosis, fistula) caused by radium irradiation.

RADIOBIOLOGICAL CONSIDERATIONS

In general, radiotherapy sequelae are divided into acute and long-term side-effects.

Acute proctitis

This is first noticed in the second or third week of a fractionated radiotherapy. Complete healing is to be expected 1–2 weeks after the end of therapy. The affected organ is the bowel mucosa. The division of crypt cells is inhibited, followed by cell loss. Consequently, water and electrolytes and much mucus are secreted to the bowel. The tolerance of the rectal mucosa concerning acute side-effects (TD 5/5, 5% intense side-effects within 5 years) is assumed[3] to be 50 Gy.

Long-term sequelae to the rectum

These occur several months after the end of radiotherapy. The aetiology consists of several factors (epithelial lesions, mechanical and peptic factors, changes of connective tissue, and vessel changes[4] in the bowel wall). The macroscopic syndrome may be rectal ulcers, bleeding, stenosis, or a fistula. Furthermore, the rectal volume is decreased and the sensoric and motoric functions of the sphincter

---

[†] deceased

may be impaired[5]. The tolerance of the rectum (TD 5/5) concerning long-term side-effects is stated to be 60 Gy in a case in which the whole rectal circumference is to be irradiated[3,6]. In practice, in a case of partial irradiation of the rectal wall, even higher doses, in the range 66–70 Gy, can be tolerated.

Consequential late effect

In general, acute and long-term side-effects are separate and have different target organs, so that it is not correct, for example, to infer the frequency of rectal ulcers from the intensity of acute proctitis. There are, however, some data indicating that patients with very intense acute side-effects may yield more late rectal sequelae (consequential late effect) than those with less acute reactions[7,8].

Predictive factors for radiation side-effects

Besides the known dependency on *total dose*, there are ample experimental and some clinical data showing that the frequency and intensity, especially of long-term sequelae, also depend on the *single dose*. According to the graph of Withers *et al.*[9] one can expect less long-term damage by lowering the daily single dose. In practice this could be achieved by decreasing the daily single dose from 2.0 to 1.8 Gy. To our knowledge there are insufficient data for even lower single doses, or hyperfractionation. Additionally, tolerance of bowel tissue is known to depend on *dose rate* in brachytherapy.

The *volume* of bowel having been irradiated is another very important prognostic factor for long-term sequelae[10]. These tend to be more frequent and intense if the irradiated volume is larger. In practice one should not irradiate the whole rectal circumference with a high dose of 60 Gy or more, in order to avoid rectal stenosis or fistula. The irradiated volume can further be limited by using conformal techniques, resulting in a lower frequency of side-effects[11].

Furthermore, patients *operated* on before radiotherapy may have a higher risk concerning sequelae because of bowel loops fixed within the target volume which thus cannot be moved outwards by the peristalsis. If radiotherapy is combined with *chemotherapy* one must expect a synergism concerning acute and late effects, especially when the two procedures are administered simultaneously[12].

CLINICAL CONSIDERATIONS

Acute side-effects

Acute proctitis occurs frequently (in 20–50% patients)[13–15]. Symptoms may begin in the second week of irradiation and may consist of diarrhoea, abdominal cramping, mucous rectal discharge, rectal pain and rectal bleeding. They usually resolve 2 weeks after completion of treatment[16]. Treatment can be by kaopectate; loperamide; tinctura opii; spasmolytics; substitution of water and electrolytes; and a diet avoiding nuts, cereals, raw vegetables, fresh fruit, alcohol, and tobacco.

Long-term side-effects

Chronic radiation sequelae to the large bowel are rare (1–12% of patients[14,17,18]). Symptoms may begin 6–18 months after the end of radiotherapy and may consist

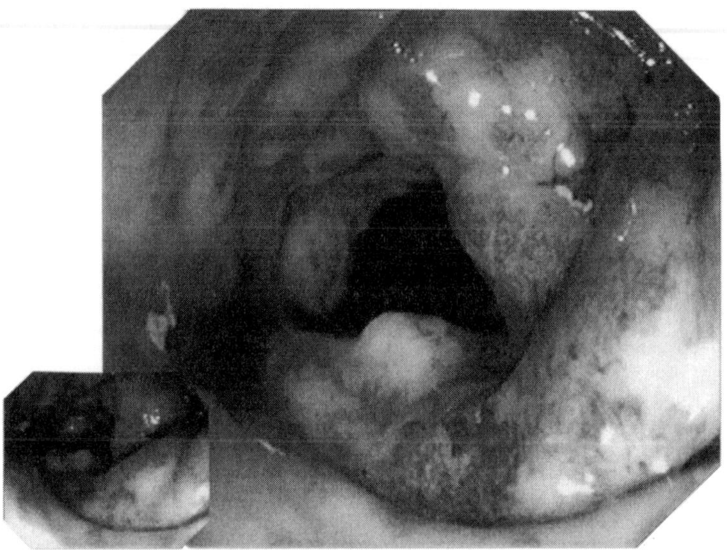

Figure 1 Long-term sequelae to the rectum with some bleeding (with kind permission from M. Menges, M.D., II. Medical Clinic of the Saarland University Hospital Homburg/Saar, Germany)

of colicky abdominal pain, bloody diarrhoea and tenesmus. Far less common are bowel obstructions, fistulas, bowel perforation and massive rectal bleeding. The shortest and most direct method of diagnosis is endoscopy (Fig. 1). Treatment will include the medical management of the patient's symptoms as mentioned in the section 'Acute side-effects'. Furthermore, anti-inflammatory or corticoid foam administered rectally may be recommendable. Some groups treat locally with sucralfat[19], formalin in 4% solution[20,21], or by argon laser coagulation[22]. Others administer hyperbaric oxygen[23].

Indication, time, and method of any surgical intervention remain the subject of debate. The rate of morbidity (anatomical dehiscence) and mortality is rather high, so that surgery should be reserved for patients in whom local therapy is not successful.

SUMMARY

Acute side-effects are frequent and almost unavoidable. They usually resolve 2 weeks after the end of radiotherapy and should be treated medically as mentioned above.

Long-term side-effects are rare; therapy is only palliative. Thus, prophylaxis is more important than therapy. This can be achieved by appropriate planning and performing of radiotherapy:

1. Prone position of the patient on a belly-board (small bowel loops are moved out of the target volume).

2. Use of conformal three- or four-field techniques and three-dimensional treatment planning.
3. Use of shrinking-field techniques.
4. Prescribing a total dose regarding the tolerance of bowel at risk (especially applying a combination of percutaneous radiotherapy and brachytherapy).
5. Reducing the daily single dose.
6. Daily treatment of all fields.

References

1. Walsh D. Deep tissue traumatism from Roentgen ray exposure. Br Med J. 1897;2:272.
2. Füth H, Ebeler F. Röntgen- und Radiumtherapie des Uteruskarzinoms. Zentralbl Gynakol. 1915; 39:217.
3. Herrmann T, Baumann M. Klinische Strahlenbiologie. 1997;3. Jena: G. Fischer Verlag, 1997.
4. Richter KK, Fink LM, Hughes BM, Shmaysani HM, Sung CC, Hauer JM. Differential effect of radiation on endothelial cell function in rectal cancer and normal rectum. Am J Surg. 1998;176:642–7.
5. Kim GE, Lim JJ, Park W *et al.* Sensory and motor dysfunction assessed by anorectal manometry in uterine cervical carcinoma patients with radiation-induced late rectal complication. Int J Radiat Oncol Biol Phys. 1998;41:835–41.
6. Schnabel K, Niewald M, Berberich W. Strahlenfolgen am Verdauungstrakt. In: Hahn E, Riemann J, editors. Klinische Gastroenterologie, 3rd edn. Stuttgart: Georg Thieme Verlag, 2000:1049–56.
7. Wang CJ, Leung SW, Chen HC *et al.* The correlation of acute toxicity and late rectal injury in radiotherapy for cervical carcinoma: evidence suggestive of consequential late effect (CQLE). Int J Radiat Oncol Biol Phys. 1998;40:85–91.
8. Denham JW, O'Brien PC, Dunstan RH *et al.* Is there more than one late radiation proctitis syndrome? Radiother Oncol. 1999;51:43–53.
9. Withers HR, Thames HD, Peters LJ. Differences in the fractionation response of acutely and late-responding tissues. In: Kärcher KH, editor. Progress in Radio-Oncology, vol. II. New York: Raven Press, 2000:287.
10. Trott KR. Chronic damage after radiation therapy – challenge to radiation biology. Int J Radiat Oncol Biol Phys. 1984;10:907.
11. Dearnaley DP, Khoo VS, Norman AR *et al.* Comparison of radiation side-effects of conformal and conventional radiotherapy in prostate cancer: a randomised trial. Lancet. 1999;353:267–72.
12. Steel G. Basic Clinical Radiobiology. London: Arnold, 1997.
13. Zeitlin SI, Sherman J, Raboy A, Lederman G, Albert P. High dose combination radiotherapy for the treatment of localized prostate cancer. J Urol. 1998;160:91–5.
14. Schultheiss TE, Lee WR, Hunt MA, Hanlon AL, Peter RS, Hanks GE. Late GI and GU complications in the treatment of prostate cancer. Int J Radiat Oncol Biol Phys. 1997;37:3–11.
15. Kovacs G, Galalae R, Loch T *et al.* Prostate preservation by combined external beam and HDR brachytherapy in nodal negative prostate cancer. Strahlenther Onkol. 1999;175 (Suppl. 2): 87–8.
16. Cancer Net. Radiation enteritis. Bethesda, MD: National Cancer Institute, 2000 <www.cancer net.nih.gov>.
17. Perez CA, Grigsby PW, Lockett MA, Chao KS, Williamson J. Radiation therapy morbidity in carcinoma of the uterine cervix: dosimetric and clinical correlation. Int J Radiat Oncol Biol Phys. 1999;44:855–66.
18. Miller AR, Martenson JA, Nelson H *et al.* The incidence and clinical consequences of treatment-related bowel injury. Int J Radiat Oncol Biol Phys. 1999;43:817–25.
19. Melko GP, Turco TF, Phelan TF, Sauers NM. Treatment of radiation-induced proctitis with sucralfate enemas. Ann Pharmacother. 1999;33:1274–6.
20. Coyoli GO, Alvarado CR, Corona BA, Pacheco PM. [The treatment of rectorrhagia secondary to postradiation proctitis with 4% formalin]. Tratamiento de la rectorragia secundaria a proctitis postradiacion con formalina al 4%. Ginecol Obstet Mex. 1999;67:341–5.

21. Mall J, Pollmann C, Myers JA. [Rectal formalin instillation – a practical and reliable therapy of hemorrhagic proctitis]. Rectale Formalininstillation – eine praktikable und sichere Therapie der hamorrhagischen Proktitis. Chirurg. 1999;70:700–4.
22. Fantin AC, Binek J, Suter WR, Meyenberger C. Argon beam coagulation for treatment of symptomatic radiation-induced proctitis. Gastrointest Endosc. 1999;49:515–18.
23. Kitta T, Shinohara N, Shirato H, Otsuka H, Koyanagi T. The treatment of chronic radiation proctitis with hyperbaric oxygen in patients with prostate cancer. BJU Int. 2000;85:372–4.

10
Radiation damage in proctology – gastroenterology

R. A. SILVA

Radiation-induced proctitis is a serious complication of pelvic radiation therapy. Acute symptoms such as abdominal pain, diarrhoea, tenesmus, and urgency are observed in about 50–75%, either during or immediately after treatment[1–3]. However, these symptoms are usually self-limited and resolve spontaneously after a 2–6-month period. Much more difficult to manage is chronic radiation injury. Indeed, in addition to the acute effects, radiation-induced injury of the colon and rectum may cause progressive submucosal fibrosis and obliterative endarteritis. These histological changes lead to varying degrees of tissue ischaemia and to serious late complications that occur among 5–20% of patients and include fistula, ulceration, strictures and bleeding[1,4–7].

Significant rectal bleeding occurs among 6–8% of patients with chronic radiation injury[5]. Although most cases resolve spontaneously, sometimes it may lead to iron-deficiency anaemia and in the more severe forms to intractable or massive bleeding, necessitating repeated hospital admissions and blood transfusions. Endoscopically, in these latter cases the irradiated mucosa appears oedematous and friable with multiple vascular telangiectasias.

Pharmacotherapy with steroids, sulphasalazine, 5-aminosalicylic acid (5-ASA) or sucralfate is generally ineffective in controlling severe rectal haemorrhage[2,8,9]. Nevertheless these treatments are still widely used as a first attempt to stop bleeding, and in a recently published study it was shown that topical sucralfate for 4–16 weeks was capable of inducing and maintaining remission in a vast majority of patients with radiation-induced proctosigmoiditis[10].

Local application of 4% formalin has also been described, and appears to be a simple and effective therapy for proctitis. After the first case report published in 1986 by Rubinstein et al.[11], several studies have shown gratifying short-term results with this form of therapy[12–15]. However, most patients will need general or regional anaesthesia, serum toxicity may be a problem depending on the method of administration and local complications such as anal ulceration, fissures and worsening of radiation-induced strictures have been reported. In addition, haemorrhagic vascular lesions extending to the sigmoid colon cannot be adequately managed with this technique.

Endoscopic therapy with both Nd:YAG and argon lasers has also been used successfully to photocoagulate the vascular lesions and stop rectal bleeding[16–18]. However, laser treatment is technically difficult, time-consuming and associated with increased risk for complications (5–15% of patients treated with Nd:YAG laser)[19–22].

Other techniques used for treating haemorrhagic radiation proctosigmoiditis include bipolar and heater probe electrocoagulation[23,24]. Jensen *et al.*[24] used both techniques to treat 21 patients with recurrent haematochezia and anaemia after radiotherapy for pelvic malignancies, reporting a statistically significant reduction in bleeding in all patients. The advantages of these thermal devices are the fact they are widely available, less expensive and more portable than lasers. However, despite all patients having less than 10 cm linear extent of vascular lesions, a mean of four treatment sessions was required for control of rectal bleeding.

Argon plasma coagulation (APC) is a new method of non-contact electrocoagulation in which high-frequency energy is delivered to the tissue through ionization of the argon gas. Its controllable depth of penetration (2–3 mm) minimizes the risk of complications, whereas the brushwork-like application provides a quick and uniform coagulation of large bleeding surfaces without the need to apply the energy point-by-point as with laser or other conventional electrocoagulation techniques[25,26]. In a recently published study[27] we reported the results of APC therapy in 28 patients with haemorrhagic radiation-induced proctosigmoiditis. Indications for treatment were anaemia in 18 patients and persistent bleeding despite pharmacotherapy in 10. The linear extent of vascular lesions ranged from 8 to 60 cm, involving the sigmoid colon in 16 patients. The severity of rectal bleeding before and after treatment was graded from 0 to 4, according to the criteria of Chuktan *et al.*[28]: 0, no blood; 1, blood on toilet paper or stool; 2, blood in toilet bowl; 3, heavy bleeding with clots; 4, bleeding necessitating transfusions. A median of 2.9 sessions per patient were performed, achieving a decrease of the mean severity score from a value of 2.96 to 0.68, with all but two patients dropping at least one point in the scale. Average haemoglobin level increased 1.2 g/dl (1.9 g/dl among anaemic patients) and no serious complications or side-effects related to the technique itself were observed. We concluded that APC appears to be a simple, safe and effective technique in the management of haemorrhagic radiation-induced proctosigmoiditis.

Surgical treatment is associated with high morbidity and mortality and should be reserved for patients who do not respond to medical or endoscopic therapies, or those with fistulas, obstruction or perforation[1,2,29].

References

1. Anseline PF, Lavery IC, Fazio VW, Jagelman DG, Weakley FL. Radiation injury of the rectum: evaluation of surgical treatment. Ann Surg. 1981;194:716–24.
2. Gilinsky NH, Burns DG, Barbezat GO, Levin W, Myers HS, Marks IN. The natural history of radiation-induced proctosigmoiditis: an analysis of 88 patients. Q J Med. 1983;205:40–53.
3. Rosen IB, Shapiro BJ. Radiation enteropathy of the small bowel. Can Med Assoc J. 1994;91:681–8.
4. Kinsella TJ, Bloomer WD. Tolerance of the intestine to radiation therapy. Surg Gynecol Obstet. 1980;151:273–84.

5. Buchi K. Radiation proctitis: therapy and prognosis. J Am Med Assoc. 1991;265:1180.
6. Cho KH, Chung KKL, Levit SH. Proctitis after conventional external radiation therapy for prostate cancer: importance of minimizing posterior rectal dose. Radiology. 1995;195:699–703.
7. Haboubi NY, Schofield PF, Rowland PL. The light and electron microscopic features of early and late phase radiation-induced proctitis. Am J Gastroenterol. 1988;83:1140–4.
8. Baum CA, Biddle WL, Miner PB. Failure of 5-aminosalicylic acid enemas to improve chronic radiation proctitis. Dig Dis Sci. 1989;34:758–60.
9. Triantafillidis JK, Dadioti P, Nicholakis D, Mericas E. High doses of 5-aminosalicylic acid enemas in chronic radiation proctitis: comparison with betamethasone enemas. Am J Gastroenterol. 1989;84:1587–8 (letter).
10. Kochar R, Sriram PVJ, Sharma SC, Goel RC, Patel F. Natural history of late radiation proctosigmoiditis treated with topical sucralfate suspension. Dig Dis Sci. 1999;44:973–8.
11. Rubinstein E, Ibsen T, Rasmussen RB, Reimer E, Sorensen BL. Formalin treatment of radiation-induced hemorrhagic proctitis. Am J Gastroenterol. 1986;81:44–5.
12. Seow-Choen F, Goh H-S, Eu K-W, Ho Y-H, Tay S-K. A simple and effective treatment for hemorrhagic radiation proctitis using formalin. Dis Colon Rectum. 1993;36:135–8.
13. Biswal BM, Lal P, Rath GK, Shukla NK, Mohanti BK, Deo S. Intrarectal formalin application, an effective treatment for grade III haemorrhagic radiation proctitis. Radiother Oncol. 1995;35:212–15.
14. Saclarides TJ, King DG, Franklin JL, Doolas A. Formalin instillation for refractory radiation-induced hemorrhagic proctitis: report of 16 patients. Dis Col Rectum. 1996;39:196–9.
15. Roche B, Chautems R, Marti MC. Application of formaldehyde for treatment of hemorrhagic radiation-induced proctitis. World J Surg. 1996;20:1092–5.
16. Ahlquist DA, Gostout CJ, Viggiano TR, Pemberton JH. Laser therapy for severe radiation-induced rectal bleeding. Mayo Clin Proc. 1986;61:927–31.
17. Carbatzas C, Spencer GM, Thorpe SM, Sargeant LR, Bown SG. Nd:YAG laser treatment for bleeding from radiation proctitis. Endoscopy. 1996;28:497–500.
18. Taylor JG, Disario JA, Buchi KN. Argon laser therapy for hemorrhagic radiation proctitis: long-term results. Gastrointest Endosc. 1993;39:641–4.
19. Hunter JG, Burt RW, Becker JM, Lee RG, Dixon JA. Colonic mucosal lesions: evaluation of monopolar electrocautery, argon laser and neodymium: YAG laser. Curr Surg. 1984;41:373–5.
20. Bown SG, Swain CP, Storey DW *et al*. Endoscopic laser treatment of vascular anomalies of the upper gastrointestinal tract. Gut. 1985;26:1338–48.
21. Gostout CJ, Bowyer BA, Ahlquist DA, Viggiano TR, Balm RK. Mucosal vascular malformations of the gastrointestinal tract: clinical observations and results of endoscopic neodymium:yttrium–aluminum garnet laser therapy. Mayo Clin Proc. 1988;63:993–1003.
22. Johnston JH. Complications following endoscopic laser therapy. Gastrointest Endosc. 1982;28:135 (abstract).
23. Maunoury V, Brunetaud JM, Cortot A. Bipolar electrocoagulation treatment for hemorrhagic radiation injury of the lower digestive tract. Gastrointest Endosc. 1991;37:492–3 (letter).
24. Jensen DM, Machicado GA, Cheng S, Jensen ME, Jutabha R. A randomized prospective study of endoscopic bipolar electrocoagulation and heater probe treatment of chronic rectal bleeding from radiation telangiectasia. Gastrointest Endosc. 1997;45:20–5.
25. Farin G, Grund KE. Technology of argon plasma coagulation with particular regard to endoscopic applications. Endosc Surg. 1994;2:71–7.
26. Grund KE, Storek D, Farin G. Endoscopic argon plasma coagulation (APC). First clinical experiences in flexible endoscopy. Endosc Surg. 1994;2:42–6.
27. Silva RA, Correia AJ, Dias LM, Viana HL, Viana RL. Argon plasma coagulation therapy for hemorrhagic radiation proctosigmoiditis. Gastrointest Endosc. 1999;50:221–4.
28. Chuktan R, Lipp J, Waye J. The argon plasma coagulator: a new and effective modality for treatment of radiation proctitis. Gastrointest Endosc. 1997;45:AB27 (abstract).
29. Browning GC, Verma JS, Smith NA, Small WP, Duncan W. Late results of mucosal proctectomy and coloanal sheeve anastomosis for chronic radiation rectal injury. Br J Surg. 1987;74:31–4.

11
Radiation injuries in urology

P. FORNARA

Urology is in the field of conflict between offender and victim in radiation therapy of the abdomen and small pelvis.

On the one hand it utilizes the proliferation-inhibiting effect of ionizing radiation on malignant degenerative tissues in radiation therapy of prostatic carcinoma, seminoma and bladder carcinoma; on the other hand the urogenital tract is one of the organ systems most often affected by typical acute and chronic side-effects of radiation therapy. Particularly the quality of life of tumour patients is impaired by side-effects of radiation therapy affecting the urogenital tract.

On the basis of side-effects associated with radiation therapy of uterus and cervix carcinomas, of retroperineal tumours, bladder carcinomas and prostatic carcinomas, the presentation will show that typical side-effects are always observed on the urinary system, although the radiation dosage is moderate and radiation technology, as well as procedures, have been improved over recent years. The most prominent side-effects include urine-transport defects due to acute inflammatory reactions or anatomical changes resulting from actinic fibroses.

The data to be presented aim at establishing an awareness that the follow-up of oncological patients with regard to the urogenital tract should be evaluated and documented according to uniform criteria.

Section IV
Inflammatory diseases
of the anorectum

12
Immunopathogenesis of inflammatory bowel disease

A. STALLMACH and M. ZEITZ

INTRODUCTION

The aetiology of inflammatory bowel disease (IBD), Crohn's disease and ulcerative colitis, remains poorly understood, although an enormous amount of data has appeared in the past few years on this matter. Most authors agree that immunological abnormalities in the local mucosa-associated immune system (MALT) are of major importance[1–4].

The intestinal lumen is populated with large numbers of bacteria, dietary antigens, and other agents. Therefore, the gut-associated immune system (GALT) has to protect the host against invasion of potential pathogens or an inappropriate immune response to luminal antigens under normal conditions[5]. Two functional compartments of the GALT can be discerned: (1) the afferent part consisting of the organized lymphoid follicles, e.g. the Peyer's patches of the ileum, and the mesenteric lymph nodes; (2) the effector part consisting of the lymphocytes located diffusely in the lamina propria (lamina propria lymphocytes, LPL) and the lymphocytes located intraepithelially above the basement membrane between the enterocytes (intraepithelial lymphocytes, IEL). It is assumed that antigens enter the intestinal mucosa via the M cells (microfolded cells) which constitute a specialized epithelium above the Peyer's patches or lymphoid follicles. In these follicles the mucosal immune response is initiated by the uptake and processing of antigenic material by macrophages and follicular dendritic cells and its presentation to T and B cells. Primed lymphocytes leave the mucosa and, after expansion in mesenteric lymph nodes, enter the circulation via the thoracic duct. Finally, they migrate back to the intestinal mucosa – a phenomenon called homing – where they exert their effector functions. Lymphocytes within the mucosal immune system differ in many respects from lymphocytes in other compartments of the body. Functionally these T cells can be characterized as differentiated effector lymphocytes which respond to triggering of the antigen-specific T cell receptor by secreting helper factors for B cells. Therefore, lamina propria T cells represent a subset of memory T cells with a unique maturational state adapted to the specific tasks in the intestinal mucosa. An antigen-specific response of intestinal lamina propria T cells, in the form of a down-regulation of proliferation and an increase in the secretion of regulatory factors, prevents potentially harmful clonal expansion of T cells in the mucosa, and at the same time allows protective immune responses, e.g. immunoglobulin secretion.

PRINCIPLES OF THE INDUCTION AND OUTCOME OF IMMUNE RESPONSES

The general principles of the induction of an immune response are similar in different organs: the initial step of an immune response is uptake and presentation of antigens by specialized antigen-presenting cells. The presentation of processed antigens in context with the major histocompatibility complex (MHC) leads to the activation of T cells. In recent years it has been shown by several groups that intestinal epithelial cells can serve as antigen-presenting cells. Antigen presentation by intestinal epithelial cells leads under physiological conditions to the stimulation of CD8-positive cells with suppressor function[6,7].

The outcome of an immune response is determined by the kind of effector cells which are stimulated by the initially activated T cells. On one hand, cyto-toxic cells (e.g. cytotoxic T cells, NK cells) may be induced (cellular immune response); on the other hand, antibody secretion by B cells rsp. plasma cells may be the major effector element (humoral immune response). At least two CD4-positive T-cell subsets with distinct patterns of lymphokine production have been identified which fundamentally influence the outcome of an inflammatory reaction[8]. One subset, referred to as T_h1 cells, produces interleukin 2 (IL-2) and interferon gamma (IFN-γ) upon activation and promotes cell-mediated effector responses (T_h1-like response). A second subset, type 2 helper T cells (T_h2), secretes IL-4, IL-5, IL-6 and IL-10, and supports antibody production by B cells or allergic reactions (T_h2-like response)[9]. A third group of T_h3-like cells, which produce transforming growth factor beta (TGF-β), is induced upon low-dose oral antigen administration, provides mucosal T helper function and down-regulates T_h1 cell function[9]. The initial events that induce the maturation of the distinct T_h cell subpopulations are unknown. Several different mechanisms have been proposed which determine differentiation of T_h0 either into T_h1 or T_h2 cells. These include locally present cytokines, type of the antigen-presenting cells, antigen characteristics, and lymphoid tissue microenvironment like cytokines and extracellular matrix components.

LYMPHOCYTE ACTIVATION AND DIFFERENTIATION IN IBD

Under physiological conditions the intestinal lamina propria contains T cells which have a distinctive phenotype and which are activated. Functionally these T cells can be characterized as differentiated effector lymphocytes which respond to triggering the antigen-specific T cell receptor by secreting helper factors for B cells. An antigen-specific response of intestinal lamina propria T cells in the form of a down-regulation of proliferation and an increase in the secretion of regulatory factors prevents potentially harmful clonal expansion of T cells in the mucosa and at the same time allows protective immune response, e.g. immunoglobulin secretion. There are indications that the tissue-specific differentiation of mucosal T cells is disturbed in IBD. The phenotype of intestinal T cells subpopulations in IBD is not significantly different from normal mucosa. However, studies investigating the state of activation of lamina propria mononuclear cells in patients with IBD have given evidence of an increased activation[10–12]. It has been shown that the number of LPL expressing CD25 or other activation markers is increased in inflamed lesions in Crohn's disease, ulcerative colitis, or pouchitis compared to non-inflamed areas or control tissue. Another finding documenting increased activation of T cells in IBD is the demonstration of higher concentrations of circulating soluble IL-2 receptors in serum of patients with active Crohn's disease compared with controls. Further, in our own studies, an increased expression of activated form of β_1-integrins on CD4$^+$ LPL in inflamed mucosa of patients with Crohn's disease and ulcerative colitis was observed (see Fig. 1). β_1-integrins, also known as very late activation (VLA) receptors, are essential for a number of physiological processes playing a prominent role in mediating diverse cell–cell and cell–matrix interactions, and act as co-stimulatory molecules (see below). It should be noted that this increased expression is not IBD-specific. Analysis of active integrins in patients with acute diverticulitis also revealed an elevation. However, these studies are a first indication of an up-regulated T cell-mediated mucosal immune response in patients with IBD.

Increased T cell proliferation in IBD

Studies investigating T cell responsiveness of mucosal T cells in IBD have confirmed unresponsiveness of normal lamina propria T cells with regard to proliferation, but have shown that T cells from inflammatory intestinal lesions from IBD patients exhibited a comparable or even higher proliferation to antigenic or CD3 stimulation compared to peripheral blood T cells[13,14]. Using antigens from the resident intestinal bacterial flora as stimulating antigens an abnormal

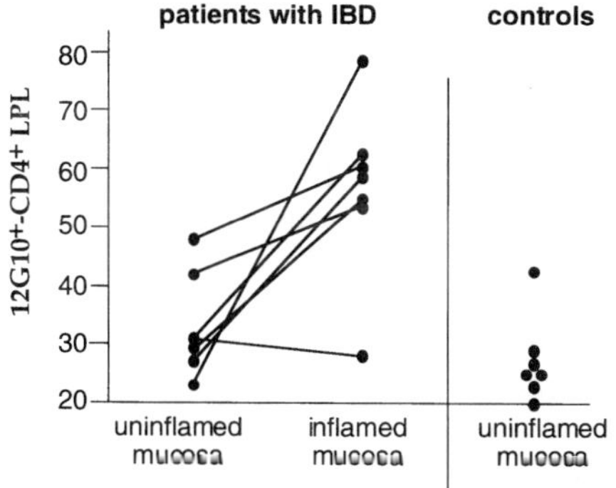

Figure 1 Increased expression of activated β_1-integrins on CD4$^+$ LPL of patients with IBD. Expression of β_1-integrins on LPL was analysed by flow cytometry. Graphs connect intra-individual values of CD4$^+$/β_1^+ LPL of inflamed and uninflamed mucosa from patients with active IBD

increase in the proliferative response of intestinal mononuclear cells from inflamed areas of IBD patients was shown[15]. Based on these observations we could demonstrate that $CD4^+$ mucosal lymphocytes proliferate vigorously in response to anti-CD3 stimulation when β_1-integrins were activated in these cells. β_1-integrin costimulation caused a 3–6-fold increase in proliferation of LPL compared with that of anti-CD3 stimulation alone. Further, co-stimulation of β_1-integrins in mucosal lymphocytes induced a significant increase of proinflammatory cytokine transcripts such as tumour necrosis factor alpha (TNF-α) or IFN-γ compared to T-cell receptor/CD3 activation alone. These data indicate that co-stimulation through β_1-integrins is of major importance to modulate LPL response after T-cell receptor stimulation, and underline the importance of increased expression of co-stimulatory molecules in inflammatory conditions.

Decreased apoptosis of T cells in IBD

It is now well recognized that induction of apoptosis, also known as activation-induced cell death or programmed cell death, is an important mechanism by which the immune system controls the overall size of cell clones undergoing expansion in response to antigenic stimuli. There are many examples of apoptosis in the immune system, programmed cell death of T cells during negative intrathymic selection of the TCR repertoire and, in the post-thymic phase, death of responsive T cells upon specific TCR/CD3 activation. Induction of apoptosis assures rapid disappearance of immune response upon antigenic clearance, avoiding the metabolic costs involved sustaining a large number of effector cells. This process may be of particular importance to a lymphocytic population that is physically close to a large and potentially stimulatory antigenic reservoir, such as that in the gastrointestinal lamina propria. In prior studies of apoptosis of mucosal T cells Boirivant and co-workers have established that, compared with peripheral blood T cells, lamina propria T cell manifest increased apoptosis when cultured in the absence of a stimulus and greatly enhanced apoptosis when cultured with a CD2 activation pathway stimulus. This increased apoptosis of lamina propria T down-regulates cell expansion and cytokine production and contributes to hyporesponsiveness after TCR/CD3 stimulation. Interestingly, T cells isolated from areas of inflammation in Crohn's disease, ulcerative colitis, and other inflammatory states manifest decreased activation-induced apoptosis. Studies of cells from inflamed Crohn's disease tissue indicate that this defect is accompanied by elevated Bcl-2 levels[16,17]. Given that β_1-integrin co-stimulation in mucosal lymphocytes results in an increase of contra-apoptotic proteins such as Bcl-xL and its various related proteins such as Bcl-2, and that activated β_1-integrins are strongly expressed on LPL in inflamed mucosa, this mechanism could contribute to the reduced activation-induced apoptosis of LPL in intestinal inflammation. These changes are probably caused by the chronic inflammation, and may aggravate the underlying disease processes that are present.

These data clearly show a different responsiveness of lamina propria T cells of IBD patients with an increased proliferation and decreased apoptosis after stimulation of the antigen-specific T cell receptor. These data indicate a breakthrough of the normally occurring tolerance towards the intestinal flora. They support the hypothesis of a disturbed differentiation of intestinal T cells in IBD.

Cytokine imbalance in IBD

Indications that cytokine imbalances in the mucosal immune system might be of major importance in the pathogenesis of IBD come from cytokine or T cell receptor mutant mice ('gene knockout mice'). Animals with non-functioning IL-2, IL-10 or T cell receptor genes develop chronic intestinal inflammation resembling IBD in several respects[18–21]. Interestingly, IL-2-deficient mice develop a disease similar to ulcerative colitis. Since IL-2 is a typical T_h1 cytokine, T_h2 cytokines dominate in these animals. In contrast, the intestinal disease in IL-10-deficient mice corresponds more to Crohn's disease. IL-10 down-regulates T_h1 cytokines, a lack of IL-10 might cause high levels of T_h1 cytokines (IL-2, IFN-γ). Corresponding to these experimental data there is some preliminary evidence in human studies that the cytokine pattern might be different in Crohn's disease (T_h1-like) and ulcerative colitis (T_h2-like)[22,23]. These findings are a first indication that the predominance of either T_h1 or T_h2 cytokines might lead to different appearances of mucosal inflammation. However, it must be critically remarked that the T_h1/T_h2 paradigm in IBD is oversimplifying the intricacies of the immune system; nevertheless it offers a useful concept for understanding chronic inflammation.

Several groups described increased levels of proinflammatory cytokines (IL-1, IL-6, IL-8) in inflamed Crohn's disease and ulcerative colitis tissue samples compared to controls[24]. Increased levels of IL-1 and IL-6 have also been described in uninvolved Crohn's disease tissue compared with control tissue. These data support the hypothesis that Crohn's disease is a panenteritis that manifests itself only in some defined areas of the gut. In addition, various groups found an increased production of TNF-α by lamina propria mononuclear cells in patients with IBD[25]. The functional importance of this cytokine in IBD is supported by several studies that showed that antibodies to TNF can be successfully used to treat intestinal inflammation in Crohn's disease[26]. Another important cytokine central to the pathogenesis of IBD could be IL-12, a cytokine produced by dendritic cells and macrophages mainly in response to bacterial products[27]. Levels of the functionally active IL-12 heteromer and increased in mucosal cells of patients with Crohn's disease but not ulcerative colitis. Since IL-12 is a potent inducer of T_h1 cell differentiation, these data suggest that IL-12 could be a key cytokine for T_h1 cell differentiation in Crohn's disease, whereas lower levels of IL-12 in ulcerative colitis favour T_h2 cell differentiation. Based on this hypothesis, Fuss et al. found a different cytokine profile of mucosal lymphocytes in IBD compared with control LPL[28]. For instance, a decreased IL-2 production of LP $CD4^+$ T cells in patients with Crohn's disease, but not with ulcerative colitis, was shown after accessory pathway stimulation. The production of IFN-γ, another T_h1 cytokine, was also analysed by several groups. Breese et al. and Autschbach et al. found an increase of IFN-γ-producing cells in Crohn's disease but not in ulcerative colitis[23,29]. Conversely, Fuss et al. demonstrated an increased production of IFN-γ by $CD4^+$ LPL in Crohn's disease but not in ulcerative colitis when cells were stimulated via accessory pathways[28]. In further studies, designed to analyse production of T_h2 cytokines in IBD, decreased production of IL-4 by LPL was found in both Crohn's disease and ulcerative colitis. This decrease of IL-4 production was associated with reduced numbers of IL-4 as shown by ELISPOT analysis. Interestingly, and in contrast to these observations, our own studies demonstrated an increased number of IFN-γ-producing cells in pouchitis in patients with ulcerative colitis. In addition, Desreumaux *et al.* demonstrated that early ileal lesions of patients with Crohn's disease were associated with a significant increase of IL-4 mRNA and a decrease of IFN-γ mRNA compared with the normal mucosa of patients with Crohn's disease or controls. The typical T_h1-type pattern was observed in this study only in chronic ileal lesions[30]. Therefore, divergent cytokine patterns may be associated with different clinical stages of IBD.

Further studies focused on production of the T_h2 cytokine IL-5 in patients with IBD. IL-5 production by $CD4^+$ LPL in Crohn's disease was normal or decreased, whereas strikingly increased production was observed in ulcerative colitis[28]. In summary, when compared to controls, lamina propria lymphocytes isolated from IBD show distinctive variation in cytokine production. In particular, Crohn's disease is characterized by an increased production of IFN-γ, while in ulcerative colitis an increased production of IL-5 is observable. However, as mentioned above, the strong T_h1/T_h2 paradigm in IBD is an oversimplification and should be used with some caution.

CONCLUSIONS

Taken together, an increased activation and a disturbed differentiation process of lamina propria T cells in IBD might lead to a different responsiveness of the T cell receptor with an inappropriate expansion of mononuclear cells in the intestinal mucosa in IBD (Fig. 2). An imbalance between helper and suppressor mechanisms in the intestinal mucosa in IBD could result in a sustained and overshooting inflammatory and immune reaction against antigens normally occurring in the intestinal lumen. Such an unchecked and excessive immune reaction in the mucosa could be responsible for the persisting and destructive nature of the inflammation in IBD patients (Fig. 3). The specific phenotype of IBD (Crohn's disease or ulcerative colitis) could be explained by a different pattern of cytokines synthesized within the mucosal immune system in the course of the overshooting immune response. However, many more studies are needed to confirm this hypothesis.

	normal conditions	IBD
activation of LPL	▲	▲▲▲
proliferation of LPL (after TCR-stimulation)	—	▲▲▲
Apoptosis	▲▲▲	▲
Secretion proinflammatory cytokines	▲	▲▲▲

Figure 2   Characteristics of LPL compared to PBL

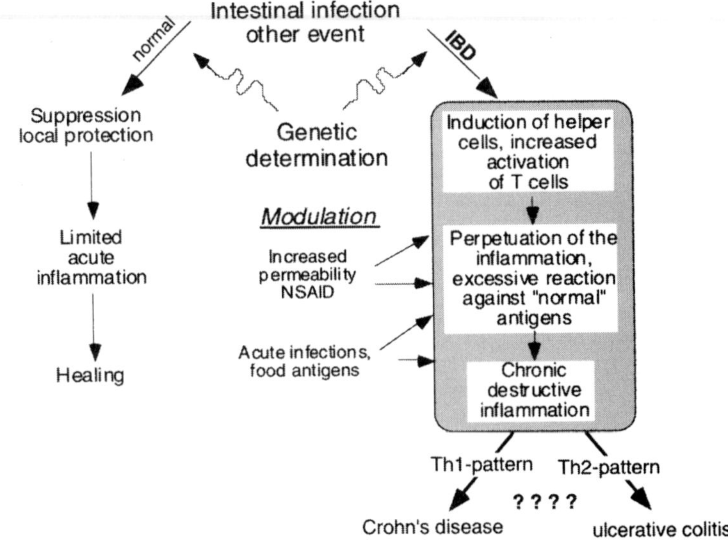

Figure 3 Proposed model of the pathogenesis of IBD based on the findings of immunoregulatory abnormalities in the local gut-associated lymphoid tissue. The highly regulated immune response in the gut is disturbed in IBD leading to an overshooting immune response with the development of destructive inflammation (for details see text)

Acknowledgements

Our studies are supported by grants from the German Research Council (DFG: Sta 295/3-1 and 4-1).

References

1. Strober W, James SP. The immunologic basis of inflammatory bowel disease. J Clin Immunol. 1986;6:415–32.
2. MacDermott RP. Alterations in the mucosal immune system in ulcerative colitis and Crohn's disease. Med Clin N Am. 1994;78:1207–31.
3. Zeitz M. Pathogenesis of inflammatory bowel disease. Digestion. 1997;58(Suppl. 1)(59):59–61.
4. Fiocchi C. Inflammatory bowel disease: etiology and pathogenesis. Gastroenterology. 1998;115:182–205.
5. Pabst R. The anatomical basis for the immune function of the gut. Anat Embryol. 1987;176:135–44.
6. Bland PW, Warren LG. Antigen presentation by epithelial cells of the rat small intestine. II. Selective induction of suppressor T cells. Immunology. 1986;58:9–14.
7. Mayer L, Shlien R. Evidence for function of Ia molecules on gut epithelial cells in man. J Exp Med. 1987;166:1471–83.
8. Mosmann TR, Coffman RL. T$_h$1 and T$_h$2 cells: different patterns of lymphokine secretion lead to different functional properties. Annu Rev Immunol. 1989;7:145–73.
9. Weiner HL, Friedman A, Miller A et al. Oral tolerance: immunologic mechanisms and treatment of animal and human organ-specific autoimmune diseases by oral administration of autoantigens. Annu Rev Immunol. 1994;12:809–37.
10. Schreiber S, MacDermott RP, Raedler A et al. Increased activation of isolated intestinal lamina propria mononuclear cells in inflammatory bowel disease. Gastroenterology. 1991;101:1020–30.

11. Ullrich R, Schneider T, Jahn HU *et al.* Altered expression of T cell differentiation antigens in T cells isolated from the large intestine of patients with Crohn's disease or ulcerative colitis. Adv Exp Med Biol. 1995;379B:1283–5.

12. Stallmach A, Schäfer F, Weber S *et al.* Increased state of activation of CD4-positive T cells and elevated interferon-γ production in pouchitis. Gut. 1998;43:499–505.

13. Pirzer U, Schonhaar A, Fleischer B, Hermann E, Meyer zum Büschenfelde K. Reactivity of infiltrating T lymphocytes with microbial antigens in Crohn's disease. Lancet. 1991;338:1238–9.

14. Qiao L, Golling M, Autschbach F, Schürmann G, Meuer SC. T cell receptor repertoire and mitotic responses of lamina propria T lymphocytes in inflammatory bowel disease. Clin Exp Immunol. 1994;97:303–8.

15. Duchmann R, Neurath M, Märker-Hermann E, Meyer zum Büschenfelde KH. Immune responses towards intestinal bacteria – current concepts and future perspectives. Z Gastroenterol. 1997; 35:337–46.

16. Boirivant M, Marini M, Di Felice G *et al.* Lamina propria T cells in Crohn's disease and other gastrointestinal inflammation show defective CD2 pathway-induced apoptosis. Gastroenterology. 1999;116:557–65.

17. Ina K, Itoh J, Fukushima K *et al.* Resistance of Crohn's disease T cells to multiple apoptotic signals is associated with a Bcl-2/Bax mucosal imbalance. J Immunol. 1999;163:1081–90.

18. Kühn R, Löhler J, Rennick D, Rajewsky K, Müller W. Interleukin-10-deficient mice develop chronic enterocolitis [See comments]. Cell. 1993;75:263–74.

19. Sadlack B, Merz H, Schorle H, Schimpl A, Feller AC, Horak I. Ulcerative colitis-like disease in mice with a disrupted interleukin-2 gene. Cell. 1993;75:253–61.

20. Kündig TM, Schorle H, Bachmann MF, Hengartner H, Zinkernagel RM, Horak I. Immune responses in interleukin-2-deficient mice. Science. 1993;262:1059–61.

21. Mombaerts P, Mizoguchi E, Grusby M, Glimcher LH, Bhan AK, Tonegawa S. Spontaneous development of inflammatory bowel disease in T cell receptor mutant mice. Cell. 1993;75: 274–82.

22. Mullin GE. Implications for T-cell lymphokine production patterns in mucosal disease. Mucosal Immunol Update. 1994;2:9–12.

23. Breese E, Braegger CP, Corrigan CJ, Walker-Smith JA, MacDonald TT. Interleukin-2- and interferon-gamma-secreting T cells in normal and diseased human intestinal mucosa. Immunology. 1993;78:127–31.

24. Isaacs KL, Sartor RB, Haskill S. Cytokine mRNA profiles in inflammatory bowel disease mucosa detected by PCR amplification. Gastroenterology. 1992;103:1587–95.

25. Reinecker HC, Steffen M, Witthoeft T *et al.* Enhanced secretion of tumour necrosis factor-alpha, IL-6, and IL-1 beta by isolated lamina propria mononuclear cells from patients with ulcerative colitis and Crohn's disease. Clin Exp Immunol. 1993;94:174–81.

26. van Dullemen HM, van Deventer SJ, Hommes DW *et al.* Treatment of Crohn's disease with anti-tumor necrosis factor chimeric monoclonal antibody. Gastroenterology. 1995;109:129–35.

27. Neurath MF, Fuss I, Kelsall BL, Stüber E, Strober W. Antibodies to interleukin 12 abrogate established experimental colitis in mice. J Exp Med. 1995;182:1281–90.

28. Fuss IJ, Neurath M, Boirivant M *et al.* Disparate CD4[+] lamina propria (LP) lymphokine secretion profiles in inflammatory bowel disease. Crohn's disease LP cells manifest increased secretion of IFN-gamma, whereas ulcerative colitis LP cells manifest increased secretion of IL-5. J Immunol. 1996;157:1261–70.

29. Autschbach F, Schurmann G, Qiao L, Merz H, Wallich R, Meuer SC. Cytokine messenger RNA expression and proliferation status of intestinal mononuclear cells in noninflamed gut and Crohn's disease. Virchows Arch. 1995;426:51–60.

30. Desreumaux P, Brandt E, Gambiez L *et al.* Distinct cytokine patterns in early and chronic ileal lesions of Crohn's disease. Gastroenterology. 1997;113:118–26.

13
The role of laboratory tests in inflammatory bowel disease

S. SCHREIBER

INTRODUCTION

The diagnosis of inflammatory bowel diseases (IBD) – ulcerative colitis (UC) and Crohn's disease (CD) – is made by a combined assessment of clinical, radiological, endoscopic and histological findings. However, laboratory evaluations may be very helpful to monitor disease activity and for the early detection of complications. The hope is that laboratory parameters may be used for prognosis of disease progression, and may sometimes even predict a relapse before clinical symptoms occur. Unfortunately, there are no specific, validated laboratory tests available to differentiate between CD and UC.

There have been several attempts to develop useful systems for describing the degree of inflammatory activity by a score. At present, disease activity in IBD is best quantified in clinical trials by using combined indices of clinical symptoms, laboratory tests, and endoscopic appearance. In clinical studies they provide the basis of an accurate comparison of patients with different degrees of disease activity and therapeutic outcomes. Although clinically useful, the first indices developed (i.e. the CDAI – Crohn's Disease Activity Index[1]) have been criticized because of their subjectivity and inter-observer variability[1–3]. Subsequently, new indices have been developed which include more laboratory parameters, in addition to clinical criteria[4,5] (see Table 1).

Table 1 Use of routine laboratory parameters as part of disease activity indices

Index	Parameter
CDAI	Haematocrit
van Hees	Serum albumin, erythrocyte sedimentation rate (ESR)
SAI	Serum albumin, haematocrit
Rachmilewitz	ESR
Truelove and Witts	ESR

Recently, several reports have also suggested various circulating mediators, e.g. proinflammatory cytokines (interleukin (IL)-1, -2, -6, -8, and tumour necrosis factor, TNF-α), as well as anti-inflammatory cytokines such as interleukin-1 receptor antagonist (IL-1ra) and interleukin-10 (IL-10), to serve as novel markers of disease activity and specificity[6–10]. Earlier reports showed an influx of inflammatory cells into the damaged mucosa and local production of proinflammatory cytokines. With recent advances in the study of IBD it has become apparent that some specific immunological factors, in particular TNF-α, may be involved in the early pathophysiology of mucosal inflammation. The utility of laboratory assessment of cytokines is a direct consequence of knowledge of the pathological processes of IBD. In experimental studies the secretion capacity for TNF-α of isolated lamina propria mononuclear cells can be used as a predictive parameter during remission of CD for a relapse in the next year following steroid induction of remission (Fig. 1). A similar phenomenon can be observed during relapse after successful therapy of CD with the TNF-binding antibody infliximab[8]. The assessment of calprotectin, which is a stable inflammatory marker that can be detected in stools, may offer a feasible alternative to use as an approach in clinical practice for the selection of high-risk patient populations[9].

For practical reasons, commonly employed, conventional serum markers of disease activity, e.g. acute-phase reactant proteins and other routinely diagnosed laboratory parameters, are separated from more, 'basic' inflammatory mediators such as cytokines. However, assessing disease activity in IBD by common

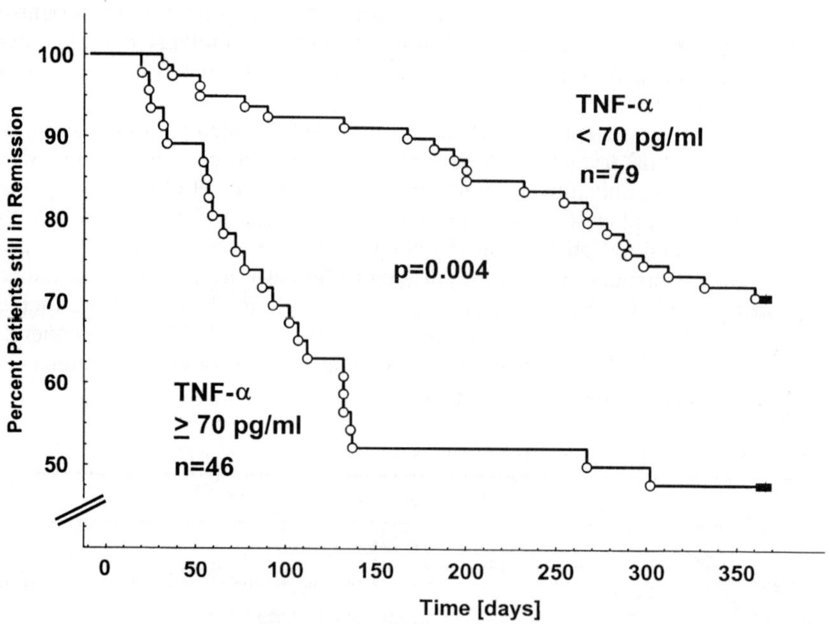

Figure 1 Secretion of tumour necrosis factor-α by lamina propria mononuclear cells predicts relapse in Crohn's disease. The group of high TNF secretors is characterized by an increased risk for relapse (reprinted from ref. 8)

laboratory activity parameters from the peripheral blood proves to be rather difficult, because 'disease activity' caused by limited mucosal inflammation may not
lead to a proportional alteration in immune activity parameters in the circulation[11].

MONITORING OF DISEASE ACTIVITY IN IBD

In both CD and UC there are two major approaches to assess inflammatory
activity by laboratory parameters: using blood tests and tests of clearances
of specific substrates into the intestinal tract (faecal excretion, respectively, gut
permeability).

State of activity in ulcerative colitis

The use of acute-phase reactant proteins, e.g. orosomucoid (an α_1-acid glycoprotein) in the assessment of the activity of UC has been repeatedly validated[12,13].
Most authors confirmed that ESR, C-reactive protein (CRP), and orosomucoid
correlate well with disease activity. According to Buckell *et al.*[14], the orosomucoid value was found to be significantly increased in acute UC patients versus
the respective groups in remission, as well as versus controls[14]. Elevated white
blood cells (WBC) are often likely to reflect disease activity; however, in
patients treated with steroids this may be difficult to interpret. Other laboratory
markers such as prealbumin, haemoglobin and α_2-globulin correlate less well
with clinical disease activity in UC[13]. To assess the extent of disease, Prantera
et al.[16] could demonstrate that a CRP > 2.8 mg/100 ml is greatly associated with
inflammation proximal the sigmoid colon, while the absence of laboratory test
alterations usually indicates a lesion below the sigmoid. Correlation between
CRP and extent of disease shows an 86% predictive value[16]. The presence of
anticolon antibodies and ANCA, which have been recognized in patients with
UC (p-ANCA particularly in UC patients with sclerosing cholangitis), or the
serum levels of nitrate oxide, respectively, do not characterize clinical severity
and extension of disease[17,19].

State of activity in Crohn's disease

Assessing disease activity in CD, determinations of thrombocytes and ESR were
found to be the best routine laboratory values, with elevations found in 70–80% of
patients with active disease[6]. In particular, serum amyloid A (SAA), orosomucoid
and CRP, were frequently increased in active disease. Andre and co-workers
demonstrated that ESR, orosomucoid and CRP are of great practical value in
assessing disease activity, and therefore defined a simple clinical index based on
these parameters[18]. The authors reported that albumin, haemoglobin, α_2-globulin,
α_1-antitrypsin, and WBC showed only a limited relationship to disease activity.
An entirely different approach is based on excretion studies: faecal excretion of
[111]In-labelled cells provided a quantitative measure of bowel inflammation[15].
The ^{111}In-faecal excretion reflected the clinical judgement and the height of the
van Hees activity index much better than did the CDAI scores. However, the
method cannot be used to localize active lesions without simultaneous scanning
by a gamma-camera. The assessment of faecal clearance of α_1-antitrypsin (α_1-
AT) is a non-radioactive method to study plasma protein loss[20]. Beeken *et al.*, as

Table 2 Value of laboratory assessments in different clinical types of IBD

Disease/type	Extent	Activity	Reoccurrence	Complications
Ulcerative proctosigmoiditis	No	No	No?	No?
Ulcerative colitis	Yes	Yes	No?	Yes?
Crohn's disease	No	Yes	Yes	Yes

well as Bjarnason *et al.*, reported increased permeability to ^{51}Cr-labelled EDTA (due to disruption of integrity of the small intestinal mucosa) to correlate well with the extent of small bowel involvement[21,22].

Prognosis of disease progression in IBD

Management of IBD patients involves repeated evaluations of the patient's condition over time. For characterization of clinical severity and inflammatory activity in UC, the disease activity index (DAI) according to Rachmilewitz[4] and the index of Truelove and Witts[3] are used. In CD the CDAI, van Hees index, and severity activity index (SAI) are commonly used (Table 1)[1–5].

One of the important functions of clinical and laboratory evaluations in IBD is the identification of those patients who become severely ill, e.g. of those who are progressing to complications (such as toxic megacolon). The value of laboratory parameters to identify patients for whom medical therapy had failed has been studied extensively. In patients with UC a study by Buckell *et al.* demonstrated that a persistent elevation of the CRP during the first days of treatment was significantly predictive of need for surgery[37]. No patient with a CRP < 25 mg/L, but most patients with CRP > 45 mg/L, required surgery. A correlation to prealbumin and α_1-acid glycoprotein has also been reported[19]. According to Charkravaty, low serum albumin levels, apart from the severity of diarrhoea, characterized patients who subsequently required colectomy[23]. However, in nearly all studies patients who succeeded in therapy had a higher haemoglobin level and lower ESR. Furthermore, Lauritsen *et al.* demonstrated elevated PGE_2 levels in rectal dialysates from asymptomatic patients who had discontinued treatment with sulphasalazine to be a predictor of relapse[24]. In long-standing UC there is an increased risk of colon cancer. No benefit exists for the systematic use of laboratory parameters to predict malignancy.

Prognosis of disease progression may be even more important in CD. The prediction of relapse for patients in clinical remission has been a crucial turning point in prevention trials. Brignola and co-workers have demonstrated that the likelihood of relapse is increased if CRP or another acute-phase reactant stays elevated despite clinical remission[25]. These workers used a complex formula to calculate risks ('prognostic index') from ESR, α_1-glycoprotein and α_2-globulin. A similar observation has been made by Wright and co-workers using orosomucoid and α_1-antitrypsin[26]. The ESR is easy to determine and has low costs, but correlates markedly less strongly to disease prognosis.

Recent studies have identified IL-6 as a serum cytokine which is linked in particular to disease activity[33]. Synthesis of CRP in the liver is to a great extent regulated by IL-6. Other studies have proposed soluble IL-2 receptor, soluble TNF

Table 3 Prognostic factors studied in Crohn's disease

Parameter	Time frame	Sensitivity (%)	Specificity (%)	Positive prediction (%)
α_1-acid glycoprotein, ESR, α_2-globulin	18 months	71	100	100
Lymphocytes, glutamine oxaloacetic acid transaminase, various clinical parameters	3 months (admission)	64	95	82
Lactulose–mannitol permeability	1 year	81	73	76
Faecal α_1-antitrypsin clearance	Post-op 1 year			100

receptors or other cytokines as objective surrogate markers of disease activity. However, none of the studies was able to demonstrate a clinical benefit resulting from the assessment of serum cytokine levels in comparison with routine clinical laboratory parameters of inflammation as discussed above. Therefore, the value of serum or plasma levels of cytokines in routine analysis has not yet been established in patients with IBD.

As outlined above, an increased mucosal production of proinflammatory cytokines (i.e. TNF-α, IL-1β) during remission is highly predictive of a relapse of Crohn's disease within the next year (Fig. 1)[7,8]. While this parameter is too complicated to routinely assess and cytokines in stools are fairly unstable, the assessment of calprotectin concentrations in stools may be a usable alternative in clinical practice[10].

COMPLICATIONS OF IBD

Local complications include the manifestation of anal lesions in CD, and the incidence of colon carcinoma in UC. Neither can be detected by laboratory assessment. About 20% of patients present with a highly acute disease, characterized by frequent episodes of diarrhoea, and generalized symptoms of inflammation. If the attack is sustained, anaemia, elevation of leucocytes, with increased neutrophils (and an increased percentage of immature cells), as well as a steep rise in acute-phase reactant proteins develop. In addition, hypoalbuminaemia, electrolyte and acid–base disorders, e.g. hypokalaemia, hyponatraemia, and metabolic alkalosis with hypochloraemia, may accompany severe diarrhoea.

Exudative enteropathy, which leads to intestinal protein loss due to extended lesions in the bowel, could be assessed by faecal α_1-antitrypsin and ^{51}Cr-labelled protein excretion. Following the nutritional state of patients, Baker and co-workers[27] have clearly demonstrated that simple bedside clinical judgement appears to be as good as measurement of complex laboratory nutritional and anthropometric assessments. Meryn et al.[28] also found that albumin, prealbumin, transferrin, and retinol-binding protein levels are associated with the nutritional status. Clinically significant malabsorption occurs in small-bowel CD; therefore, several tests have been assessed to measure intestinal absorptive capacity. Kruis et al.[29] demonstrated that the presence of fistulas was greatly associated with extended disease involvement and malnutrition of the patient.

Extraintestinal manifestions may involve eyes, skin, liver, kidney, bone, blood, and blood vessels. The most common haematological manifestations associated with IBD are: anaemia, thrombocytosis, leucocytosis, and thromboembolic disease because of possible hypercoagulability[34].

Elevated cholestatic liver enzymes (e.g. alkaline phosphatase, gamma glutamyl transpeptidase, and glutamate dehydrogenase) can be indicative of primary sclerosing cholangitis (commonly p-ANCA are positive). In cases of nephrolithiasis urinary oxalate excretion and urine status should be tested. Serum creatinine can be used to screen for a manifest injury of the glomeruli. According to Zehnter et al.[30] and Schreiber et al.[31] the excretion of tubular membrane proteins as detected by SDS-PAGE indicated possible clinical involvement of the kidneys in the inflammatory process, but may also reflect the impact of chronic medication with 5-ASA. Mahmud et al.[32] reported that patients with active IBD showed higher urinary excretion of albumin than did patients in remission.

WHAT TO ASSESS IN DAILY CLINICAL PRACTICE

As laboratory parameters of inflammation in general are redundant and of little influence for everyday treatment decisions, we would recommend the assessment of stable molecules and the use of inexpensive tests. In our routine practice it has been proven useful to assess thrombocyte counts and CRP in addition to the clinical index. In the expectation of complications, frequent and repetitive determinations of other parameters (i.e. haemoglobin, leucocyte count or others) may be warranted. However, with the continuing validation of prognostic indices we expect that future clinical trials and daily clinical practice will be able to utilize stool parameters[7-9] to identify those patients who are at particular risk either for development of highly active and complicated disease or of developing a relapse after only a short period of remission. The future will see stable molecular genetic markers being defined, which will help to perform risk assessments for the course of disease or for therapeutic responses on the basis of the individual genetic make-up of patients[35,36].

References

1. Best WR, Becktel JM, Singleton J, Kern F Jr. Development of Crohn's disease activity index. Gastroenterology. 1976;70:439–44.
2. van Hees PA, van Elteren PH, van Lier HJ, van Tongeren JH. An index on inflammatory activity in patients with Crohn's disease. Gut. 1980;21:279–86.
3. Truelove SC, Witts LJ. Cortisone in ulcerative colitis: final report on a therapeutic trial. Br Med J. 1955;2:1041–8.
4. Rachmilewitz D. Coated mesalazine (5-aminosalicylic acid) versus sulphasalazine in the treatment of active ulcerative colitis: a randomized trial. Br Med J. 1989;298:82–6.
5. Goebell H, Wienbeck M, Schomerus H, Malchow H. Evaluation of Crohn's disease activity index (CDAI) and the Dutch index for severity and activity of Crohn's disease. Med Klin. 1990;10:573–6.

6. Niederau C, Backmerhoff F, Schumacher B, Niederau C. Inflammatory mediators and acute phase proteins in patients with Crohn's disease and ulcerative colitis. Hepato-gastroenterology. 1997;44:90–107.

7. Schreiber S, Nikolaus S, Hampe J et al. Tumor necrosis factor-α and interleukin 1β in relapse of Crohn's disease. Lancet. 1999,353:459–61.

8. Nikolaus S, Kühbacher T, Sfikas N, Raedler A, Fölsch UR, Schreiber S. Mechanisms in failure of infliximab for Crohn's disease. Lancet. 2000;356:1475–9.

9. Tibble JA, Sigthorsson G, Bridger S, Fagerhol MK, Bjarnason I. Surrogate markers of intestinal inflammation are predictive of relapse in patients with inflammatory bowel disease. Gastroenterology. 2000;119:15–22.

10. Schreiber S, Heinig T, Thiele HG, Raedler A. Immunoregulatory role of interleukin 10 in patients with inflammatory bowel disease. Gastroenterology. 1995;108:1434–44.

11. Singleton JW. Clinical activity assessment in inflammatory bowel disease. Dig Dis Sci. 1987; 32:42–5S.

12. Dearing WH, McGuckin WF, Elveback LR. Serum α1-acid glycoprotein in chronic ulcerative colitis. Gastroenterology. 1969;56:295–303.

13. Weeke B, Jarnum S. Serum concentrations of 19 serum proteins in Crohn's disease and ulcerative colitis. Gut. 1969;12:292–303.

14. Buckell NA, Lennard-Jones MA, Hernandez MA et al. Measurements of serum proteins during attacks of ulcerative colitis as a guide to patient management. Gut. 1979;20:22–7.

15. Fischbach W, Becker W. Clinical relevance of activity parameters in Crohn's disease estimated by the faecal excretion of ^{111}In-labeled granulocytes. Digestion. 1991;50:149–52.

16. Prantera C, Davoli M, Lorenzetti R et al. Clinical and laboratory indicators of extent of ulcerative colitis. J Clin Gastroenterol. 1988;10:41–5.

17. Oudkerk Pool M, Ellerbroek PM, Ridwwan BU et al. Serum antineutrophil cytoplasmic auto-antibodies in inflammatory bowel disease are mainly associated with ulcerative colitis. A correlation study between perinuclear antineutrophil cytoplasmic autoantibodies and clinical parameters, medical and surgical treatment. Gut. 1993;34:46–50.

18. Andre C, Descos L, Andre F et al. Biological measurement of Crohn's disease activity – a reassessment. Hepato-gastroenterology. 1985;32:135–7.

19. Travis SP, White J, Jewell DP. Are serum concentrations of nitrate oxide metabolites useful for predicting the clinical outcome of severe ulcerative colitis? Eur J Gastroenterol Hepatol. 1995;7:227–30.

20. Meyers S, Wolke A, Field SP, Feuer EJ, Johnson JW, Janowitz HJ. Faecal antitrypsin measurement: an indicator of Crohn's disease activity. Gastroenterology. 1985;89:13–18.

21. Beeken WL, Busch HJ, Sylwester D. Intestinal protein loss in Crohn's disease. Gastroenterology. 1972;62:207–15.

22. Bjarnason I, O'Morain C, Levi AJ, Peters TJ. Absorption of [51]chromium labeled ethylenediaminetetra-acetate in inflammatory bowel disease. Gastroenterology. 1983;85:318–22.

23. Charkravaty BJ. Predictors and the rate of medical treatment failure in ulcerative colitis. Am J Gastroenterol. 1993;88:852–5.

24. Lauritsen K, Laursen LS, Bukhave K, Rask-Madsen J. Use of colonic eicosanoid concentration as predictor of relapse in ulcerative colitis: a double-blind placebo-controlled study in sulphasalazine maintenance treatment. Gut. 1988;29:1316–21.

25. Brignola C, Campieri M, Bazzocchi G, Farruggia P, Tragnone A, Lanfranchi GA. A laboratory index for predicting relapse in asymptomatic patients with Crohn's disease. Gastroenterology. 1986;91:1490–4.

26. Wright JP, Alp MN, Young GO, Tilger-Wybrandi N. Predictors of acute relapse of Crohn's disease: a laboratory and clinical study. Dig Dis Sci. 1987;32:164–70.

27. Baker JB, Detsky AS, Wesson DE et al. Nutritional assessment, a comparison of clinical judgement and objective measurements. N Engl J Med. 1982;306:969–72.

28. Meryn S, Lochs H, Bettelheim P, Sertl K, Mulak K. Serumproteinkonzentration – Parameter für die Krankheitsaktivität bei Morbus Crohn. Leber Magen Darm. 1985;15:160–4.

29. Kruis W, Scheuchenstein AM, Scheurlen C, Weinzierl M. Risikofaktoren für die Entstehung von Fisteln bei Morbus Crohn. Z Gastroenterol. 1989;6:313–16.

30. Zehnter E, Dörhöfer H, Ziegenhagen DJ, Scheurlen C, Baldamus CA, Kruis W. Renal damage in patients with inflammatory bowel disease treated with 5-aminosalicylic acid and sulphasalazine. Gastroenterology. 1995;100:A264 (abstract).

31. Schreiber S, Hämling J, Zehnter E *et al.* Renal tubular dysfunction in aminosalicylate treated patients with inflammatory bowel disease. Gut. 1997;40:761–6.
32. Mahmud N, O'Connell MA, Stinson J, Goggins MG, Weir DG, Kelleher D. Tumour necrosis factor-alpha and microalbuminuria in patients with inflammatory bowel disease. Eur J Gastroenterol Hepatol. 1995;7:215–19.
33. Gross V, Andus T, Cesar I, Roth M, Scholmerich J. Evidence for continuous stimulation of interleukin-6 production in Crohn's disease. Gastroenterology. 1992;32:1531–4.
34. Lake AM, Stauffer JQ, Stuart MJ. Hemostatic alterations in inflammatory bowel disease – response to therapy. Am J Dig Dis. 1978;10:897–902.
35. Schreiber S, Hampe J. Genomics and inflammatory bowel disease. Curr Opin Gastroenterol. 2000;16:297–305.
36. Schreiber S, Hampe J, Eickhoff H, Lehrach H. Functional genomics in gastroenterology. Gut. 2000;47:601–7.
37. Buckell NA, Lennard-Jones JE, Hernandez MA, Kohn J, Riches PG, Wadsworth J. Measurement of serum proteins during attacks of ulcerative colitis as a guide to patients' management. Gut. 1979;20:22–7.

14
Inflammatory diseases of the anorectum: diagnostic procedures: endoscopy and other imaging

A. FORBES

INTRODUCTION

Important diagnostic information comes from the clinical history and from a general examination of the patient. Inflammatory bowel disease is usually responsible for diarrhoea and, when the colon is involved, the rectal passage of blood. Depending on severity and the particular site(s) affected there may also be weight loss, anorexia and fatigue, or other systemic features such as tachycardia and pyrexia. Features that point towards Crohn's disease or ulcerative colitis reflect, on the one hand, the relative frequency of rectosigmoid involvement and, on the other, the malabsorptive effects of small bowel involvement in Crohn's disease. The history alone will occasionally remove any significant differential diagnosis. A young adult Caucasian patient presenting with several months' diarrhoea, weight loss and right iliac fossa pain might well be considered to have Crohn's disease until proved otherwise. Equally, gastrointestinal infection must always be considered and especially so when the history is short. We still have a long way to go given the continuing reports of prolonged delay between first symptom and a definitive diagnosis; in a large multicentre European study patients had symptoms for a mean period measured in years[1]!

Examination

The general examination will often contribute little, beyond confirming aspects of the history, but evidence of perianal disease suggests Crohn's disease – affecting upwards of 15% of patients. One study put the frequency of perianal fistula in Crohn's disease as high as 33%, but was probably biased towards those with more severe disease, as all had been inpatients for at least a month at some point[2]. It would, however, be a mistake to consider that perianal disease is pathognomonic of Crohn's disease, since around 10% of all perianal disease associated with inflammatory bowel disease is in patients with ulcerative colitis.

Severe perianal disease is nonetheless mainly confined to patients with Crohn's disease.

Up to a third of patients who finally prove to have predominantly distal colitis may, despite a clear history of diarrhoea, be constipated to abdominal palpation. One study has suggested that this proximal stasis is actually the cause of acute relapse in up to 10% of cases[3].

Bleeding

Bleeding is generally a feature of ulcerative colitis and distal Crohn's disease, but catastrophic bleeding from Crohn's disease also occurs – at a lifetime frequency of under 1%. Although most of the information is in the form of case reports, 34 patients collected from a single Belgian centre allow some generalizations to be drawn[4]. Most of the patients had an established diagnosis of Crohn's disease (mean > 5 years) but in only a third did the bleeding occur during a time of active disease. No less than 95% of the patients had a causative ulcer, the left colon being the most frequent site. This is consistent with impressions from the literature and from collections available only in abstract form.

DIFFERENTIAL DIAGNOSIS

Functional disorders compared to inflammatory bowel disease

Distinction from functional bowel disorders may be obvious in inflammatory bowel disease patients with bleeding, but in more subtle cases weight loss or the presence of night-time symptoms sufficient to wake the patient from sleep may be strong pointers to an organic aetiology. There may also be differences in underlying personality type between the two principal forms of inflammatory bowel disease. Patients with Crohn's disease were found in one study to be more extrovert and with a greater psychoticism score than those with ulcerative colitis, but with no differences in respect of neuroticism[5]. A degree of caution is needed in interpreting these data as prevalent cases were studied; the possibility that the course of the disease may have affected the prevailing personality state remains open (also relatively small numbers were studied, including only 27 with ulcerative colitis).

Other differential diagnosis

The differential diagnosis of apparent acute colitis includes infection, non-steroidal drug-related, and acute, self-limiting colitis (which may itself be infective), as well as inflammatory bowel disease. The most likely organisms – *Shigella, Campylobacter, Escherichia coli* 0157, *Entamoeba*, and to a lesser extent as bleeding is less frequent, *Salmonella, Aeromonas, Yersinia* and rota virus – are all fairly readily identified (or excluded) by conventional laboratory microbiological examination of the stools. More rigorous microbiological attention is required if the patient is immunodeficient. Pseudomembranous colitis from *Clostridium difficile* infection should be sought, by culture and by examination for its cytotoxin, especially if the patient has recently been exposed to antibiotics. Also, patients with inflammatory bowel disease may present acutely because of a secondary gastrointestinal infection. In the patient presenting for the first time the differential diagnosis is rather wider and includes colorectal carcinoma, ischaemic colitis and radiation enteritis if there is rectal bleeding, and intestinal tuberculosis, irritable bowel syndrome and a variety of malabsorptive and other gastrointestinal conditions, if diarrhoea is unaccompanied by bleeding. When the history does not provide obvious pointers it is then reasonable to proceed with investigation as for inflammatory bowel disease.

IMAGING

The traditional radiological methods of imaging the bowel have been increasingly challenged by newer modalities. Few would now argue that even the most carefully conducted double-contrast barium enema is superior to competent colonoscopy, but they remain complementary investigations[6] (see also below). The alternatives to barium-based examination of the small intestine are less established. The principal competition now comes from magnetic resonance imaging (MRI), but enteroscopy and white-cell scanning have important roles. Use of reconstructive three-dimensional computerized tomography, better known as virtual endoscopy, and of newer methods of more specific isotopic imaging, have not yet been exploited to the full in inflammatory bowel disease.

Plain abdominal radiograph

The plain abdominal radiograph is now undervalued and underused in many gastrointestinal centres. It will often be obvious from a supine film that the patient has faecal loading in the proximal colon (effectively excluding a diagnosis of total colitis) and, on the contrary, total colitis becomes an important possibility when there appears to be no faecal residue at any site.

Abdominal ultrasonography

The modest abdominal ultrasonographic scan has also been under-utilized. Apart from its role in detection and assessment of abscesses, it will often identify a loop of thickened, inflamed bowel with proximal distension and fluid retention, and not infrequently make possible a strong case for a diagnosis of Crohn's disease in the newly presenting patient with abdominal pain.

Modern ultrasound technology permits ready evaluation of the intestine at most sites in the abdomen, and radiologists and gastroenterologists are becoming more skilled at interpreting the findings. Using a very simple single criterion to determine postoperative recurrence – namely the presence of a bowel wall thickness of greater than 5 mm – ultrasonography proved nearly as reliable as full ileo-colonoscopy in a blinded study of over 40 Crohn's disease patients, and was possible in all patients; unlike the endoscopy, which was prevented by disease or its location in 13%[7]. With this criterion alone there was a sensitivity of 81% and a positive predictive value of 96%; full ileo-colonoscopy can legitimately be reserved for those with negative or uncertain results given the negative predictive value of 57%. Endoscopic ultrasonography will be dealt with separately in this volume.

Barium radiology

Contrast radiology is the longest-established imaging modality for diagnosis of inflammatory bowel disease. Barium sulphate is appropriately radiodense, is essentially inert, and is not normally absorbed from the gut. However, extraluminal barium creates a vigorous and potentially fatal inflammatory reaction in the peritoneum with a high risk of subsequent devastating fibrosis. Barium should be avoided where free perforation is a possibility, using instead a water-soluble contrast agent. Inferior definition is then to be expected, not least because many water-soluble media have a potent osmotic effect and tend to be diluted by resultant intestinal secretions.

The classical appearances of ulcerative colitis and Crohn's disease are well documented, and reference texts and atlases allow perusal of the variation in extent and severity and the more subtle aspects of radiological diagnosis.

Barium enema

Although controlled comparisons of colonoscopy and barium enema favour colonoscopy, which of course offers the advantage of permitting histological sampling, there remains a case for barium radiology. There is potential value of the unprepared or 'instant' enema in fulminant colitis, and it retains a role in the early assessment of a new patient with colitic symptoms in whom the extent of the disease will have an immediate influence on management.

The radiological distinction between different forms of colitis is based on the distribution, depth, and presence/absence of complications. It is usually possible to draw a confident interpretation from the combination of the radiological signs and the clinical features. The double-contrast enema, using both air and barium, has superseded the single-contrast examination (except for the 'instant' enema described above). In early/mild colitis there may be only a granularity of the mucosa which, in ulcerative colitis, will almost always be continuous from the rectum upwards. At a relatively early stage the space between the rectum and the sacrum (the retrorectal space) becomes enlarged. It is probable that this reflects both thickening of the rectal wall and the beginnings of rectal shortening as the bowel becomes fibrotic. The so-called hosepipe colon is now infrequently seen (perhaps the result of better medical therapy or earlier surgery), but when present is strongly supportive of a diagnosis of chronic fibrotic ulcerative colitis.

Crohn's colitis may mimic ulcerative colitis but usually declares itself from deeper ulceration (the rose-thorn ulcer), and a more patchy or asymmetrical distribution (with a strong tendency to affect the mesenteric border preferentially). In mild disease the halo appearance of aphthoid ulcers is characteristic. The presence of fistulous connections with other structures makes for a sure distinction from ulcerative colitis.

When polyps are demonstrated the radiologist may be confident that 'bridging' seen between polyps (also referred to as filiform polyposis) is the result of past inflammation, but will usually choose to defer to colonoscopic/histological assessment, since it is not possible to make a clear distinction between the inflammatory polyp and the adenoma.

Despite its limitations the barium enema still provides information that cannot be obtained by other means in every centre. The proximal colon of a patient with a tight stricture can often be assessed adequately, and radiological recognition of abnormal distensibility and contour of the bowel may be the earliest signs of malignant transformation in the long-standing colitic.

The radiological differential diagnosis for conditions other than inflammatory bowel disease includes ischaemia, which is patchy like Crohn's disease, but usually affects the vascular watershed zones such as at the splenic flexure. Infective colitides may be confused with inflammatory bowel disease (usually when the history is deficient). The classic cone-shaped caecum of chronic amoebiasis is rarely seen in Western centres, and tends to yield a differential diagnosis of neoplasia rather than of inflammatory bowel disease when it appears. Pseudomembranous colitis poses more of a challenge as it may complicate underlying inflammatory bowel disease, but the radiological features of plaque formation and proximal distension may be helpful if there has not already been clinical or endoscopic suspicion.

All of the remaining roles of barium enema in inflammatory bowel disease are likely soon to be overtaken by developments in virtual colonoscopy, which is less invasive and which should be at least as informative as the best conventional enema.

Barium studies of the small bowel

Barium studies of the small bowel are currently more secure, clinical experience continuing to support their use in the investigation of patients with symptoms potentially attributable to the small bowel[8] even when a centre has special expertise in colonoscopic ileoscopy[9]. There is some debate as to the relative place of the traditional follow-through and the small bowel enema or enteroclysis in which the barium is instilled through a nasal tube placed into the jejunum. The former tends to give better visualization of the lower small bowel (very often the area of greater interest in inflammatory bowel disease), and it is generally possible to compress the contrast-filled bowel, in turn helping to permit separation of superimposed intestinal loops[10]. The more distended bowel created in the adequately filled bowel at enteroclysis may be more difficult or painful to compress. It may be helpful to use anticholinergics, not only for their influence on intestinal motility, but also because patients often find that the examination is then appreciably less uncomfortable[11]. A follow-through examination can be performed as an adjunct to assessment of the more proximal gastrointestinal tract (the meal and follow-through), but this is almost always second-best for both parts of the examination as the ideal density and quantity of barium differs for the different purposes: it is not recommended.

It may be helpful, especially for comprehensive visualization of the terminal ileum, to introduce air into the colon (or to use an oral effervescent agent) to obtain partially double-contrast views. This is distinct from the retrograde examination of the small bowel obtained at barium enema when the ileocaecal valve is incompetent or absent, and which is not an investigation of choice for the ileum. Retrograde examinations are nevertheless valuable in patients with an ileostomy, especially so when there is proximal stenosis or when the patient is unwilling or unable to retain oral barium.

The radiological features of small bowel Crohn's disease reflect its pathological nature and distribution. The early changes include granularity, aphthous ulcers, and fold thickening, progressing with increasing severity to nodularity, frank focal ulceration, fissuring and stenosis. The asymmetry, typical of all aspects of Crohn's disease, is usually manifest as a disproportionate involvement of the mesenteric border of the gut. The classical 'string' sign, in which lengths of bowel appear narrowed and irregular, is as much the result of inflammation as of fibrous stricturing, and the separation of adjacent loops indicates that one is dealing with thickening of the bowel. In a dynamic examination it should be possible to make a distinction between motile but severely inflamed loops and those in which there is fixed stenotic scarring. This has clear therapeutic implications. 'Cobblestones' reflect the presence of deep and intersecting transverse and longitudinal ulcers and are rarely seen in other conditions. The presence of spontaneous fistulas, either between intestinal loops or from intestine to other structures, is almost pathognomonic of Crohn's disease in developed countries.

Although involvement of the terminal ileum is characteristic, it is by no means inevitable in small bowel Crohn's disease: in a recent survey nine of 71 patients with small bowel disease had a normal terminal ileum[9]. Patients with extensive Crohn's disease may also exhibit the characteristic malabsorption pattern of barium dilution and flocculation; a modest diffuse dilatation of the intestine may be seen. There tends to be a loss of the intestinal fold pattern in the proximal jejunum (and sometimes an increase more distally, although this is more a feature of non-Crohn's disease malabsorption).

Differential diagnosis for small bowel barium studies

Intestinal tuberculosis poses special problems in the differential diagnosis at centres in developed countries because of its relative rarity. The converse problem for patients with Crohn's disease in populations in which tuberculosis is more endemic is less worrying given the relative therapeutic implications of a wrong diagnosis. The radiologist may help by distinguishing the characteristic multiple transverse ulcers, the classic funnelled caecum, gross thickening of the intestinal wall and fixity of the terminal ileum, or from other manifestations of tuberculosis, not least of these being the chest radiograph – although this is abnormal in only about 50% of those with intestinal tuberculosis[12]. A continued high index of suspicion is needed if early infection is to be identified and late complications avoided.

The differential diagnosis for terminal ileitis includes previous irradiation, Behçet's syndrome, and yersinial infection. Intestinal lymphoid hyperplasia (idiopathic or related to a variety of acute and chronic infections) may be over-interpreted as Crohn's disease in young patients with gastrointestinal symptoms, but the experienced radiologist will usually be confident of the correct interpretation when associated ulceration is absent. Contrast examinations are increasingly performed in patients with intestinal ischaemia; focal and segmental ischaemia can be difficult to distinguish from active Crohn's disease.

Fistulography

Fistulas are poorly demonstrated by endoscopic techniques, and the degree of filling at intraluminal contrast studies is often inadequate for their full anatomy to be discerned. CT scanning may be of some limited help in the assessment of the patient with enterocutaneous fistulas, but until MRI methodology is a little more mature it is unlikely that the traditional 'fistulogram' will be superseded. Introduction of water-soluble contrast directly into the cutaneous opening will usually permit adequate demonstration of the fistula track and the site of its origin from the bowel. The tendency of the contrast to spill back can be overcome by its introduction through a balloon-tipped catheter which seals the skin opening. As relatively high pressures may be required the caution of an experienced operator is advised to avoid damage and maintain the reputation of fistulography as a safe technique.

CT scanning

CT scanning has mostly been used in the evaluation and management of complications of inflammatory bowel disease rather than in diagnosis of new patients with lower gastrointestinal symptoms, but more modern scanners with helical/spiral image capturing permit detailed assessment of the entire alimentary tract. In Crohn's disease the thickening of the bowel loops and their approximate location are easily identified, and further information in respect of significant stenoses and fistulous connections is now beginning to be of comparable reliability to that of barium follow-through. CT appearances will reliably differentiate between ulcerative colitis and Crohn's colitis in most cases, and may occasionally avoid colonoscopy[13]. The analysis of small bowel abnormalities can often differentiate causes other than Crohn's disease, such as ischaemia and Behçet's[14,15]. The need for histological samples remains, nonetheless. Enhanced CT scans are good at evaluating the retroperitoneum and ilio-psoas region in patients with suspected abdominal sepsis, these areas often proving inaccessible to ultrasonography. Abscesses appear as relatively low density spaces with enhancing walls, and can often be shown to contain gas (or previously administered contrast material).

Virtual colonoscopy

Virtual colonoscopy utilizes reconstructive techniques that permit the creation of images that apparently equate to the three-dimensional intraluminal view of the colon at colonoscopy. This is beginning to take on a service role in the assessment of the colon for neoplasia in the pioneer centres[16], but the resolution and pseudo-colour are still substantially inferior to colonoscopy. It is not yet clear that there will be a major place in inflammatory bowel disease work, but the speed at which improvements are emerging indicates that this may be just a question of time. There is no conceptual reason why the same approach should not be used to perform pseudo-endoscopy of the upper gastrointestinal tract or small intestine. It is unlikely, however, that therapeutic roles or means of obtaining biopsies will arise so as to render the comparable endoscopic routes obsolete. All forms of CT expose the patient to high radiation dose, and it is more likely that CT virtual endoscopy will itself be vanquished by equivalent reconstructions using MRI.

Magnetic resonance imaging

MR scanning permits non-invasive three-dimensional imaging of the abdomen and pelvis, and the speedier image acquisition of modern equipment reduces earlier difficulties associated with artefact from respiratory and intestinal movement. As long ago as 1994 MR outperformed the visual diagnosis made at colonoscopy in a small controlled study[17]. MR images are particularly helpful in the pelvis – a difficult area for most other forms of imaging – where unenhanced spin echo sequences can be invaluable in identifying and distinguishing inflammation/sepsis from surrounding normal tissues. Its application to patients with Crohn's disease has not been overlooked, but constraints of finance and availability have precluded gastroenterologists in many centres from developing adequate degrees of familiarity with its strengths and weaknesses.

MR enhanced by gadolinium (intravenously) and barium (orally), has been compared blindly with similarly enhanced, state-of-the-art CT scanning in 26 patients with Crohn's disease[18] with the subsequent knowledge of all other investigations to provide a gold standard. Depiction of mural thickening was superior on the MR images, which showed over 80% of 65 abnormal bowel segments, compared to helical CT, which showed only 63% ($p < 0.05$). Most of this gain was in the better recognition by MR of mildly diseased segments.

In the general context of pelvic sepsis and anorectal fistulas, anal endosonography has, however, proved the best modality, a primacy that is retained in Crohn's disease in which it out-performed MRI to a sensitivity of 89% versus only 48% for the MRI[19], but MR technology has already moved on to some extent, and it is possible that the deficit has by now been largely eliminated, and with less dependence on a specially skilled operator than is required for the sonographic technique.

MR scanning may prove to be of value in sequential imaging in Crohn's disease – a small blinded study having demonstrated good correlation between gadolinium-enhanced MR and a 'gold standard' derived from a composite of conventional radiography, endoscopy and/or surgery[20]. Increased bowel wall thickness and increased signal intensity on T1- and on T2-weighted images were seen (only) in affected parts of the small and large intestine. All three parameters improved significantly with successful steroid treatment.

There has been less use of axial imaging in the monitoring of ulcerative colitis, but this may be about to change if early data from the use of a new negative superparamagnetic oral contrast agent (ferumoxil) are substantiated by other centres. D'Arienzo *et al.* achieved identical diagnostic information from ferumoxil-enhanced MR scanning to that achieved from colonoscopy, with useful information about extent and severity of disease in each colonic segment[21]. An initial need for histological confirmation nonetheless remains.

It is clear that as MR scanning becomes faster, and with a wider selection of contrast agents, it will replace many, if not all, of the CT scans and barium examinations currently performed for inflammatory bowel disease.

White cell scanning, SPECT and E-selectin scanning

Radiolabelled white cell scanning identifies areas of inflammation and has the potential to yield quantitative assessments. When autologous leucocytes are returned to the host circulation they migrate preferentially to areas of inflammation or, in the absence of inflammation, mainly to the bone marrow and spleen. Labelled neutrophils re-injected into patients with inflammatory bowel disease tend to localize to areas of bowel currently involved in the disease. Initial work with 111-indium permitted a distinction between patients with active and inactive disease, and the radioactivity of timed faecal collections gave an 'excretion index' score. Indium has been superseded in most centres by labelling with 99^m-technetium which is cheaper, more readily available, has a shorter half-life, lower expected radiation exposure, and gives images more quickly and of better resolution. The usual carrier, hexamethyl propylene amine oxime (HMPAO), is lipophilic and easily able to enter white cells for labelling, but then becomes converted intracellularly to a hydrophilic form which cannot escape, leaving it and its associated technetium fixed within the cell. Crohn's disease activity and its predominant site(s) can be reliably documented[22]. It is possible to quantify disease activity, but there is difficulty in judging the accuracy and sensitivity of HMPAO scanning.

The distinction between currently active Crohn's disease – amenable to steroid therapy or other non-surgical method – and fibrostenotic disease – that can only be expected to respond to surgical resection or repair – is an important one. The radiologist may be able to make an informed judgement from barium images but will often acknowledge that a trial of therapy is a better indication of the predominant problem. White cell scanning has a logical role in this context – a normal scan in a symptomatic patient with known radiological abnormalities ought to constitute a strong indication for surgery. Unfortunately, although this is true at a statistical level, it appears not to hold good for the individual patient in whom a therapeutic decision is required[23], and a barium image is often still needed alongside the scan to obtain the full picture.

White cell scanning can be refined further by its combination with software developed for computerized tomography to allow creation of single-photon-emission-CT (SPECT) images, in which a three-dimensional reconstruction becomes possible[24]. All of the variants of white cell scanning expose the patient to a great deal less ionizing radiation than barium imaging and X-ray CT, with typical doses in the region of that of a standard chest radiograph (but more than from MRI). Many inflammatory bowel disease centres do not find HMPAO scanning clinically useful, despite the claimed quantitative reproducibility and undoubted low invasiveness[25]. It is especially disappointing, given the aim of minimizing irradiation, that scintigraphy was found to be unreliable in Birmingham children[26].

E-selectin scanning has emerged from experiences with labelled white cell scintigraphy. The selectin is over-expressed in endothelial cells at sites of inflammation and can be detected following the intravenous administration of a radiolabelled anti-E-selectin antibody. It has the theoretical advantages of studying a more fixed entity that (unlike white cells) will not be shed into the bowel lumen, and is applicable in the neutropenic patient. Preliminary data indicate an accuracy comparable to that of HMPAO scanning[27]; if indium as radiolabel can be switched to the more user-friendly technetium it could prove to have a clinical role.

ENDOSCOPY

Proctoscopy

At proctosigmoidoscopy the confluent erythema and ulceration of ulcerative colitis is, when typically exhibited, distinguishable from more characteristic aphthoid ulceration, serpiginous ulcers, and generally patchy distribution of Crohn's diseases. In a patient with a history suggestive of inflammatory bowel disease, and in whom the rectum appears normal, a Crohn's disease diagnosis is supported. It is most unusual for ulcerative colitis to present with a normal-appearing rectum (and still less with a histologically normal rectum) unless topical therapy has already been utilized, but most authorities allow that this scenario very rarely occurs. Confluent proctitis is of course seen also in Crohn's disease.

Colonoscopy and ileoscopy

Endoscopic assessment of the intestine is most helpful in inflammatory bowel disease, but full colonoscopy is not always required: the high proportion of the needed information that can be obtained from simple sigmoidoscopy and biopsy is sometimes now underestimated. The characteristic appearances of confluent inflammation will permit the experienced endoscopist to diagnose ulcerative colitis with some confidence. Needless to say this is substantially less reliable than the equivalent information from the pathologist and no firm conclusion should be drawn without histological support. Colonoscopy comes into its own in ulcerative colitis in determining the proximal extent of disease and in surveillance for neoplasia. The upper limit of disease at colonoscopy tends to be somewhat more proximal than predicted by concurrent barium enema, and is often very well defined.

A curious exception to the confluence of ulcerative colitis exists, however, in respect of the caecum. For years colonoscopists have worried about the significance of minor areas of inflammation around the caecal pole in patients who otherwise seemed to have ulcerative colitis, and it is probable that some patients have been labelled as having Crohn's disease on this criterion alone. In a prospective study of 20 patients with established 'left-sided ulcerative colitis' Rutgeerts' group has clarified and reassured things in this area[28]. The upper margin of inflammation was sharply demarcated in six patients and gradual in 14, but there was then proximal segmental inflammation, separated from the distal inflamed segment by apparently uninvolved mucosa, in no less than 75%, which always included the area around the appendiceal orifice. There were no other reasons to doubt the prior diagnosis of ulcerative colitis and the histology from all sites was concordant. The caecal patch or skip lesion may thus be considered a normal feature of distal ulcerative colitis; there are no good grounds for considering that this warrants these patients being considered to have extensive colitis.

In surveillance the endoscopist will be alert to focal areas of more abnormal mucosa and to mass lesions. The oddly termed 'dysplasia-associated lesion or mass' (DALM) has especial prognostic significance, but in the main the examination serves to permit the collection of a series of biopsies from around the colon (at least 10 biopsies for a reasonable chance of representative sampling).

Distal endoscopy is less helpful in Crohn's disease than in ulcerative colitis, but it is always worth taking a mucosal biopsy even of normal-looking mucosa when the differential diagnosis includes Crohn's disease, as a single characteristic granuloma can lend substantial weight to the diagnostic process. Full colonoscopy is proportionately more valuable in diagnosis than in ulcerative colitis given the potential for patchy disease expression, and also because of the possibility of examining (and biopsying) the terminal ileum in a majority of cases.

Optical coherence tomography

A number of centres have become interested in extending the sensitivity of colonoscopy by including optical coherence tomography (OCT). This can permit high-resolution, cross-sectional imaging of the microstructure of biological tissues. It is somewhat analogous to ultrasound, but instead of measuring the intensity of back-reflected sound waves it utilizes infrared light. OCT could in theory be performed through a conventional endoscope and can already provide two- and three-dimensional images of tissues *in situ*. The image resolution approaches the cellular level, and is to a depth similar to a conventional biopsy. There are preliminary clinical data suggesting that apparent rigidity and dilatation of terminal capillaries as detected by the technique is a feature peculiar to ulcerative colitis, but there are no fully published series as yet. Pitris *et al.* have nonetheless provided important data confirming its value in distinguishing colitis from both normal and from neoplastic tissue in an *ex-vivo* context[29]. If this can be replicated *in vivo* it may prove an important addition to surveillance methodology.

Laser-induced fluorescence

Laser-induced fluorescence is another technique with a strong laboratory pedigree that is now being assessed clinically. An argon laser is used to provoke fluorescence, and yields a range of fluorescence patterns with almost complete correlation, in stained tissue sections, with histological presence or absence of dysplasia[30]. It is not yet clear that this could be of sufficient sensitivity for the distinction of dysplasia from inflammation *in vivo*.

Other endoscopy

Upper gastrointestinal endoscopy is helpful in patients with proximal symptomatology (see below), and enteroscopy has the potential to assist in the diagnostic work-up of patients in whom more standard investigations are inconclusive or contradictory. As long ago as 1993 one group was finding routine per-operative enteroscopy valuable in the full assessment of their patients with Crohn's disease[31], and the non-operative use of push enteroscopy (with the inherent advantage over sonde enteroscopy of being able to take biopsies) in difficult Crohn's disease is now relatively routine in some centres[32].

THERAPEUTIC ENDOSCOPY

Endoscopic stricture dilatation

Anorectal strictures have been dilated by surgeons and patients since mythological times with good results. There is always concern that strictures of the large bowel complicating inflammatory bowel disease have neoplastic potential, but with initial and periodic histological assessment their dilatation can also be routinely undertaken with the expectation of good results[33]. More proximal strictures can now be reached endoscopically and with reliable, modern, through-the-scope balloons, endoscopic therapy became a technical possibility. The problem with earlier balloons was not so much their small calibre, but their short length which led to them slipping proximally or distally as the balloon was inflated. Now that balloons of 5 cm or more in length, and up to 25 mm in diameter, are routinely available, this is much less of a problem. Virtually all colonic and anastomotic strictures are theoretically accessible. There is still a technical failure rate (stricture too tight or its distal opening too angled for access), and a perforation rate, both in the region of 5–10% depending on selection criteria. There are no clear comparative data for long-term results from dilatation. My clinical impression has been that patients with inactive disease and entirely or mainly fibrous stricturing can achieve good and long-lasting results, but those with any degree of inflammatory activity obtain little benefit, apart perhaps from a placebo response which is lost after 2 or 3 weeks. Accordingly it may be logical to reserve this approach for patients with negative inflammatory markers and negative white cell scans. The literature is a little more positive but inclusion criteria are not uniform and there has been no controlled trial. Papers inevitably come from endoscopy enthusiasts, and there may be a publication bias towards better results. The Leuven group probably have most experience, and reported on their technical success in dilating 16 of 18 strictures in 1992[34]. Their more recent review includes 55 patients with 59 strictures (average length 40 mm) treated on 78 occasions[35]. All of these patients were considered resistant to medical therapy and would otherwise have been treated surgically. Dilatation, with a water-filled balloon, was to 18 mm, and to 25 mm in the more recent patients. It was possible to pass a colonoscope through 73% of the strictures after dilatation, and a further 17% of procedures were considered technical successes. There were six perforations, only two of which necessitated laparotomy and resection; there was no mortality. Kaplan–Meier estimation of recurrence-free survival time indicated that around 40% of patients remained well to 3 years, and that surgery had been avoided in more than 60% at 3 years. The results compare favorably with those to be expected from surgical stricturoplasty[36], but there are important identifiable differences between the patients included in surgical and endoscopic series, not least the higher frequency of multiple strictures in the former. There is a continuing case for both forms of intervention in appropriately selected patients.

Endoscopic stenting for benign disease

Stenotic Crohn's disease can, despite dilatation and stricturoplasty, still be difficult to manage. Surgical resection is often inappropriate in the patient who has received substantial previous resection, and a small group of patients remains for whom a more permanent endoscopic solution is sought. There is a convincing literature for the use of metal stents in malignant colonic obstruction, which is either for life-long palliation in the patient with disseminated disease, or as a short-term measure to allow full resuscitation in the patient who is unfit for surgery at the time of presentation and who goes on to a potentially curative resection (complete with the stent) once stable. Neither scenario is naturally applicable in Crohn's disease or ulcerative colitis as the conditions are not fatal, and there would be little expectation that the patient in whom the procedure would be considered would become suitable for surgery at a later date. It is not surprising therefore that the literature is scant. Matsuhashi *et al.* have reported their short- and medium-term happiness with the procedure[37], and it is legitimate to consider it a technical option for a small number of carefully selected patients in whom a dominant stricture is within endoscopic range and in whom there is an acceptance that the risk of permanent foreign-body placement is outweighed by the expected benefits. These current anxieties may diminish with the further development of biodegradable stent materials as currently under evaluation in cardiological practice.

References

1. Moum B, Ekbom A, Vatn MH *et al.* Inflammatory bowel disease: re-evaluation of the diagnosis in a prospective population based study in south eastern Norway. Gut. 1997;40:328–32.
2. Maeda K, Okada M, Yao T *et al.* Intestinal and extra-intestinal complications of Crohn's disease: predictors and cumulative probability of complications. J Gastroenterol. 1994;29:577–82.
3. Allison MC, Vallance R. Prevalence of proximal faecal stasis in active ulcerative colitis. Gut. 1991;32:179–82.
4. Belaiche J, Louis E, D'Haens G *et al.* Acute lower gastrointestinal bleeding in Crohn's disease: characteristics of a unique series of 34 patients. Belgian IBD Research Group. Am J Gastroenterol. 1999;94:2177–81.
5. Barrett SML, Standen PJ, Lee AS, Hawkey CJ, Logan RFA. Personality, smoking and inflammatory bowel disease. Eur J Gastroenterol Hepatol. 1996;8:651–5.
6. Dijkstra J, Reeders JW, Tytgat GN. Idiopathic inflammatory bowel disease: endoscopic–radiologic correlation. Radiology. 1995;197:369–75.
7. Andreoli A, Cerro P, Falasco G, Giglio LA, Prantera C. Role of ultrasonography in the diagnosis of postsurgical recurrence of Crohn's disease. Am J Gastroenterol. 1998;93:1117–21.
8. Chernish SM, Maglinte DD, O'Connor K. Evaluation of the small intestine by enteroclysis for Crohn's disease. Am J Gastroenterol. 1992;87:696–701.
9. Halligan S, Saunders B, Williams C, Bartram C. Adult Crohn disease: can ileoscopy replace small bowel radiology? Abdom Imaging. 1998;23:117–21.
10. Bartram CI. Barium radiology. Scand J Gastroenterol. 1994;203(Suppl.):20–3.
11. Halligan MS, Jobling JC, Bartram CI. Benefit of intravenous muscle relaxants during barium follow through. Clin Radiol. 1994;49:179–82.
12. Palmer KR, Patil DH, Basran GS, Riordan JF, Silk DB. Abdominal tuberculosis in urban Britain – a common disease. Gut. 1985;26:1296–305.
13. Philpotts LE, Heiken JP, Westcott MA, Gore RM. Colitis: use of CT findings in differential diagnosis. Radiology. 1994;190:445–9.
14. Horton KM, Corl FM, Fishman EK. CT of non-neoplastic diseases of the small bowel: spectrum of disease. J Comput Assist Tomogr. 1999;23:417–28.
15. Meyers MA, McGuire PV. Spiral CT demonstration of hypervascularity in Crohn disease: 'vascular jejunization of the ileum' or the 'comb' sign. Abdom Imaging, 1995;20:327–32.
16. Kay CL, Kulling D, Hawes RH, Young JW, Cotton PB. Virtual endoscopy – comparison with colonoscopy in the detection of space-occupying lesions of the colon. Endoscopy. 2000;32:226–32.
17. Shoenut JP, Semelka RC, Magro CM, Silverman R, Yaffe CS, Micflikier AB. Comparison of magnetic resonance imaging and endoscopy in distinguishing the type and severity of inflammatory bowel disease. J Clin Gastroenterol. 1994;19:31–5.
18. Low RN, Francis IR, Politoske D, Bennett M. Crohn's disease evaluation: comparison of contrast-enhanced MR imaging and single-phase helical CT scanning. J Magnet Reson Imaging. 2000;11:127–35.

19. Orsoni P, Barthet M, Portier F, Panuel M, Desjeux A, Grimaud JC. Prospective comparison of endosonography, magnetic resonance imaging and surgical findings in anorectal fistula and abscess complicating Crohn's disease. Br J Surg. 1999;86:360–4.

20. Madsen SM, Thomsen HS, Schlichting P, Dorph S, Munkholm P. Evaluation of treatment response in active Crohn's disease by low-field magnetic resonance imaging. Abdom Imaging. 1999;24:232–9.

21. D'Arienzo A, Scaglione G, Vicinanza G *et al.* Magnetic resonance imaging with ferumoxil, a negative superparamagnetic oral contrast agent, in the evaluation of ulcerative colitis. Am J Gastroenterol. 2000;95:720–4.

22. Lantto E, Jarvi K, Krekala I *et al.* Technetium-99m hexamethyl propylene amine oxime leukocytes in the assessment of disease activity in inflammatory bowel disease. Eur J Nucl Med. 1992;19:14–18.

23. McCarthy M, Dutton J, Hirst J, Rottenberg G, Sanderson J. Can technetium white cell scintigraphy predict response to medical therapy in stricturing ileal Crohn's disease? Gut. 1999;45 (Suppl. V):A129.

24. Bicik I, Bauerfeind P, Breitbach T, Von Schulthess GK, Fried M. Inflammatory bowel disease activity measured by positron-emission tomography. Lancet. 1997;350:262.

25. Weldon MJ, Lowe C, Joseph AEA, Maxwell JD. Review article: Quantitative leucocyte scanning in the assessment of inflammatory bowel disease activity and its response to therapy. Aliment Pharmacol Ther. 1996;10:123–32.

26. Murphy MS, Grahnquist L, Romani P, Chapman S. ^{99m}Tc-HMPAO scintigraphy in paediatric IBD: a systematic comparison with barium follow-through, upper GI endoscopy and colonoscopy. Gut. 1999;45(Suppl. V):A129.

27. Bhatti M, Chapman P, Peters M, Haskard D, Hodgson HJ. Visualising E-selectin in the detection and evaluation of inflammatory bowel disease. Gut. 1998;43:40–7.

28. D'Haens G, Geboes K, Peeters M, Baert F, Ectors N, Rutgeerts P. Patchy cecal inflammation associated with distal ulcerative colitis: a prospective endoscopic study. Am J Gastroenterol. 1997;92:1275–9.

29. Pitris C, Jesser C, Boppart SA, Stamper D, Brezinski ME, Fujimoto JG. Feasibility of optical coherence tomography for high-resolution imaging of human gastrointestinal tract malignancies. J Gastroenterol. 2000;35:87–92.

30. Romer TJ, Fitzmaurice M, Cothren RM *et al.* Laser-induced fluorescence microscopy of normal colon and dysplasia in colonic adenomas: implications for spectroscopic diagnosis. Am J Gastroenterol. 1995;90:81–7.

31. Smedh K, Olaison G, Nyström PO, Sjödahl R. Intraoperative enteroscopy in Crohn's disease. Br J Surg. 1993;80:897–900.

32. Perez-Cuadrado E, Macenlle R, Iglesias J, Fabra R, Lamas D. Usefulness of oral video push enteroscopy in Crohn's disease. Endoscopy. 1997;29:745–7.

33. Linares L, Moreira LF, Andrews H *et al.* Natural history and treatment of anorectal strictures complicating Crohn's disease. Br J Surg. 1988;75:653–6.

34. Breysem Y, Janssens JF, Coremans G, Vantrappen G, Hendrickx G, Rutgeerts P. Endoscopic balloon dilation of colonic and ileo-colonic Crohn's strictures: long-term results. Gastrointest Endosc. 1992;38:142–7.

35. Couckuyt H, Gevers AM, Coremans G, Hiele M, Rutgeerts P. Efficacy and safety of hydrostatic balloon dilatation of ileocolonic Crohn's strictures: a prospective longterm analysis. Gut. 1995; 36:577–80.

36. Tjandra JJ, Fazio VW. Stricturoplasty without concomitant resection for small bowel obstruction in Crohn's disease. Br J Surg. 1994;81:5661–3.

37. Matsuhashi N, Nakajima A, Suzuki A, Yazaki Y, Takazoe M. Long-term outcome of non-surgical strictureplasty using metallic stents for intestinal strictures in Crohn's disease. Gastrointest Endosc. 2000;51:343–5.

15
What can we expect from rectal endosonography in inflammatory bowel diseases?

P. GAST

INTRODUCTION

Rectal endosonography (RE) in inflammatory bowel diseases (IBD) has two fields of application: the colorectal wall and the anoperineal region.

RESULTS OF ENDOSONOGRAPHIC EXAMINATION OF THE WALL

In the 1990s, authors were mostly interested in identification of endosonographic criteria for differential diagnosis between Crohn's disease (CD) and ulcerative colitis (UC). Hildebrandt *et al.* in 1992[1] observed two endosonographic patterns of the rectal wall in chronic colitis. In the first one the normal five-layer stratification was preserved. This pattern was correlated to mucosal inflammation; in other words to UC. In these patients they also observed that the submucosa was thickened. In the second pattern the normal five-layer stratification was replaced by a three- or four-layer structure. Correlation to transmural inflammation (CD) was established. Later, Dägli *et al.*[2] and Soweid *et al.*[3] used and confirmed the Hildebrandt criteria to differentiate UC from CD. However, the differential diagnosis between CD and UC based on the number of wall layers does not seem to be applicable in all cases, as demonstrated in the following publications. Cellier *et al.*[4] did not report any differences in the wall pattern of UC compared to CD, but they observed significantly more lymph nodes around the rectum in UC. Shimizu *et al.*[5], particularly interested in correlating the endosonographic pattern of UC wall and the severity of the disease, described five different patterns, and in the fifth one the interface between mucosa and submucosa almost disappeared. This resulted in a four-layer wall structure in seriously ill UC patients. Soweid *et al.*[3] observed a normal five-layer stratification in 50% of their CD patients. Prediction of UC or CD according to the number of wall layers, then, is probably dependent on intramural extension of inflammation, and can be inadequate in severe UC or in mild CD.

We performed RE in a blinded study in 36 acute IBD patients and compared their results with those of 20 normal subjects and 16 with acute colitis[6]. We used Olympus EUM 3 and EUM 20. The following protocol was used: we systematically measured wall thickness (WTh) and submucosal thickness (STh); looked for perirectal lymph node (nLN) and intrasubmucosal vessels (nV); and analysed the wall stratification (WSt).

In IBD patients the rectal wall appeared thicker than in normals and those with acute colitis. The normal five-layer stratification was lost in 88.8% of IBD patients and replaced by a wall composed of three layers in 18 patients, or of four layers in 14 (cf. Table 1). The population of IBD patients also showed other differences: we observed several lymph nodes (LN) around the rectum in 21 patients, and enlarged vessels (V) in the submucosa of 10 patients; these abnormalities were absent in normal subjects and in those with acute colitis. LN and V were rarely seen in the same patient. We reanalysed the results after having separated UC ($n=20$) and CD ($n=16$). In UC we observed significantly more LN (5.5) than in CD (0.25), and less vessels (0.1) than in CD (1.13) (cf. Table 2). We observed abnormal wall stratification in UC as well as in CD. In our study LN were specifically correlated to UC and vessels to CD. In multivariate analysis the best endosonographic parameter differentiating UC from CD was the LN, with a threshold of two LN predicting UC.

Following these results we performed three confirmation studies. In the first one we used a Doppler echoendoscope and confirmed that hypoechoic images seen around the rectum of UC patients were not cross-sections in vessels. We also confirmed the presence of vessels in the submucosa of CD patients. Twice we performed the same study in a population of IBD patients independent from the first one, to test the sensitivity and specificity of the UC-predicting value of two LN. In the population 72% of the 28 UC patients had two or more LN, and

Table 1 Mean wall thickness (WTh), mean submucosal thickness (STh), in IBD ($n=36$), in normal subjects ($n=20$), and in acute colitis ($n=16$)

	IBD ($n=36$)	Normal subjects ($n=20$)	Acute colitis ($n=16$)
WTh	5.84	3.4	2.9
STh	2.78	1.45	1

Table 2 Endosonographic results in CD ($n=16$) and in UC ($n=20$)

	CD	UC	p-Value
WTh	5.94	5.75	n.s.
STh	2.81	2.45	n.s.
nLN	0.25	5.55	0.0001
nV	1.13	0.1	0.005

none of the 12 CD patients had any LN, showing that the specificity of the method was excellent! The third study consisted in performing a full-length endosonographic examination in three colonic surgical specimens. Endosonography showed numerous LN against the colonic wall, and an anatomopathologist observed a mean number of 15 LN between the wall and the first centimetre of fat and a mean number of 13 LN beyond this limit. Endosonographically, and on the entire length of the colon, we observed that the wall never had five layers, but three or four. In an area of three layers an anatomopathologist concluded there was loss of the mucosa, the submucosa lying bare; and in an area of four layers the submucosa was separated from the mucosa by a dense inflammatory exudate. In our study, observation of at least two LN around the rectum seems to be specifically correlated to UC, and observation of a wall with less than five layers does not exclude UC!

During recruitment of acute colitis patients we made two original observations[7]. RE performed in two patients with well-documented infectious diarrhoea showed LN, while the 16 previous patients with the same causal agents showed none. They also had a thicker wall and a modified wall structure. After treatment, clinical conditions (diarrhoea with blood and fever) did not improve, in spite of negative cultures. Endoscopy was at that time compatible with UC, but anatomopathology concluded there was infectious colitis. Change of treatment (mesalazine in one patient and methylprednisolone in the second one) was necessary to obtain improvement. Several months later we achieved a final diagnosis of UC in both patients. Observation of LN in acute colitis of difficult diagnosis could suggest UC.

We performed RE in eight patients with unclassified chronic colitis lasting for more than 12 months at the time of the examination. The endosonographic results are presented in Table 3. The last evaluation took place 2–3 years after the RE. Five patients were definitively classified as UC. None of these five patients had two or more lymph nodes, so the UC-predicting criteria were not applicable to this population. The patients were chronically treated and not necessarily examined in acute phase; these two conditions could have interfered with observations of LN, as we will see below. Except for the study of

Table 3 Endosonographic results in unclassified chronic colitis: wall thickness (WTh) in mm, wall stratification (WSt) normal or abnormal (abn), number of lymph nodes (nLN), number of vessels (nV)

Patient no.	WTh	WSt	nLN	nV	Final diagnosis
1	4	abn	0	1	UC
2	4	abn	1	0	UC
3	4	abn	0	0	UC
4	4	abn	0	0	UC
5	4	abn	0	2	UC
6	5	abn	1	1	?
7	4	abn	0	1	?
8	4	abn	0	1	?

Hildebrandt *et al.*[1], there is no other publication concerning unclassified chronic colitis.

Prediction of remission in UC has been studied by Dägli *et al.*[2] and Tsuga *et al.*[8] In acute UC, Dägli *et al.* determined that the wall had to be equal to or thicker than 5.4 mm, mucosa equal to or thicker than 2.2 mm, and submucosa equal to or thicker than 2.3 mm. Tsuga *et al.* proposed an endosonographic score of activity and correlated this one to endoscopy. In patients in whom endoscopy was better, they observed a better endosonographic score in 44%, the same score in 48%, and a worse one in 8%. In our study[6], wall thickness and number of lymph nodes showed only a tendency to decrease (cf. Table 4). We calculated the predicting activity threshold of WTh: $\geqslant 4$ mm; and the predictive activity threshold of nLN: $\geqslant 1$. LN had the tendency to disappear in remission, although in the Cho *et al.* study[9] LN were still visible in remission.

There is no other study concerning prediction of remission in CD. In our study[6] we have observed a significant reduction of wall thickness in 23 remitting patients compared to 16 acute patients (respectively, 4.35 mm versus 5.94 mm, $p < 0.005$). We also observed a tendency to normalization of the wall stratification: 94% of the patients had an abnormal stratification in the acute phase and 43.5% had a normal wall stratification in remitting patients (cf. Table 5). Vessels were always visible in remission. Enlarged vessels in CD seem to be a diagnostic variable independent of activity.

In UC, endosonographic parameters have been correlated to different clinico-biological or endoscopic indices or scores to predict the severity of the disease. Cellier *et al.*[4] observed a correlation between mucosal thickness and lymph node diameter and clinical activity. Cho *et al.*[9] observed a correlation between wall

Table 4 Prediction of remission in UC

	Acute UC *(n=20)*	Remitting UC *(n=6)*	p-Value
WTh	5.75	4.5	0.062
STh	2.75	2.33	n.s.
nLN	5.55	2.67	0.056
nV	0.1	0.5	n.s.
Abn WSt*	85%	66%	n.s.

*abnormal wall stratification

Table 5 Prediction of remission in CD

	Acute CD *(n=16)*	Remitting CD *(n=23)*	p-Value
WTh	5.94	4.35	<0.005
STh	2.81	2.22	n.s.
nLN	0.25	0.04	n.s
nV	1.13	0.95	n.s.
Abn WSt	94%	56.5%	<0.05

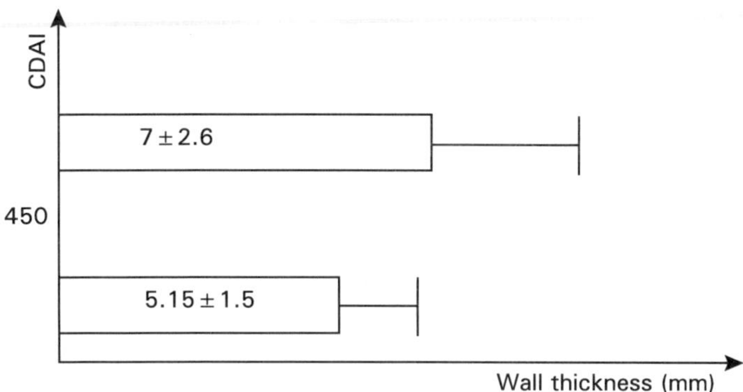

Figure 1   Correlation between wall thickness and CDAI in CD

thickness and Matts endoscopic classification, and Truelove and Witts classification. Shimizu *et al.*[5] observed five endosonographic patterns of the colonic wall (type 1 to type 5: according to wall thickness, mucosal and submucosal echogenicity), and correlated them to endoscopy and histology. Patients with mild disease had a type 1 or 2, patients with moderate disease had a type 3 or 4, patients with severe disease had a type between 2 and 5. Type 5, however, was present only in the more severe diseases. A prediction of the response to treatment was also suggested according to the type of endosonographic pattern. Shimizu *et al.* observed no correlation between severity and number of lymph nodes, although lymph nodes were more frequent in seriously ill patients. Soweid *et al.*[3] obtained a negative correlation between persistence of the five layers and severity of the disease, and a positive but mild correlation between wall thickness and histological severity. Tsuga *et al.*[8], using a catheter probe, observed six different patterns of the colonic wall according to thickness, and aspect of the boundaries between mucosa and submucosa, and between muscularis propria and submucosa. Correlating their results with the endoscopic correlation of Matts, they observed a thicker wall in the most seriously ill patients. In the most serious cases the boundaries between mucosa and submucosa had a tendency to disappear. In our study[6] we observed no significant correlation between wall thickness or number of lymph nodes and endoscopic score of activity in 35 patients. Even after exclusion of the 19 proctitis patients we did not find any correlation between endosonographic parameter and clinical or endoscopic scores of severity.

There are fewer studies concerning activity in CD: Soweid *et al.*[3] observed a negative correlation between number of layers and severity of the disease, and a mild positive correlation between wall thickness and histological criteria of severity. In our study[6] we observed a good correlation between wall thickness and CDAI. The thicker walls (>7 mm to 11 mm) were observed in patients with CDAI greater than 450 (cf. Fig. 1).

RESULTS FROM ANOPERINEAL REGION EXAMINATIONS

Publications have demonstrated that endosonography was able to detect perianal abscesses with a high level of concordance with surgery (100% in Cataldo *et al.*[10]).

Perianal abscess appears as a hypoechoic area surrounded by a hyperechoic border. Detection of perianal fistulas also seems good, with 80% concordance with surgery in the experience of Choen et al.[11] Fistula is described as a narrow line crossing the muscle. Endosonography does not give additional results to the clinical examination in the case of simple tracks. The performance of the technique is not so good in supralevator extensions[12]. Endosonographic detection of internal opening is poor, with only 28% of cases in the experience of Cataldo et al.[10] Internal opening, when recognized, appears as a break in the normal balloon–mucosa interface, or as disruption of the mucosa. An important point is the ability of endosonography to simultaneously assess the sphincter's integrity, and this allows discussion of the most appropriate treatment.

Publications on magnetic resonance imaging (MRI) give excellent results for the method, mainly with endo-anal coils. However, endosonography is of easier access and is cheaper. The best indications of MRI are anal stenosis or painful lesions. MRI also seems to be superior to endosonography in differentiating scarring from acute inflammation and in identifying supralevator extension, and it provides an easy-to-read three-dimensional reconstruction of images[13-19].

Recently, improvements in the endosonographic technique have been proposed. Sultan et al.[20] and Poen et al.[21] have demonstrated that endovaginal examination could add important information in 25% of cases (better identification of anterior lesions), could provide a study of the anal region without distortion by the probe, and could be an alternative method in cases of stenosis or painful lesions. It also provides a more frequent recognition of internal openings.

Cheong et al.[22] and Poen et al.[21] proposed enhancement of images by injection of 1–2 ml of hydrogen peroxide in the external opening. This enables better identification of extension of fistulas, and recognition of the connection between primary and secondary tracks. Internal openings are clearly identified (but not more frequently?). This also makes possible the differentiation between acute inflammation and scarring. Injection is not useful in simple low fistulas because of immediate bubbling in the anal region.

To remain a competitive method compared to MRI, endosonography needs:

1. a perfect knowledge of cross-section anatomy at different levels when using a rotative echoendoscope;
2. a systematic endovaginal examination in women;
3. the infusion of hydrogen peroxide whenever possible.

Recognition of high pelvic abscesses still needs radiology. Three-dimensional reconstruction is always difficult with endosonography.

In December 1999 we began an endosonographic study of what happens in patients treated with Infliximab® (chimaeric monoclonal antibody to tumour necrosis factor) for refractory perianal lesions of Crohn's disease. Present et al.[23] and Ouraghi et al.[24] reported closure of all fistulas in 44–56% of patients after three infusions of 5 mg/kg. However, D'Haens et al.[25] reported recurrence in 80% of patients at 12 months. To date there is no published morphological study of the evolution of the tracks after Infliximab. Five patients had an endosonographic examination before the first infusion, to exclude an undraining abscess, and after the third infusion. We used 'Olympus GFUM20', performed a systematic endovaginal examination in women, and injected hydrogen peroxide whenever possible. The second examination was performed blind to the protocol fo the first one. Four patients showed complete closure of all fistulas and one patient did not respond at all (rectovaginal fistula). In all five patients the second examination demonstrated the same location of fistulas. The only difference between the two examinations in good responders seemed to be the disappearance of bright spots in the tracks at control. This could suggest that tracks were still present, but without exudate[26]. Three additional patients have been examined. One had incomplete clinical response and air inclusions (bright spots) were still visible at endosonography. The last two patients were followed endosonographically after the third infusion; the clinical response was complete in both and fistulous tracks completely disappeared with time.

Further examinations are needed for confirmation, and more time to observe what happens when there is a recurrence.

CONCLUSIONS

Endosonography in IBD has shown interesting results in different areas of application such as differential diagnosis, prediction of remission, or prediction of severity. Clinical usefulness needs to be evaluated, but it is clear that the method cannot take the place of clinicobiological or endoscopic scores. In our experience we reserve the method for difficult chronic or acute cases, when traditional means of diagnosis have failed. In anoperineal lesions of CD endosonography is able to assess correctly the topography of fistulas, even in cases of complex tracks. However, the technique is more difficult and operator-dependent than is MRI. Nevertheless, in our experience endosonography was equal or superior to MRI.

References

1. Hildebrandt U, Kraus J, Ecker KW *et al.* Endosonographic differentiation of mucosal and transmural nonspecific inflammatory bowel disease. Endoscopy. 1992;24:359–63.
2. Dägli U, Over H, Tezel C *et al.* Transrectal ultrasound in the diagnosis and management of inflammatory bowel disease. Endoscopy. 1999;31:152–7.
3. Soweid A, Chak A, Katz J *et al.* Catheter probe-assisted endoluminal US in inflammatory bowel disease. Gastrointest Endosc. 1999;50:41–6.
4. Cellier C, Chaussade S, Roseau G *et al.* Endosonographic features in ulcerative colitis. Gastrointest Endosc. 1993;39:A301
5. Shimizu S, Tada M, Kawai K. Value of endoscopic ultrasonography in the assessment of inflammatory bowel disease. Endoscopy. 1992;24:354–8.
6. Gast P, Belaïche J. Rectal endosonography in inflammatory bowel disease: different diagnosis and prediction of remission. Endoscopy. 1999;31:158–67.
7. Gast P. Endorectal ultrasound in infectious colitis may predict development of chronic colitis. Endoscopy. 1999;31:265–8.
8. Tsuga K, Haruma K, Fujimura J *et al.* Evaluation of the colorectal wall in normal subjects and patients with ulcerative colitis using an ultrasound catheter probe. Gastrointest Endosc. 1998;48:477–84.
9. Cho E, Yasuda K, Nakajima M. Endoscopic ultrasonography in the diagnosis of ulcerative colitis. Gastroenterology. 1990;98:164 (abstract).
10. Cataldo PA, Senagore A, Luchtefeld MA. Intrarectal ultrasound in the evaluation of perirectal abscesses. Dis Colon Rectum. 1993;36:554–8.
11. Choen S, Burnett S, Bartram CI *et al.* Comparison between anal endosonography and digital examination in the evaluation of anal fistulae. Br J Surg. 1991;78:445–7.

12. Law PJ, Talbot RW, Bartram CI *et al.* Anal endosonography in the evaluation of perianal sepsis and fistula in ano. Br J Surg. 1989;76:742–5.
13. de Souza NM, Hall AS, Puni R *et al.* High resolution magnetic resonance imaging of the anal sphincter using a dedicated endoanal coil: comparison of magnetic imaging with surgical findings. Dis Colon Rectum. 1996;39:926–34.
14. Luniss PJ, Barker PG, Sultan AH *et al.* Magnetic resonance imaging of fistula-in-ano. Dis Colon Rectum. 1994;37:708–18.
15. Stoker J, Hussain SM, Lameris JS. Endoanal magnetic resonance imaging versus endosonography. Radiol Med. 1996;92:738–41.
16. Schäfer A, Enck P, Fürst G *et al.* Anatomy of the anal sphincters: comparison of anal endosonography to magnetic resonance imaging. Dis Colon Rectum. 1994;37:777–81.
17. Cyna-Gorse F, Attal P, Contou JF *et al.* Interet de l'imagerie par resonance magnetic dans les atteintes ano-perineales de la maladie de Crohn. Gastroenterol Clin Biol. 1994;18:B254.
18. Bodnar D, Dubreuil A, Valette PJ *et al.* Imagerie par resonance magnetique des suppurations ano-perineales. Gastroenterol Clin Biol. 1994;18:A37.
19. Koelbel G, Schmiedl U, Majer MC *et al.* Diagnosis of fistulae and sinus tracts in patients with Crohn disease: value of MR imaging. Am J Radiol. 1989;152:999–1003.
20. Sultan AH, Loder PB, Bartram CI *et al.* Vaginal endosonography; new approach to image the undisturbed anal sphincter. Dis Colon Rectum. 1994;37:1296–9.
21. Poen AC, Felt-Bersma RJ, Cuesta MA *et al.* Vaginal endosonography of the anal sphincter complex is important in the assessment of faecal incontinence and perianal sepsis. Br J Surg. 1998;85:359–63.
22. Cheong DM, Nogueras JJ, Wexner SD *et al.* Anal endosonography for recurrent anal fistulas: image enhancement with hydrogen peroxyde. Dis Colon Rectum. 1993;36:1158–60.
23. Present DH, Rutgeerts P, Targan S *et al.* Infliximab for treatment of fistulas in patients with Crohn's disease. N Engl J Med. 1999;340:1398–405.
24. Ouraghi A, Quandalle P, Mougenelle JI *et al.* Traitement par anticorps anti-TNF (Remicade®) des lésions anopérinéales de la maladie de Crohn. Gastroenterol Clin Biol. 2000;24:A55.
25. D'Haens G, Aerden I, van Hogezand R *et al.* Duration of response following cessation of Infliximab therapy for active or fistulizing Crohn's disease. Gastroenterology. 1999;116:A696 (abstract).
26. Gast P, Bilaïche J, Louis E. Endosonographic prediction of non-response to Infliximab in perianal fistulae of Crohn's disease: a pilot study. Gut. 2000;47 Suppl 3.

16
Established conservative treatment of inflammatory bowel diseases

E. F. STANGE

INTRODUCTION

The standards of treatment are well established for both inflammatory bowel diseases (IBD), Crohn's disease and ulcerative colitis. In most instances and for most situations the standards were developed on the solid base of randomized, controlled and double-blinded trials. In Germany, two consensus conferences sponsored by the German Society of Digestive and Metabolic Diseases have dealt with both diseases, and the results were published recently[1,2]. The second conference, focusing on diagnosis and treatment of ulcerative colitis, was evidence-based since it included a systematic literature search and graded all recommendations according to common standards based on the level of evidence. The English versions are available on the internet (www.prous.com). For an extensive list of references the reader is referred to these sources. The present brief review is not fully referenced and is designed only to provide an overview of current medical standards in IBD.

STANDARDS OF THERAPY IN ULCERATIVE COLITIS

The standards in ulcerative colitis are listed in Table 1. It is a general rule to prefer topical to systemic therapy if the *location* is distal. It should also be noted that aminosalicylate topical therapy proved to be superior to corticosteroid topical therapy[3], although the opposite appears to be true for the systemic medication. Further differentiation according to *severity* is also important, especially if disease becomes fulminant and requires in-hospital treatment with immunosuppressive drugs such as cyclosporine or tacrolimus. Chronic active disease should be treated with azathioprine or 6-mercaptopurine, whereas for maintenance of remission in intermittent disease 5-aminosalicylates are usually sufficient. A new approach based on controlled trials is the use of *E. coli* Nissle, which proved to be equivalent to aminosalicylates in two trials[4,5].

Table 1 Therapeutic standards in ulcerative colitis

Mild to moderate flare	
Distal colitis	
Standard	Aminosalicylates (topically): 0.5–1.5 g/day suppositories (proctitis) or 1–4 g/day enemas (left-sided colitis)
Alternative	Corticosteroids (topically) as foam or enema, e.g. budesonide 2 mg/day
Extensive colitis	
Standard	Aminosalicylate (orally): 3–4 g/day plus aminosalicylates (topically)
Alternative	Corticosteroids (orally), 40–60 mg/day prednisone or equivalent
Severe or fulminant flare	
Distal colitis	
Standard	Corticosteroids (orally or parenterally): 40–100 mg/day prednisone or equivalent plus aminosalicylates (topically)
Extensive colitis	
Standard	Corticosteroids (orally or parenterally): 40–100 mg/day prednisone or equivalent plus aminosalicylates (topically)
If steroid-refractory	Additional:
Standard	Cyclosporine (continuous infusion): 4 mg/kg body weight for 24 h
Alternative	Tacrolimus (continuous infusion): 0.01 mg/kg body weight for 24 h
Chronic active disease	
Standard	Azathioprine or 6-mercaptopurine (orally): 2–2.5 and 1 mg/kg body weight, respectively, per day
Maintenance of remission	
Standard	Aminosalicylates (orally): 1–2 g/day
If ineffective/intolerant	*E. coli* Nissle (orally): 200 mg/day

STANDARDS OF THERAPY IN CROHN'S DISEASE

The standards in Crohn's disease are listed in Table 2. Again, both location and severity of disease are of importance when tailoring therapy to an individual case. Although corticosteroids are still the mainstay of therapy in an acute flare, the troublesome side-effect profile argues against their regular use. Although either budesonide or aminosalicylates may substitute in mild to moderate acute disease, budesonide is probably the superior choice in ileocaecal Crohn's disease[6]. In severe relapse corticosteroids are unavoidable since the new TNF-antibody is usually reserved for the steroid-refractory situation[7].

Unfortunately, despite overwhelming evidence supporting the use of azathioprine-type immunosuppressants in chronic active disease[8], most gastroenterologists are reluctant to administer these potentially toxic drugs. It must be emphasized that their benefit largely outweighs any risk including lymphoma[8,9] with nine out of 10 patients tolerating the drug. The alternative drug is methotrexate[10], whereas the benefit of mycophenolate is controversial[11,12]. The effectiveness of aminosalicylates in maintaining remission in Crohn's disease is much more limited than in ulcerative colitis; its use is indicated preferentially in the postoperative situation[13]. The conservative treatment of fistulas is often disappointing and a simple seton may be more helpful than

Table 2 Therapeutic standards in Crohn's disease

Mild or moderate flare

Standard	Corticosteroids (orally) 40–80 mg/day prednisone or equivalent
Ileocaecal disease	Budesonide (orally) 9 mg in the morning
Alternative	Aminosalicylates (orally) 4 g/day
Small intestinal disease	Enteral polymeric diet
Distal Crohn's colitis	Aminosalicylates (topically) 1–4 g/day
Alternative	Corticosteroids (topically), i.e. budesonide 2 mg/day

Severe flare

Standard	Corticosteroids (orally or intravenously) 40–100 mg/day prednisone or equivalent
If steroid refractory	Infliximab (TNF-antibody) 5 mg/kg body weight intravenously
Alternative	Cyclosporine (continuous infusion) 4 mg/kg body weight for 24 h
Distal Crohn's colitis	Additional aminosalicylates (topically)
Alternative	Budesonide (topically)

Chronic active disease

Standard	Azathioprine or 6-mercaptopurine (orally 2–2.5 or 1 mg/kg body weight per day, respectively)
Alternative	Methotrexate (intramuscular) 25 mg per week
If therapy-refractory	Infliximab (TNF-antibody) 5 mg/kg body weight intravenously

Fistulas

Standard	Metronidazole (orally) 2–3 × 400 mg per day
If chronic	Azathioprine (orally) 2–2.5 mg/kg body weight per day
If therapy-refractory	Infliximab (TNF-antibody) 5 mg/kg body weight intravenously
Alternative	Cyclosporine (parenterally)

Maintenance of remission

Standard	Azathioprine or 6-mercaptopurine (orally) 2–2.5 or 1 mg/kg body weight per day, respectively
Alternative	Methotrexate (intramuscularly) 25 mg per week
If therapy-refractory	Infliximab (TNF-antibody) at 8–12-weekly intervals or on demand
If postoperative	Aminosalicylates (orally) 2–3 g/day

expensive infliximab infusions. Metronidazole and azathioprine, are established; infliximab should be restricted to otherwise therapy-refractory problem cases.

CONCLUSION

It may be concluded that the majority of drug interventions in inflammatory bowel diseases are evidence-based and therefore rational. Nevertheless, novel treatments, including cytokines such as IL-10 or IL-11, are urgently needed if they prove to spare steroids and, above all, causal treatment is still not on the horizon.

References

1. Stange EF, Schreiber S, Raedler A *et al*. Therapy of Crohn diseases – results of Consensus Conference of the German Society of Digestive and Metabolic Diseases. Z Gastroenterol. 1997;35:541–54.

2. Stange EF, Riemann J, von Herbay A *et al*. Diagnostik und Therapie der Colitis ulcerosa – Ergebnisse einer evidenz-basierten Konsensuskonferenz der 'Deutschen Gesellschaft für Verdauungs- und Stoffwechselkrankheiten'. Z Gastroenterol. 2001;39:19–72.
3. Marshall JK, Irvine EJ. Rectal corticosteroids versus alternative treatments in ulcerative colitis: a meta-analysis. Gut. 1997;40:775–81.
4. Kruis W, Schutz E, Fric P *et al*. Double-blind comparison of an oral *Escherichia coli* preparation and mesalazine in maintaining remission of ulcerative colitis. Aliment Pharmacol Ther. 1997;15:853–8.
5. Rembacken BJ, Snelling AM, Hawkey PM *et al*. Non-pathogenic *Escherichia coli* versus mesalazine for the treatment of ulcerative colitis: a randomised trial. Lancet. 1999;21:635–9.
6. Thomsen OO, Cortot A, Jewell D *et al*. and the International Budesonide-Mesalamine Study Group. A comparison of budesonide and mesalamine for active Crohn's disease. N Engl J Med. 1998;339:370–4.
7. Targan SR, Hanauer SB, von Deventer SJ *et al*. A short-term study of chimeric monoclonal antibody cA2 to tumor necrosis factor alpha for Crohn's disease. N Engl J Med. 1997;337:1029–35.
8. Stange EF. Immunosuppressive therapy. In: Emmrich J, Liebe S, Stange EF, editors. Innovative Concepts in Inflammatory Bowel Disease. Dordrecht: Kluwer; 1998:297–303.
9. Lewis JD, Schwartz JS, Lichtenstein GR. Azathioprine for maintenance of remission in Crohn's disease: benefits outweigh the risk of lymphoma. Gastroenterology. 2000;118:1018–24.
10. Feagan BG, Fedorak RN, Irvine EJ *et al*. and the North American Crohn's Study Group Investigators. A comparison of methotrexate with placebo for the maintenance of remission in Crohn's disease. N Engl J Med. 2000;342:1627–32.
11. Neurath MF, Wanitschke R, Peters M *et al*. Randomised trial of mycophenolate mofetil versus azathioprine for treatment of chronic active Crohn's disease. Gut. 1999;44:625–8.
12. Fellermann K, Steffen M, Stein J *et al*. Mycophenolate mofetil: lack of efficacy in chronic active inflammatory bowel disease. Aliment Pharmacol Ther. 2000;14:171–6.
13. Camma C, Giuntana M, Rosselli *et al*. Mesalamine in the maintenance treatment of Crohn's disease: a meta-analysis adjusted for confounding variables. Gastroenterology. 1997;113:1465–73.

17
Efficacy, tolerance, and acceptance of 5-aminosalicylic acid foam in the treatment of distal ulcerative colitis

S. ARDIZZONE, S. BOLLANI, E. COLOMBO,
V. IMBESI and G. BIANCHI PORRO

INTRODUCTION

Ulcerative colitis is an inflammatory disease primarily affecting the colonic mucosa; the extent and severity of colon involvement are variable. In its most limited form it may affect only the rectum, whereas in its most severe form the entire colon is involved. However, more than half of patients present with disease extending from the rectum to the splenic flexure. Thus, although ulcerative colitis may be classified as proctitis, proctosigmoiditis or left-sided colitis, the term 'distal colitis' is a working classification, which implies that the inflammation is amenable to topical treatment by intrarectal drug administration.

The use of rectal therapy in ulcerative colitis has two potential advantages. First, locally instilled medication is delivered directly to the site of inflammation, and second, the potential for mucosal drug absorption is less than with oral preparations: this may diminish the systemic toxicity of the drugs employed.

EFFICACY OF TOPICAL 5-AMINOSALICYLIC ACID (5-ASA) IN THE TREATMENT OF DISTAL ULCERATIVE COLITIS

Topical treatment with 5-ASA is considered to be a primary choice for patients with distal ulcerative colitis, because it delivers a large amount of the drug to the rectum and distal colon with good response, low systemic drug absorption, and minimal side-effects[1,2].

A meta-analysis of reported randomized, controlled trials assessing topical 5-ASA, in enema or suppository formulation, for the treatment of distal ulcerative colitis, has been published[3]. In this analysis, in mild to moderately active disease, the proportion of patients who improved symptomatically with rectal 5-ASA (in dosages varying from 1 to 4 g/day) ranged from 60% to 94%, compared with 14–42% in the placebo groups. Rates of symptomatic remission varied between 31–80% in 5-ASA-treated groups and 7–11% in those receiving placebo. Comparing 5-ASA with placebo, symptomatic improvement and remission rates were consistently higher than the endoscopic rates which were, in contrast, more favourable than the rates calculated using histology.

In quiescent disease, rectal 5-ASA was compared with placebo or with an oral 5-ASA preparation. Dosage regimens varied considerably among the studies (from 1 to 4 g/day). The rate of remission maintenance ranged between 54–80% in patients receiving the active treatment and 15–20% in those treated with placebo.

The long-term use of 5-ASA enemas is also effective in inducing remission in patients with left-sided ulcerative colitis who are unresponsive to, or intolerant of, conventional therapy, wih an 80% remission rate by week 34, thus allowing patients to reduce or discontinue glucocorticoid treatment[4].

As shown by a recent meta-analysis[5], when compared with rectal steroid administration, rectal 5-ASA was significantly better than conventional rectal corticosteroids in inducing symptomatic, endoscopic, and histological remission with a pooled odds ratio of 2.42 (95% CI 1.72–3.41), 1.89 (95% CI 1.29–2.76), and 2.03 (95% CI 1.28–3.20), respectively. The two trials which compared rectal 5-ASA with budesonide suggested that 5-ASA is at least as effective in producing disease improvement and remission.

Finally, it is also well established that rectal administration is more effective than oral administration of 5-ASA in the treatment of distal ulcerative colitis[6].

USE OF 5-ASA FOAM IN THE TREATMENT OF DISTAL ULCERATIVE COLITIS

Background

Although effective in the treatment of distal ulcerative colitis, rectal therapy is not well tolerated in all patients, since it interferes with daily activities and this may reduce compliance. In particular, enemas seem to impair patients' quality of life (QoL). Therefore, in an effort to increase the benefits of 5-ASA rectal therapy, improving the delivery of large amounts of the drug to the diseased colonic tract, and enhancing QoL and patient acceptance, several galenic formulations (suppositories, gel, and foams) of rectal 5-ASA are available in clinical practice for patients with distal ulcerative colitis. In particular, foam formulations seem to be better tolerated than enemas since they can be applied without the need for the patient to actively hold the drug in the colon by manoeuvres such as lying on the left side or active sphincter contraction. For example, in a study aiming to evaluate the effect on symptoms and QoL of a comparative trial of hydrocortisone acetate foam and prednisolone 21-phosphate enemas, in patients suffering from distal ulcerative colitis, foam was associated with less interference with general activities than enema treatment, differences being significant for work or social activities, sexual relationships, and occupational activities[7].

Colonic spreading and distribution

In order to evaluate whether 5-ASA foam delivers an adequate quantity of locally active drugs to the distal colon, Campieri *et al.*[8] have undertaken a study to compare the scintigraphy colonic distribution of 4 g 5-ASA foam versus 4 g 5-ASA in 100 ml liquid enema in 10 patients with ulcerative colitis, most of them with active disease, using a crossover randomized design. Both preparations were labelled with 100 Mbq [^{99m}Tc] sulphur colloid before administration. Activity, expressed as a percentage of total radioactivity, was measured in the rectum, sigmoid, descending, transverse and ascending colon. Six patients had the same extent of spread with the two formulations; a greater spread was observed in three patients with foam and in one patient with enema. The foam reached the upper limit of disease in all cases, while enema failed in two cases. The maximum spread with foam was observed within 30 min in nine out of 10 patients, compared with seven of 10 after enema. Thus, compared to enema, foam distributed more uniformly and seemed to persist longer in the descending and sigmoid colon.

Similar results were obtained in patients with quiescent distal ulcerative colitis[9].

Clinical efficacy, tolerance and acceptance

The clinical efficacy, tolerance and acceptance of 5-ASA foam were evaluated in five controlled trials.

The efficacy, tolerance and acceptance of a 5-ASA colonic foam (Asacol® foam) were compared in 233 patients with active distal ulcerative colitis from 12 outpatient clinics in Italy, against those of a liquid enema formulation of the same drug, for 3 weeks[10]. Patients were subdivided into two arms. In arm 1, 117 patients with mild attacks received 2 g of 5-ASA as foam or enema at bedtime. In arm 2, 116 patients with moderate attacks were given 4 g of 5-ASA as foam or enema at bedtime. Endpoints were defined as complete relief of symptoms and endoscopic and histological evidence of remission or improvement. In patients with mild relapse, 34 of 63 (54%) treated with foam were in clinical remission after only 10 days, compared with 17 of 51 (31%) treated with enemas ($p < 0.05$). However, there was no statistically significant difference between foam (83%) and enema (74%) after 3 weeks. In patients with moderate relapse a higher proportion of patients achieved complete clinical remission in the foam group (63%) compared with the enema group (52%) after 3 weeks. No significant differences were observed in endoscopic or histological evaluation of colonic mucosa between treatment groups in both arms. Analysis of the data collected showed that a higher proportion of patients receiving foam reported good acceptance (81%), in comparison with enema treatment (49%) ($p < 0.01$). Among patients treated with foam, 81% preferred the new formulation over the previous use of enema, because foam was more comfortable, more practical, easier to retain and caused less interference with daily life.

In a second multicentre Italian study[11], 87 patients with mild to moderate active distal ulcerative colitis were randomized to receive 5-ASA rectal foam at different dosages (2 and 4 g) in comparison with suspension enemas. After 20 days a clinical, endoscopic and histological improvement was seen in both groups and at both dosages. However, the rectal foam provided a higher endoscopic remission rate (foam >40% vs enemas >30%), that was associated with a rapid clinical improvement.

A randomized, multicentre, investigator-blind, parallel-group trial was conducted in the United Kingdom[12], in which patients presenting with a relapse of distal ulcerative colitis were randomly allocated to treatment with 5-ASA foam enema (Asacol®) ($n = 149$ evaluable patients) and prednisolone foam enema ($n = 146$ evaluable patients) for 4 weeks. It was found that, after 4 weeks of treatment, clinical remission was achieved by 52% of 5-ASA-treated patients and 31% of patients treated with prednisolone ($p < 0.001$). There was a trend in favour or more patients in the 5-ASA group achieving sigmoidoscopic remission (40% vs 31%, $p = 0.10$). Histological remission was achieved in 27% and 21% of patients receiving 5-ASA and prednisolone, respectively. Symptoms improved in both treatment groups, and both treatments were well tolerated.

To compare the efficacy, tolerance and overall acceptance of a new 5-ASA rectal foam (Salofalk® foam) with 5-ASA enema in the treatment of active distal ulcerative colitis, 195 patients were enrolled in another multicentre Italian study, coordinated by our IBD unit[13]. Patients were randomly assigned to receive, in open-label fashion, either 5-ASA foam 2g twice a day or 5-ASA enema (2 g/60 ml twice a day) for 3 weeks. Patients who did not achieve remission after 3 weeks continued the study receiving the alternative galenic formulation for a further 3 weeks. After 3 weeks of treatment, 112 patients were in remission and only 59 patients entered the second treatment phase, thus providing data on acceptability (Figs 1 and 2). Remission was achieved after 3 weeks in 54% of patients treated with foam and in 67% of those treated with enema. At the end of the second treatment phase, 70% of the patients switched to foam were in remission vs 65% switched to enema. Out of the 59 patients interviewed at the end of the crossover phase, 39 (66%) preferred enema to the foam, while 20 (34%) preferred the foam or had no preference. Accordingly, on the basis of the QoL index, 33 (56%) preferred the enema or had no preference, whereas 26 (44%) favoured the use of foam. The initial concept of this study was to change patients, not yet in remission after 3 weeks, on to the alternative treatment. However, due to a high remission rate in the first period, only a small number of patients actually switched to the crossover group. Thus, the main aim of comparing patients' acceptance using each patient as his own control was not really achieved.

Finally, in another multicentre, randomized, double-blind, parallel-group study[14], 111 patients with mildly to moderately active proctitis, proctosigmoiditis or left-sided ulcerative colitis received 5-ASA foam enema or placebo enema (2 g/day) for 6 weeks. Clinical remission was more frequent in the 5-ASA group than in the placebo group (65% vs 40%; $p = 0.0082$), particularly in patients with mild disease and patients with proctosigmoiditis. The frequency of patients with an endoscopic remission was higher in the 5-ASA group (57%) than in the placebo group (37%). Similarly, 59% of patients receiving 5-ASA, but only 41% of those receiving placebo, showed an improved histological index. The foam enemas were generally well tolerated, and no treatment-related changes in laboratory variables or vital signs were noted. Among the 55 patients who had previous experience with liquid enema formulations of 5-ASA, 24 (44%) preferred the new foam formulation, 23 (42%) patients had no preference, and only eight (15%) patients preferred the enema formulation (Table 1).

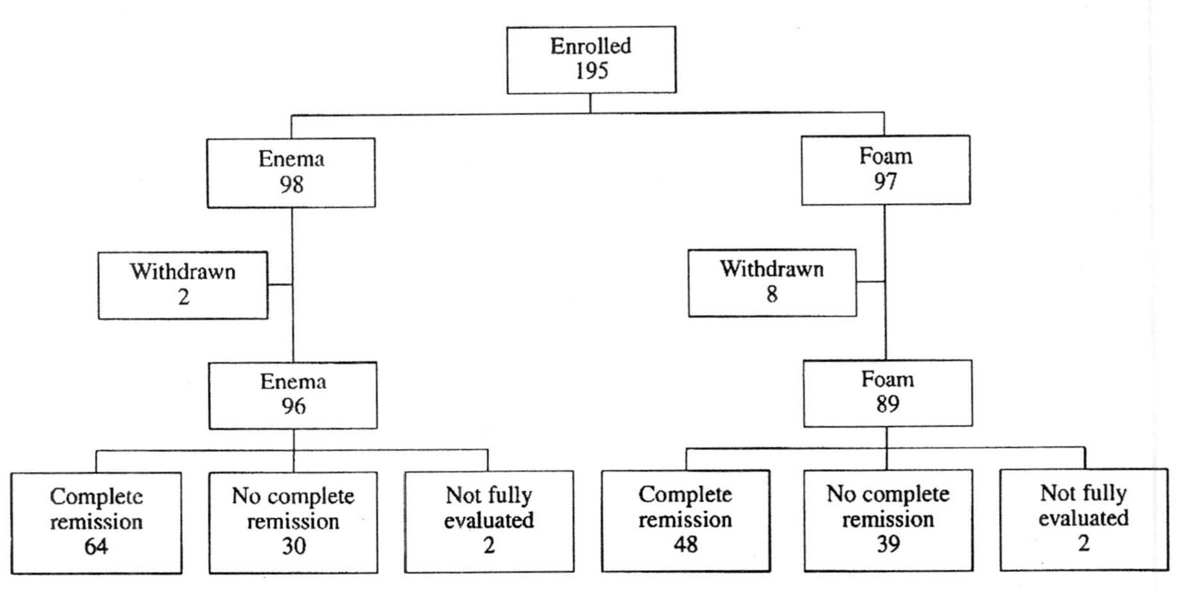

Figure 1   Trial-profile: treatment phase 1

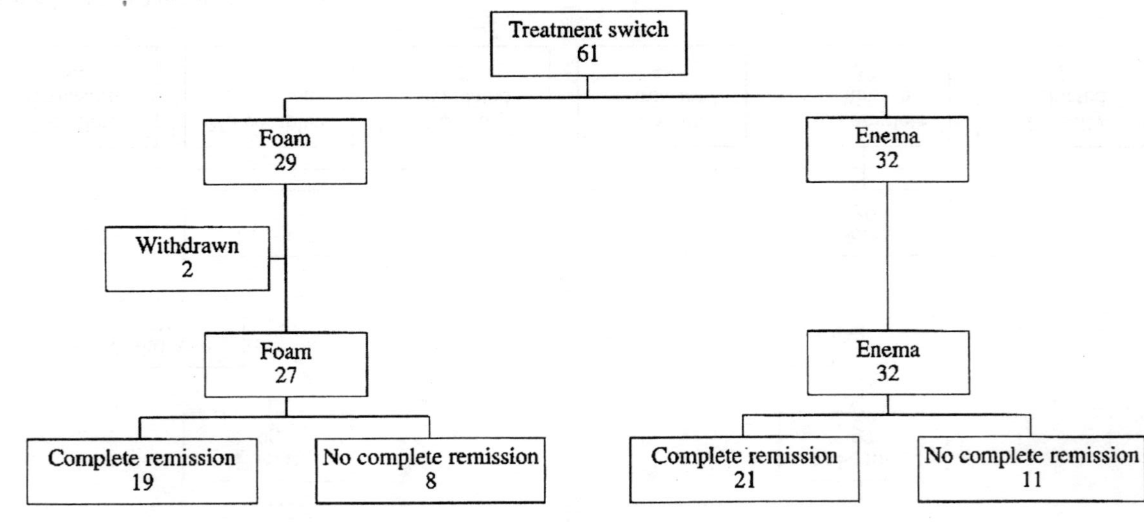

Figure 2 Trial profile: treatment phase 2

Table 1 Patient acceptability of therapy

Which formulation do you prefer?	
Preferred the foam	24/55 (44%)
Preferred the enema	8/55 (15%)
No preference	23/55 (42%)

CONCLUSIONS

5-ASA foam and 5-ASA enema are therapeutically equivalent in the treatment of proctitis, proctosigmoiditis and left-sided colitis.

5-ASA foam represents an alternative formulation which may be better appreciated by patients who had a difficult or unsatisfactory experience with 5-ASA enema. However, for some patients the application device of the foam is less than optimal, as indicated by the complaints of anal burning, burning and meteorism. The foam applicator is still relatively inconvenient and needs to be improved in order to allow patients to enjoy their obvious advantages, such as lack of active retention manoeuvres and leaking. Thus, questions of improving QoL and tolerance of this kind of treatment are of major importance[15].

Further and better-designed trials are necessary to improve patients' satisfaction.

References

1. Ardizzone S, Bianchi Porro G. The topical treatment of distal ulcerative colitis. Eur J Gastroenterol Hepatol. 1996;8:599–602.
2. Ardizzone S, Bianchi Porro G. A practical guide to the management of distal ulcerative colitis. Drugs. 1998;55:519–42.
3. Marshall JK, Irvine EJ. Rectal aminosalicylate therapy for distal ulcerative colitis: a meta-analysis. Aliment Pharmacol Ther. 1995;9:293–300.
4. Bidle WH, Miner PB. Long-term use of mesalamine enemas to induce remission in ulcerative colitis. Gastroenterology. 1990;99:113–18.
5. Marshal JK, Irvine EJ. Rectal corticosteroids versus alternative treatments in ulcerative colitis: a meta-analysis. Gut. 1997;40:775–81.
6. Andreoli A, Spinella S, Levenstein S, Prantera C. 5-ASA enema versus oral sulphasalazine in maintaining remission in ulcerative colitis. Ital J Gastroenterol. 1994;26:121–5.
7. Sommerville KW, Langman JJS, Kane SP, MacGilchrist AJ, Watkinson G, Salmon P. Effect of treatment on symptoms and quality of life in patients with ulcerative colitis: comparative trial of hydrocortisone acetate foam and prednisolone 21-phosphate enemas. Br Med J. 1985;291:866.
8. Campieri M, Corbelli C, Gionchetti P et al. Spread and distribution of 5-ASA colonic foam and 5-ASA enema in patients with ulcerative colitis. Dig Dis Sci. 1992;37:1890–7.
9. Wilding IR, Kenyon CJ, Chauhan S et al. Colonic spreading of a non-chlorofluorocarbon mesalazine rectal foam enema in patients with quiescent ulcerative colitis. Aliment Pharmacol Ther. 1995;9:161–6.
10. Campieri M, Paoluzi P, D'Albasio G, Brunetti G, Pera A, Barbara L. Better quality of therapy with 5-ASA colonic foam in active ulcerative colitis. A multicenter comparative trial with 5-ASA enema. Dig Dis Sci. 1993;38:1843–50.
11. Lanfranchi GA, Tragnane G, Bazzocchi G et al. Efficacy and tolerability of new 5-ASA formulation 'rectal foam' in active distal ulcerative colitis (UC): multicenter controlled randomized trial. Gastroenterology. 1995;108 (Suppl.):A857.
12. Lee Fi, Jewell DP, Keighley MRB et al. A randomised trial comparing mesalazine and prednisolone foam enemas in patients with acute distal ulcerative colitis. Gut. 1996;38:229–33.

13. Ardizzone S, Doldo P, Ranzi T *et al.* and the SAF-3 study group. Mesalazine foam (Salofalk® foam) in the treatment of active distal ulcerative colitis. A comparative trial vs Salofalk® enema. Ital J Gastroenterol Hepatol. 1999;31:677–84.

14. Pokrotnieks J, Marlicz K, Paradowski L, Margus B, Zaborowski P, Greinwald R. Efficacy and tolerability of mesalazine foam enema (Salofalk foam) for distal ulcerative colitis: a double-blind randomized, placebo-controlled study. Aliment Pharmacol Ther. 2000;14:1191–8.

15. Schölmerich J. Treament of distal ulcerative colitis: now the patients have the choice. Ital J Gastroenterol Hepatol. 2000;31:685–7.

18
Budesonide foam in the treatment of proctosigmoiditis

S. BAR-MEIR

Ulcerative colitis is a chronic inflammatory bowel disease of unknown origin that is characterized by short- and long-term inflammation of the bowel. The proximal extent of the colonic mucosal inflammation varies among individuals, but always involves the rectum[1]. Oral administration of medication is justified for patients with extensive involvement of the colon. However, for patients with localized disease, rectal administration of medication is advantageous because a higher concentration of the drug is obtained at the rectal mucosa with fewer systemic adverse effects. 5-ASA administered rectally for patients with proctosigmoiditis has been shown to be efficacious[2].

Several modalities are available for topical medical therapy of inflammatory diseases of the anorectum. These include suppositories, foam, enema and colonic-release oral tablets. These differ in the extent of their retrograde spread. Suppositories spread into the rectum, whereas foam reaches the sigmoid colon[3] and enema reaches the splenic flexure[4]. The more extensive the disease, the more extensive is the spread of medication[4]. Larger volumes increase the retrograde spread of an enema, but have no effect on the spread of a foam[3].

Budesonide is a synthetic steroid with high affinity for the steroid receptor; 15-fold higher than that of hydrocortisone. After intestinal absorption, 90% of the drug undergoes first-pass metabolism in the liver and the systemic bioavailability is therefore only about 10%[5]. The metabolites have an intrinsic glucocorticoid activity which is 100-fold lower than that of budesonide.

The pharmacokinetics of budesonide depends on its mode of administration. The systemic bioavailability of budesonide is better, and absorption faster, when administered per rectum rather than orally[6]. Budesonide therapy administered as a foam in patients with proctosigmoiditis is highly effective[7]. The foam, however, is better tolerated, and patients claim an improvement in quality of life using the foam rather than the enema. There are two steroid foams available: the hydrocortisone and the budesonide. At the present time there is no study available comparing the efficacy and adverse reactions of the two foams.

Such a study was conducted as a multinational, multicentre, randomized, controlled trial. In this study the efficacy of budesonide (Budenofalk) foam 2 mg was compared to hydrocortisone acetate (Colifoam) foam 100 mg. Both medications were given once daily for 8 weeks to patients with proctitis or proctosigmoiditis confirmed by endoscopy and histology. Ages ranged between 18 and 70 years and the disease activity index (DAI) was four or higher[8]. Patients were excluded from the study if their colitis was of less than 2 weeks duration, and definitely if an infectious agent could be isolated. Patients with lesions proximal to the sigmoid colon, and those who received either steroids within 1 month or immunosuppressant within 3 months prior to their possible enrolment into the study, were excluded. Patients were assessed at the beginning of the study and 2, 4 and 8 weeks later. On each visit each patient's general feeling was assessed, a physical examination performed and blood for chemistry, complete blood count and cortisol was obtained. Compliance was determined by the weight of the containers returned by the patients. DAI, sigmoidoscopy and histology were obtained at the beginning of the study and at weeks 4 and 8. Patients were included in the intention-to-treat analysis if they took at least one dose of the study medication. In order to be included in the per-protocol analysis patients had to follow the inclusion–exclusion criteria and to be compliant for at least 2 weeks.

Two hundred and fifty-one patients were enrolled in the study; 248 qualified for intention-to-treat analysis and 179 for per-protocol analysis. Eighty-eight patients were randomized to receive budesonide foam and 91 to receive hydrocortisone foam. Thirty-two patients in the budesonide group and 37 in the hydrocortisone group were excluded because of major protocol violations, in most cases at about two violations per patient. Violations included non-compliance with study medications, concomitant intake of prohibited medications, and failure to show up for the last visit by more than 5 days. The two groups were similar in their baseline characteristics. Their DAI at the time of enrolment was 7.2 ± 1.9 and 7 ± 2 for the budesonide and hydrocortisone respectively.

Remission rate, defined as DAI of 3 or less, at the end of therapy was 55% and 51% for the budesonide and hydrocortisone group, respectively. The rate of improvement was similar for both groups and by the end of 8 weeks the DAI decreased from 7.2 and 7.0 to 3.5 and 4.1 in the budesonide and hydrocortisone groups, respectively. A similar rate of improvement was noticed when endoscopic and histological criteria were used. The rate of subjective improvement was higher; 66% and 70% for the budesonide and hydrocortisone groups, respectively. Thus, between 15% and 20% of patients felt well, even though their endoscopic appearance and their histology indicated active disease.

Side-effects were negligible; acne occurred in two patients in the budesonide group and in one in the hydrocortisone group. None developed hirsutism. Adrenal suppression occurred in 7% of the budesonide group and in 1% of the hydrocortisone group. The slightly higher adrenal suppression seen in the budesonide group may be the result of budesonide absorption through the inferior and middle rectal veins directly into the systemic circulation without passing through the liver.

It is concluded that budesonide foam for 8 weeks for patients with ulcerative proctosigmoiditis is of similar efficacy to hydrocortisone acetate foam, safe and with minimal adrenal suppression.

References

1. Kirsner JB. The historical basis of the idiopathic inflammatory bowel diseases. Inflamm Bowel Dis. 1995;1:2–26.
2. Campieri M, Gionchetti P, Belluzzi A. Optimum dosage of 5-aminosalicylic acid as rectal enema in patients with ulcerative colitis. Gut. 1991;32:929.
3. Farthing MJG, Rutland MD, Clark ML. Retrograde spread of hydrocortisone containing foam given intrarectally in ulcerative colitis. Br Med J. 1979;2:822–4.
4. Jay M, Digenis GA, Foster TS, Antonow DR. Retrograde spreading of hydrocortisone enema in inflammatory bowel disease. Dig Dis Sci. 1986;31:139–44.
5. Brattsand R. Overview of the newer glucocorticoid preparations for IBD. Can J Gastroenterol. 1990;4:407–14.
6. Dahlstrom K, Edsbacker S, Kallen A. Rectal pharmacokinetics of budesonide. Eur J Clin Pharmcol 1996;49:293–8.
7. Sclottmann K, Bregenzer N, Caesar I *et al*. Open randomized multicenter trial comparing safety and efficacy of budesonide foam with betamethasone enema in patients with active distal ulcerative colitis. Gastroenterology. 1998;114:A1078.
8. Sutherland LR, Martin F, Greer S *et al*. 5-Aminosalicylic acid enema in the treatment of distal ulcerative colitis, proctosigmoiditis, and proctitis. Gastroenterology. 1987;92:1894–98.

19
Therapeutic strategies for managing inflammatory diseases of the anorectum: 6-MP cyclosporin, methotrexate and anti-TNFα

D. H. PRESENT

Although one-third of all patients with Crohn's disease have complicating fistulization, there have been only two therapeutic control trials which have randomized for this complication. Therefore data are limited, and we must unfortunately rely on uncontrolled reports. The incidence of perianal complications will vary from 20% to 85% depending upon the definition of what type of abnormalities are seen in the perianal area. More recent literature suggests that about 35% of perianal problems are symptomatic and usually associated with colonic disease. In the approximately one-third of patients who have fistulization this occurs from transmural inflammation producing fissuring and fistulization through the bowel wall. We can define fistula as internal (ileo-ileal, ileocolic, ileovesical, gastrocolic, etc.) or external, which would be in either the perianal area or perivaginal or to the abdominal wall.

If one reviews the literature, there are no studies using the 5-aminosalicylates (5-ASA) (sulphasalazine, mesalamine) in looking at the response of fistulization. Likewise, in the initial controlled trials looking at steroids in the treatment of Crohn's disease, patients were not randomized for this complication[1,2]. The only deaths that occurred in the two large control trials looking at steroids concerned patients who had internal fistulization and developed an abscess with sepsis, after being treated with prednisone.

I try to avoid using steroids in the majority of my patients; however, I have had the anecdotal experience in my patients who were treated with either 5-ASA drugs and/or antibiotics who did well and who, on relapse, were placed on steroids by another physician, and then quickly went on to develop a major fistula and abscess. It is my personal feeling that Crohn's disease patients who are 'genetically' prone to developing fistula may do worse with the use of steroids.

Metronidazole has been studied in Crohn's disease and several control trials have shown efficacy in active disease when compared to sulphasalazine[3] or in high or low doses compared to placebo. Colonic disease seems to respond better, but none of the control trials mentioned fistula in the design or the results. Several uncontrolled studies have shown that metronidazole is initially effective in the vast majority of patients with fistula[4,5]; however, when the dose is lowered or the drug withdrawn, relapse usually occurs rapidly. The long-term use of metronidazole has many problems because of toxicity. In my personal experience about 30% of patients cannot tolerate the drug because of nausea, anorexia, bad taste in the mouth, and often the development of neuropathy, especially when the dose of metronidazole exceeds 1 g daily. On the other hand, I have had some success in maintaining fistula patients on doses as low as 500–750 mg daily.

The first study to randomize for fistulization was our paper using 6-mercaptopurine (6-MP) in the treatment of chronic active Crohn's disease[6]. In that study we closed 31% of fistulas while patients were taking the active drug and the placebo patients closed only 6%. Healing was seen in another 18% with placebo and 24% with 6-MP. A subsequent paper was published by Korelitz and Present[7], reviewing 34 patients in whom closure was seen in 39% and improvement in another 26%. The mean time to respond was 3.1 months, but it could take as long as 8 months to show closure of a fistula. The paper also reported that if patients stayed on the drug the fistula remained closed, but if they stopped the drug, relapse was evident in about 50% of patients. Restarting the drug reclosed the majority of patients. We have in practice demonstrated closures of all types of fistula, including gastrocolic and ileovesical fistulas. We have also demonstrated that these patients can stay closed long-term with maintenance therapy with 6-MP and the concurrent use of a 5-ASA.

Methotrexate has been studied in a controlled manner by Feagan and co-workers in terms of inducing remission and maintaining remission[8,9]. A dose of 25 mg weekly was used for induction and 15 mg weekly for maintenance. Although the drug has been shown to be effective in both parameters, there is no mention of fistula in these papers. Several other papers have been published in an uncontrolled manner, and the only study that has looked at fistula was that of Mahadevan *et al.*[10] In this study of 33 patients, fistula closed in four of 16 (25%) and improved in five of 16 (31%). This provides an overall response of 56%; however, relapse was frequent.

Cyclosporin has been reported in several uncontrolled studies as showing efficacy in Crohn's fistula[11,12]. When using 4 mg/kg of intravenous cyclosporin (which is comparable to 8–10 mg orally), the response rate was 86%, with complete closure observed in 61%. Mean response time was 4–7 days; however, relapse occurred on oral cyclosporin in about 42%. The long-term toxicity of cyclosporin is uncertain; therefore, when using intravenous cyclosporin to close fistulas, it is mandatory that patients be maintained with either 6-MP/azathioprine, or methotrexate if the patients cannot tolerate 6-MP/azathioprine.

As we have noted, most of the fistula studies are uncontrolled; however, a recently completed control trial was carried out looking at infliximab in the treatment of fistulas of Crohn's disease[13] In this trial 84 patients were randomized with either single or multiple draining enterocutaneous fistulas. Stable concomitant medications were permitted, and these included 6-MP/azathioprine, antibiotics, 5-ASA or steroids. An intravenous infusion was administered at weeks 0, 2, and 6 in doses of either 5 mg/kg, 10 mg/kg or placebo.

The primary endpoint was that of >50% closure of fistulas for two consecutive visits (which would be a minimum of 4 weeks). Secondary endpoints included complete closure of all fistulas, the Crohn's Disease Activity Index, a patient's global assessment, as well as a prior reported perianal disease activity index. A fistula was considered closed if it was no longer draining despite gentle finger compression. The results indicated that both infliximab treatment groups (5 and 10 mg/kg) had a statistically greater number of patients achieving the primary endpoint (62%) compared to the placebo group of 26%. Although there was a trend to a greater response with 5 mg/kg, this was not statistically significant.

Most impressive was the fact that 55% of fistulas closed completely with 5 mg/kg compared with 13% of placebo-treated patients. Closure of the fistulas occurred rapidly, usually within 2 weeks and, if a patient was going to respond, almost all responded before the third infusion was given.

In looking at an odds ratio analysis of subgroups there was no differentiating response when considering the number of fistulas prior to therapy, any prior surgery, age, disease duration, site of disease, etc. In a study of patients with active disease there was a trend towards maintenance of response when patients were also receiving 6-MP/azathioprine[14]; however, this combination was not evaluated in the fistula study.

Overall, the study concluded that the primary endpoint was observed in 60% of patients and slightly over 50% of patients had complete closure of all fistulas. The dose of 5 mg/kg produced a higher degree of benefit which lasted at least 3 months.

Since the initial studies I have looked at my open-label experience in the treatment of perianal fistula in 38 patients. I have seen complete closure in 39% with partial closure in another 39%. Once again the vast majority of patients respond before the third infusion is given, and it would appear that this infusion is required for maintenance rather than closure. Relapse was seen in one-third of the patients who closed and in another third of those patients who responded. There were no differences in fistula closure when stratifying for immunomodulatory agents, antibiotics, or steroids. It has been my personal preference to use antibiotics concordantly when trying to close fistula, since the infliximab may work too rapidly and produce closure of the skin without complete healing of the underlying process.

There are many unresolved issues in using infliximab for fistulous Crohn's disease. They include the question of how many infusions are really required, and how frequently maintenance infusions should be given? What is the role of the concurrent use of steroids, will they prevent healing, and are antibiotics and 6-MP/azathioprine needed to prevent relapse? Can infliximab effectively close rectovaginal fistulas, as well as major internal fistulas? Is infliximab a first-line therapy? Can we predict who will respond? Finally, what is the long-term toxicity?

Several recent studies have appeared with other agents showing efficacy, both controlled and uncontrolled, in the treatment of Crohn's disease. CDP571, a more humanized anti-tumour necrosis factor agent, has shown efficacy in clinical response, steroid sparing and fistula healing[15]. Uncontrolled studies have shown fistula healing with thalidomide and FK506[16,17].

The role of surgery is also important in the management of perianal fistula in Crohn's disease. When a patient has a complex fistula it is our practice to refer

Table 1   Response of Crohn's fistula to medical therapy

Drug	Closure	Some response	Study comments
5-Aminosalicylates	?	?	No studies
Steroids	?	?	No studies ?Worse in subgroups
Antibiotics (metronidazole)	?50%	?30–40%	Short term – uncontrolled
6-MP/azathioprine	35–40%	25%	Controlled and uncontrolled
Methotrexate	25%	31%	Uncontrolled
Cyclosporin	61%	25%	Uncontrolled
Infliximab	55%	13%	Controlled
CDP571	50%	?	Controlled
FK506*	63%	37%	Uncontrolled – plus 6-MP/azathioprine
Thalidomide	30–40%	?	Uncontrolled

* Controlled trial under way

him/her to an experienced surgeon for an examination under anaesthesia to drain any residual abscesses and often to place a seton. Once we are assured that the patient is well drained then we will institute anti-fistula therapy. In the year 2000 it would appear that standard therapy after development of a perianal fistula includes antibiotics and adequate drainage if necessary. If there is no healing, then 6-MP should be started, although a case can be made for starting 6-MP and infliximab together. If the fistula does not heal with 6-MP alone, then infliximab should be added. If there is no response then consideration should be given to the use of intravenous cyclosporin, or if FK506 proves to be effective, this would be the earlier drug of choice. Temporary ostomies in my experience have no long-term efficacy in the management of fistula.

A review of medical therapy in fistula is noted in Table 1.

References

1. Summers RW, Switz DM *et al.* National Cooperative Crohn's Disease Study: Results of drug treatment. Gastroenterology. 1979;77:847–69.
2. Malcow H, Ewe K *et al.* European Cooperative Crohn's Disease Study: Results of drug treatment. Gastroenterology. 1984;86:249–66.
3. Ursing BO, Alm T *et al.* A comparative study of metronidazole and sulfasalazine for active Crohn's disease: the Cooperative Crohn's Disease Study in Sweden. Gastroenterology. 1982;83:550–62.
4. Bernstein LH, Frank MS *et al.* Healing of perineal Crohn's disease with metronidazole. Gastroenterology. 1980;79:357–65.
5. Brandt LJ, Bernstein LH *et al.* Metronidazole therapy for perineal Crohn's disease: a follow-up study. Gastroenterology. 1982;83:383–7.
6. Present DH, Korelitz BI *et al.* Treatment of Crohn's disease with 6-mercaptopurine: a long-term randomized, double-blind study. N Engl J Med. 1980;302:981–7.
7. Korelitz BI, Present DH. Favorable effect of 6-mercaptopurine on fistula of Crohn's disease. Dig Dis Sci. 1985;1:58–64.
8. Feagan BG, Rochon J *et al.* Methotrexate for the treatment of Crohn's disease. N Engl J Med. 1995;332:292–7.
9. Feagan BG, Fedorak RN *et al.* A comparison of methotrexate with placebo for the maintenance of remission in Crohn's disease. N Engl J Med. 2000;342:1627–32.

10. Mahadevan U, Marion J *et al*. The place for methotrexate in the treatment of refractory Crohn's disease. Gastroenterology. 1997;112A:1031.
11. Present DH, Lichtiger S. Efficacy of cyclosporine in treatment of fistula of Crohn's disease. Dig Dis Sci. 1994;39:374–80.
12. Hanauer, SB, Smith MB. Rapid closure of Crohn's disease fistulas with continuous intravenous cyclosporine. Am J Gastroenterol. 1993;88:646–9.
13. Present DH, Rutgeerts P *et al*. Infliximab treatment of fistulas in patients with Crohn's disease. N Engl J Med. 1999;340:1398–405.
14. Rutgeerts P, D'Haens *et al*. Efficacy and safety of retreatment with anti-tumor necrosis factor antibody to maintain remission in Crohn's disease. Gastroenterology. 1999;117:761–9.
15. Feagan BG, Sandborn WJ *et al*. A randomized, double-blind placebo controlled multicenter trial of the engineered human antibody to TNF (CDP 571) for steroid sparing and maintenance of remission in patients with Crohn's disease. Gastroenterology. 2000;118:A655.
16. Ehrenreis ED, Kane SV *et al*. Thalidomide therapy for patients with refractory Crohn's disease: an open-label trial. Gastroenterology. 1999;117:1271–7.
17. Lowry PW, Weaver AL *et al*. Combination therapy with oral tacrolimus (FK506) and azathioprine or 6 mercaptopurine for treatment refractory Crohn's disease perianal fistula. Inflamm Bowel Dis. 1999;5:239–45.

20
Inflammatory diseases of the anorectum: surgical therapy

S. A. STRONG

INTRODUCTION

Proctitis appears as endoscopic inflammation that is limited to the distal ~15 cm of large bowel mucosa. However, proctosigmoiditis may represent a more appropriate term because biopsies often reveal inflammation and crypt distortion affecting the sigmoid colon and rectum. Proctitis and proctosigmoiditis are occurring more often, especially in the urban population, and the accompanying symptoms are sometimes difficult to manage with an increasing prevalence of refractory cases[1]. Proximal extension of the disease is frequent and may occur late after the original diagnosis. Operative treatment is reserved for those patients whose disease is refractory to appropriately aggressive medical therapy and those who develop disease complications. Total proctocolectomy with ileal pouch–anal anastomosis is the procedure of choice for persons requiring operative treatment of their ulcerative proctitis or proctosigmoiditis. Although a sphincter-sparing procedure can be considered in select individuals with Crohn's disease, patients are usually relegated to a proctectomy with permanent stoma.

INCIDENCE AND EXTENSION OF DISEASE

Epidemiological studies of ulcerative colitis have reported that 25–55% of cases initially present with disease confined to the rectum[2–4]. Many clinicians feel this more limited inflammation represents the early stages of a disease continuum. However, during the past few decades the incidence of ulcerative proctitis has been increasing, whereas the incidence of more extensive colitis has remained unaltered in most geographic regions. This phenomenon has led some investigators to hypothesize that ulcerative proctitis is a distinct clinical entity despite reports of proximal disease extension in many patients (Table 1).

The cumulative rate of proximal disease extension is 20% at 5 years, 54% at 10 years, and 84% at 20 years[4]. For extension beyond the sigmoid colon and

Table 1 Proximal extension of ulcerative proctitis

	Number of patients	Study period	Patient population	Proximal disease extension (%)
Leijonmarck et al.[5]	397	1955–84	Community	24
Farmer et al.[6]	516	1960–83	Referral	46
Meucci et al.[4]	341	1989–94	Community	27

splenic flexure the corresponding rates are 8% and 30%, 56% and 4%, and 10% and 40%, respectively. Overall, more than half of patients will experience disease progression but the inflammation does not typically migrate beyond the sigmoid colon, and the incidence of disease proximal to the splenic flexure is only 10% at 10 years. The risk factors for disease extension vary between series but include early disease onset, specific presenting symptoms, tobacco use, and relapsing clinical course[4,6,7]; others have refuted these associations[8].

The 5-year cumulative colectomy rate is 8–20%, and the 10-year rate is 11–28% for patients with ulcerative colitis[5]. If an individual has total colonic involvement when diagnosed with ulcerative colitis, the likelihood of colectomy is higher than if the disease is limited to the rectum or left side of the colon. However, the majority of patients who undergo colectomy after initially presenting with proctitis will be found to have pan-colonic inflammation at the time of resection. Only 10% of patients undergoing resection for ulcerative colitis will have disease limited to the distal bowel[9,10].

Crohn's disease of the anorectum

Farmer and colleagues of the Cleveland Clinic were among the first to describe Crohn's disease according to its anatomical pattern of disease distribution and make comparisons based upon these divisions[11]. The incidence of each of the anatomical disease patterns is as follows: small bowel (29%); ileocolic (41%); large bowel (30%). Of the patients with large bowel disease, only ~25% will have disease of the entire colon and rectum; the distal bowel is the most commonly affected site in the remainder. The anatomical pattern of Crohn's disease can be further stratified based upon disease behaviour as follows: inflammatory disease; stricturing disease; penetrating disease.

Anoperineal disease affects 40–90% of patients with Crohn's disease during their lifetime. Disease manifestations are more common with persons affected by colonic disease (47–92%) than individuals with small bowel disease (26–74%). The various forms of anoperineal disease can be classified as follows: skin lesions (i.e. maceration, erosion, ulceration, skin tags); anal canal lesions (i.e. fissure, ulcer, stenosis); fistulas and abscesses.

OPERATIVE INDICATIONS AND OPTIONS

The severity and chronicity of the anorectal inflammation influences the management of ulcerative colitis and Crohn's disease with surgery indicated because

Table 2   Indications for operative treatment

Disease complication	Failure of medical therapy
Haemorrhage	Unresponsive disease
Perforation	Incomplete response
Malignancy	Excessive steroid requirements
Obstruction	Complications due to medications
Growth retardation	Non-compliance with medications
Extraintestinal manifestations	

Table 3   Operative options for inflammatory bowel disease of the anorectum

Ulcerative proctitis	Crohn's disease of the anorectum
Proctectomy and end-ileostomy	Proctocolectomy and end-ileostomy
Proctocolectomy and continent ileostomy	Proctectomy and colostomy
Proctocolectomy and ileal pouch–anal anastomosis	Rectal sleeve advancement and procto-anal anastomosis
	Proctectomy and colo-anal anastomosis

of disease complications or for failed medical therapy (Table 2). The choice of operative procedure is affected by multiple factors and must be tailored to the individual patient (Table 3).

Disease complications

Acute complications

Haemorrhage.   Massive bleeding that requires repeated transfusions rarely occurs in persons with inflammatory disorders of the anorectum. The bleeding is most often secondary to erosion of mesenteric ulcers into the underlying submucosal vessels. Local measures are often the first-line therapy; if bleeding persists despite disease control, or excessive transfusions are required, resection is warranted.

Perforation.   Perforation occurs infrequently but is encountered more commonly in patients with Crohn's disease than individuals with ulcerative proctitis. A mortality rate of 20–40% emphasizes the need for emergent surgical intervention.

Chronic complications

Malignancy.   Patients with ulcerative colitis are at increased risk for the development of colorectal cancer compared with the general population[12]. This risk positively correlates with greater extent of involvement, duration of disease, and young age at onset of symptoms. Patients with extensive colitis have a higher relative risk of developing cancer (4.3 29.0) compared with those with left-sided colitis (1.5–3.0). Contrarily, ulcerative proctitis is not associated with any substantial increase in risk. However, adenocarcinoma and its precursor, dysplasia, can complicate proctitis and are the principal indication for operative treatment in 15% of patients with distal ulcerative colitis[9].

The relative risk of colorectal cancer in Crohn's disease has been reported in several population-based and case–control series, and ranges from 1.1 to 86[12]. Uncertainty of disease extent and a relatively high resection rate confound interpretation of the risk. However, when patients with ulcerative colitis and Crohn's proctocolitis of similar anatomical extent are followed in a comparable manner, the two diseases share a similar risk for colorectal cancer.

Obstruction. Obstruction is a well-recognized complication of anorectal Crohn's disease with narrowing commonly located at the proximal aspect of the anorectal ring. These strictures are typically benign, usually respond to simple dilatation, and rarely require resection. Contrarily, rectal stenosis in a patient with long-standing ulcerative proctitis more likely represents concomitant malignancy. Therefore, once a stricture is discovered in this instance, regardless of its radiographic, endoscopic, or histological appearance, operative therapy is suggested.

Growth retardation. The disease chronicity, nutritional deficiencies, and effects of steroids can cause severe growth retardation in children with proctitis. Prednisone therapy that exceeds $5\,mg/m^2$ per day for more than 6 months can significantly retard growth. Resection of their disease, before the epiphyseal fusion associated with puberty, will typically evoke a tremendous growth spurt.

Extraintestinal manifestations. Approximately 30% of patients with ulcerative colitis or Crohn's disease will demonstrate extraintestinal stigmata of their disease. With the exception of sclerosing cholangitis and ankylosing spondylitis, these will usually regress with resection of all intestinal disease. Therefore, if any of the responsive manifestations cause significant problems despite control of gut symptoms by medical therapy, operative treatment is warranted.

Failure of medical management

Most flares of ulcerative proctitis respond to medical therapy with topical mesalamine or corticosteroids. Recalcitrant disease may require oral steroids while severe disease warrants hospitalization and intravenous hydrocortisone or cyclosporine. Of patients achieving only a partial response, some tolerate their long-term symptoms while others do not, and require operative treatment. Once a disease flare is controlled, the steroid therapy is tapered with or without the use of steroid-sparing immunosuppressives. If the steroids cannot be discontinued or weaned to a minimal dosage, surgery is indicated. Less commonly, a patient will develop side-effects, intolerance, or complications related to the medication that mandates its discontinuation with a resultant disease recrudescence. In a meta-analysis by Cohen and colleagues, mesalamine suppositories achieved clinical improvement and remission in a duration-dependent but not dose-dependent response, with higher rates of remission than associated with topical steroids[13]. Maintenance of remission ranged from 75–90% at 6 months to 61–90% at 12 months for mesalamine agents. Reported adverse events were most common for mesalamine foam but affected only 8% of patients, and withdrawal from therapy rarely (< 2%) occurred.

Management of anorectal Crohn's disease can be much more difficult because anoperineal sepsis may complicate coexisting proctitis. The proctitis is treated with topical, oral, and parenteral medications similar to those used for ulcerative proctitis. Concomitant perineal or fistulizing disease requires individual or combination therapy with antibiotics such as metronidazole, immunomodulators including azathioprine, 6-mercaptopurine, or cyclosporine, and biological agents such as Infliximab.

Operative options

Ulcerative proctitis

Three operations are available for patients with ulcerative proctitis requiring elective operative therapy; these are: proctocolectomy and end-ileostomy; proctocolectomy and continent ileostomy; and proctocolectomy and ileal pouch–anal anastomosis.

Proctocolectomy and end-ileostomy. Proctocolectomy and end-ileostomy became the standard elective operation for ulcerative proctitis or proctosigmoiditis in the early 1950s with the advent of the Brooke ileostomy. This relatively safe and simple operation provides satisfactory results in over 90% of patients. Therefore, despite the development of sphincter-sparing operations, proctocolectomy and end-ileostomy still has a role in the operative treatment of patients with advanced age, significant co-morbid conditions, poor sphincter function, failed ileal pouch–anal anastomosis, or distal rectal carcinoma. An endoanal proctectomy without complete mesorectal excision is acceptable unless dysplasia or a distal rectal malignancy is confirmed. Utilizing this technique, Leicester and colleagues reported only a 4% incidence of permanent ejaculation difficulty without any instances of parasympathetic dysfunction[14].

In the absence of malignancy or dysplasia the rectum is mobilized so as to avoid damage to the lateral pelvic sidewall structures, including the autonomic innervation of the bladder and reproductive organs. The superior rectal vessels are identified at the level of the sacral promontory, carefully sweeping the presacral sympathetic nerves posteriorly; following ligation and division of the vessels the areolar space between the fascia propria of the mesorectum and the presacral fascia is entered. Sharp dissection continues distally in this plane dividing the rectosacral ligament as the levator hiatus is approached. Laterally, the reflections of the parietal peritoneum are incised to the depths of the genitorectal cul-de-sac, remaining close to the rectal wall. The anterior peritoneal reflection is incised dorsal to Denonvilliers' fascia, thereby protecting the seminal vesicles and prostate or vagina. The dissection cones down onto the muscularis propria of the rectum at the superior aspect of the lateral stalks. Distal to this point, the lateral and anterior mobilization continues on the rectal wall because inadvertent wandering out to the pelvic sidewalls risks needless injury to the nervi erigentes. The neurovascular structures of the fatty lateral stalks are divided using electrocautery to maintain haemostasis and reduce the potential for a postoperative pelvic abscess. Any bleeding that cannot be controlled with cauterization is stopped with suture ligation. Once the levator ani muscles are reached, the abdominal portion of the dissection is complete.

Following transabdominal mobilization of the rectum, an intersphincteric (endoanal) anorectal excision is advised. Perianal sutures efface the anal canal and expose the intersphincteric groove. Using electrocautery, a circumferential incision is made just outside the anoderm entering the intersphincteric plane. The dissection is carried cephalad to the level of the levators, meeting the previous point of transabdominal mobilization. The specimen, including internal sphincter, is delivered from the operative field. Primary closure of the perineal wound is recommended because it hastens the recovery associated with healing by secondary intention.

Proctocolectomy and continent ileostomy. In 1969 Kock described the continent ileostomy as an alternative to an-end ileostomy in persons requiring proctocolectomy for their disease[15]. Using the nipple valve as a continent mechanism the early results were promising. However, with time, 10–20% of patients needed revisional surgery for slippage or reduction of the intussuscepted valve. Like the Brooke ileostomy, the continent ileostomy has been replaced in large part by the sphincter-sparing operations. At present the procedure is recommended in select patients who abhor the notion of an existing or impending end-ileostomy; this would include patients with poor sphincter function, failed ileal pouch–anal anastomosis, or distal rectal cancer.

Proctocolectomy and ileal pouch–anal anastomosis. The pelvic reservoir operation is currently the procedure of choice for most patients requiring an elective operation for their ulcerative proctitis or proctosigmoiditis. This continence-preserving procedure has gained popularity as surgical experience has lessened the likelihood of patient dissatisfaction and pouch failure. Controversy stems from management of the anal transitional zone mucosa and the routine use of a temporary diverting loop ileostomy. While disagreement persists over the effect of mucosectomy on functional results and malignancy, few would argue the necessity of mucosectomy when dysplasia, malignancy, or poor follow-up compliance complicates ulcerative proctitis or proctosigmoiditis. Diversion of the faecal stream is suggested for most surgeons performing ileal pouch–anal anastomoses; however, the experienced surgeon may avoid an ileostomy if the operation has proceeded without event and the patient is not being treated with high dosages of prednisone (>20 mg/day) or immunosuppressives. Patients suffering from co-morbid conditions, obesity, or regionally advanced (stage II, III), proximal rectal cancer are best treated by an alternative procedure with preservation of the anal canal; an ileal pouch–anal anastomosis can be created at a later operation when the concomitant problem has resolved or been adequately managed. Alternatively, the procedure can be primarily performed in patients with ulcerative proctitis or proctosigmoiditis over the age of 50 years, or those harbouring a locally contained (stage I), proximal rectal cancer.

Crohn's disease of the anorectum

Four operations are available for patients with Crohn's disease of the anorectum requiring elective operative therapy; these are: proctocolectomy and end-ileostomy;

proctectomy and end colostomy; proctectomy and colo-anal anastomosis, and rectal sleeve advancement and procto-anal anastomosis.

Proctocolectomy with the creation of an ileal pouch and continent ileostomy or pouch–anal anastomosis is contraindicated in a patient with a preoperative diagnosis of Crohns's disease, regardless of the disease distribution. Deutsch and colleagues from the University of Toronto published their experience on five patients found to have histological evidence of Crohn's disease after the creation of a pelvic reservoir[16]. With nearly 3 years of surveillance, two of the patients have lost their ileal pouches because of severe perianal disease while the other three patients remain asymptomatic. The Mayo Clinic's experience in 37 patients with a median follow-up of 10 years reveals a 45% pouch failure rate[17]. Hyman and colleagues at the Cleveland Clinic were able to stratify their 24 patients treated by ileal pouch–anal anastomosis in whom the postoperative pathological diagnosis was reported as Crohn's colitis[18]. In the nine people with preoperative symptoms or signs suggestive of Crohn's disease, eight ultimately needed pouch excision or proximal diversion. Of the remaining 15 patients who lacked suspicious symptoms, only one had lost his pouch with an average follow-up period of 3 years.

Contrary to the attitude shared by most major centres, Panis *et al.*, from the Hopital Lariboisiere in Paris, intentionally performed a pelvis reservoir procedure in 31 patients with recognized Crohn's disease[19]. None of these patients manifested symptoms or signs of anoperineal or small bowel disease. After a mean follow-up of 52 months, six (19%) of the patients had late complications related to their underlying Crohn's disease but only two (6.5%) have undergone pouch excision or permanent pouch defunctioning.

Proctocolectomy and end-ileostomy. Proctocolectomy with end-ileostomy is indicated in those patients with Crohn's proctitis whose disease mandates operative treatment. The procedure is conducted in a manner similar to that described for ulcerative proctitis except for management of the perineal wound. In all cases the levators and puborectalis are closed, abscesses are drained with mushroom catheters, and fistulas are unroofed and curetted. If perineal sepsis is absent the external sphincter and perianal skin are also approximated; otherwise the remaining wound is packed with gauze.

Prior to abdominal wound closure, an attempt is made to fill the pelvic dead space. The pelvic parietal peritoneum is left open and the small bowel adequately mobilized so that it might migrate into the pelvis. A pedicle of omentum based on the left gastroepiploic vessel can be created and secured at the level of the levator hiatus. A suction drain is positioned in the depths of the pelvis to prevent the collection of serosanguineous fluid, an ideal culture medium for bacteria. The purpose of these manoeuvres is to avoid the unfortunate complication of an unhealed perineal wound with recalcitrant sinus. However, despite careful operative technique, some wounds will not readily heal. The majority of these wounds do not require early reoperation because many of them will heal gradually over the ensuing 6–12 months.

Instead of primary proctectomy, Sher and colleagues previously advocated a low Hartmann's closure of the rectum to allow regression of the anoperineal disease, thereby allowing subsequent perineal proctectomy to be performed in less inflamed tissues[20]. Of 25 patients treated by a low Hartmann's pouch, 10 continued to demonstrate anoperineal sepsis that required intersphincteric perineal proctectomy. In a follow-up report the remaining 15 patients underwent surveillance proctoscopy[21]. One patient developed squamous-cell carcinoma of the anal canal, underwent resection and adjuvant therapy, and was disease-free. Two patients developed adenocarcinoma of the rectum requiring resection and adjuvant therapy; one patient died and the other developed a recurrence. Therefore, the group now recommends interval perineal proctectomy in all patients undergoing low Hartmann's procedure for severe anorectal Crohn's disease. Surveillance proctoscopy with random and directed biopsies is also recommended to exclude occult malignancies.

Proctectomy and colostomy. In patients with Crohn's disease and large bowel inflammation limited to the rectum, Ritchie and Lockhart-Mummery suggested disease resection with end-colostomy[22]. However, the colostomy should be constructed as an ileostomy with precise siting and spigot configuration, anticipating the high-volume, liquid effluent associated with Crohn's disease. Moreover, proctectomy alone should be avoided if other colonic segments are involved, as pancolonic disease will ensue. Therefore unless significant small bowel has been resected, or older age necessitates sparing of the large intestine's absorbing surface, proctocolectomy with end-ileostomy is preferred over proctectomy and colostomy.

Proctectomy and colo-anal anastomosis. Although severe Crohn's disease of the rectum warrants proctectomy and permanent stoma in the majority of patients, select patients may be candidates for proctectomy with colo-anal anastomosis[23]. These persons must be highly motivated, lack anoperineal disease, possess adequate sphincter function, and demonstrate sparing of the remaining large bowel. The procedure entails transabdominal resection of the diseased segment with primary anastomosis and diverting loop ileostomy; a colonic reservoir is not employed.

Rectal sleeve advancement and procto-anal anastomosis. In the event that the rectal mucosa is minimally inflamed, and the patient suffers from stenosis of the anorectal ring that is not amenable to dilatation, a rectal sleeve advancement with temporary ileostomy may be recommended[24,25]. This operation is a more extensive version of the rectal mucosal advancement flap whereby the full thickness of the rectum is circumferentially mobilized followed by excision of the strictured segment. A formal procto-anal anastomosis is performed in combination with diverting loop ileostomy. Although the mobilization can be done transanally in the majority of cases, the patient must be cautioned that transabdominal mobilization is sometimes necessary.

OPERATIVE OUTCOME

Ulcerative proctitis

Proctocolectomy and ileal pouch–anal anastomosis has become the procedure of choice for most patients requiring operative treatment of their ulcerative colitis.

The procedure safely resects the diseased large bowel, restores intestinal continuity, and, in the presence of a normally functioning anal sphincter, preserves faecal continence. For patients with extensive colitis the procedure provides a quality of life comparable to patients in remission with mild disease[26]; other studies suggest the quality of life is similar to that of the general population[27]. An increasing number of patients with severe or refractory ulcerative colitis involving only the rectum, or rectum and sigmoid colon, are being offered the procedure.

Patients undergoing proctocolectomy and ileal pouch–anal anastomosis for distal disease have been compared to those with more extensive disease[9]. The incidence (35%) and range of early operative morbidity, and the functional outcome, were similar between the two groups. After an average follow-up of more than 2 years the two groups experienced the same number of daytime and nocturnal stools with minor faecal incontinence equally unlikely (18%).

Brunel and associates assessed the impact of proctocolectomy and ileal pouch–anal anastomosis on patients with distal disease, comparing bowel function and quality of life before and 12 months following the procedure[10]. Postoperatively the daytime and nocturnal stool frequency was significantly reduced, as was the number of patients with urgency to defaecate. Of the 27 patients, social life was improved in 26 persons, professional life in eight, and sex life in eight. Overall satisfaction with the operation was high; 19 patients were completely satisfied, six were well satisfied, one was little satisfied, and one person with continued urgency was not satisfied. Interestingly, 25 of the 27 patients wished that they had received the operation earlier in their disease course.

Crohn's disease of the anorectum

Stoma procedures

One of the most common components of Crohn's disease that manifests itself following proctocolectomy and ileostomy is recurrence of disease in the ileostomy or remaining small bowel. Scammell and associates reported a 24% and 35% cumulative reoperative rate for recurrence at 5 and 10 years, respectively[28]. The majority (89%) of recurrences occurred within 25 cm of the stoma. Although the rates vary, these values largely agree with the experience of others (Table 4). Similarly, recurrent disease complicates proctectomy and colostomy. In a series of 26 typically older patients treated in this fashion, a single occurrence was noted after 7 years of follow-up (22).

Table 4 Operative recurrence following proctocolectomy and ileostomy for Crohn's disease

	Number of patients	*Follow-up (years)*	*Recurrence rate (%)*
Lock *et al.*[29]	26	11.5	15
Goligher[30]	162	15.0	15
Andrews *et al.*[31]	110	8.2	24

Sphincter-sparing procedures

Thirteen patients underwent proctectomy with colo-anal or low-colorectal anastomosis at the Cleveland Clinic for Crohn's disease of the rectum; 11 of the persons had a diverting ileostomy constructed at the time of resection and one of these has not yet undergone elective stoma closure[23]. After 28 months of follow-up, two patients have required resection for recurrent disease. One person underwent resection of bowel remote from the anastomotic site and another individual required a completion colectomy with creation of a permanent ileostomy. Of the 11 patients with restored bowel continuity, nine rate their faecal continence as good or excellent.

The rectal sleeve advancement with procto-anal anastomosis is most commonly performed for an anal fistula with anorectal stricturing secondary to Crohn's disease. In this difficult group of patients, the procedure ameliorated symptoms in eight of 13 (62%) persons after 15 months of recovery[32]. The success of this operation would undoubtedly be improved in the absence of concomitant fistulous disease that negatively impacts outcome.

CONCLUSIONS

Operative treatment of anorectal inflammatory diseases is reserved for those patients whose symptoms are refractory to appropriately aggressive medical therapy and those who develop disease complications. Total proctocolectomy with ileal pouch–anal anastomosis is the procedure of choice for persons requiring operative treatment of their ulcerative proctitis or proctosigmoiditis. Candidates for the operation should be counselled about the 35% morbidity rate as well as the high likelihood of improved bowel function and enhanced quality of life. Although a sphincter-sparing procedure can be considered in select individuals with Crohn's disease, patients are usually relegated to a proctectomy with permanent stoma. The stoma procedures are associated with a lower operative recurrence rate, but the impact of an ileostomy or colostomy on the individual's quality of life has not been studied in this patient population.

References

1. Present DH, Banks PA. What is the best initial treatment and maintenance therapy for distal ulcerative colitis? Inflam Bowel Dis. 1996;2:308–9.
2. Bjornsson S, Johansson JH, Oddsson E. Inflammatory bowel disease in Iceland, 1980–89: a retrospective nationwide epidemiologic study. Scand J Gastroenterol. 1998;33:71.
3. Russel MG, Dorant E, Volovics A *et al.* High incidence of inflammatory bowel disease in The Netherlands: results of a prospective study. The South Limbourg IBD Study Group. Dis Colon Rectum. 1998;41:33–40.
4. Meucci G, Vecchi M, Astegiano M *et al.* The natural history of ulcerative proctitis: a multi-center, retrospective study. Am J Gastroenterol. 2000;95:469–73.
5. Leijonmarck CE, Persson PG, Hellers G. Factors affecting colectomy rate in ulcerative colitis: an epidemiologic study. Gut. 1990;31:329–33.
6. Farmer RG, Easley KA, Rankin GB. Clinical patterns, natural history and progression of ulcerative colitis: a long-term follow-up of 1116 patients. Dig Dis Sci. 1993;38:1137–46.
7. Langholz E, Munkholm P, Davidsen M, Binder V. Course of ulcerative colitis: analysis of changes in disease activity over years. Gastroenterology. 1994;107:3–11.

8. Ayers RC, Gillen CD, Walmsley RS *et al*. Progression of ulcerative proctosigmoiditis: incidence and factors influencing progression. J Gastroenterol Hepatol. 1996;8:555–8.

9. Samarasekera DN, Stebbing JF, Kettlewell MGW, Jewell DP, Mortensen NJMcC. Outcome of restorative proctocolectomy with ileal reservoir for ulcerative colitis: comparison of distal colitis with more proximal disease. Gut. 1996;38:574–7.

10. Brunel M, Penna C, Tiret E, Balladur P, Parc R. Restorative proctocolectomy for distal ulcerative colitis. Gut. 1999;45:542–5.

11. Farmer RG, Whelan G, Fazio VW. Long-term follow-up of patients with Crohn's disease. Gastroenterology. 1985;88:1825–33.

12. Lewis JD, Deren JJ, Lichtenstein GR. Cancer risk in patients with inflammatory bowel disease. Gastroenterol Clin N Am. 1999;28:459–78.

13. Cohen RD, Woseth DM, Thisted RA, Hanauer SB. A meta-analysis and overview of the literature on treatment options for left-sided ulcerative colitis and ulcerative proctitis. Am J Gastroenterol. 2000;95:1263–76.

14. Leicaster RJ, Ritchie JK, Wadsworth J, Thompson JPS, Hawley PR. Sexual function and perineal wound healing after intersphincteric excision of the rectum for inflammatory bowel disease. Dis Colon Rectum. 1984;27:244–8.

15. Kock NJ. Intraabdominal 'reservoir' in patients with permanent ileostomy: preliminary observations on a procedure resulting in fecal 'continence' in five ileostomy patients. Arch Surg. 1969;99:223–31.

16. Deutsch AA, McLeod RS, Cullen J, Cohen Z. Results of the pelvic-pouch procedure in patients with Crohn's disease. Dis Colon Rectum. 1991;34:475–7.

17. Sagar PM, Dozois RR, Wolff BG. Long-term results of ileal pouch–anal anastomosis in patients with Crohn's disease. Dis Colon Rectum. 1996;39:893–8.

18. Hyman NH, Fazio VW, Tuckson WB, Lavery IC. Consequences of ileal pouch–anal anastomosis for Crohn's colitis. Dis Colon Rectum. 1991;34:653–7.

19. Panis Y, Poupard B, Nemeth J, Lavergne A, Hautefeuille P, Valleur P. Ileal pouch/anal anastomosis for Crohn's disease. Lancet. 1996;347:854–7.

20. Sher ME, Bauer JJ, Gorfine S, Gelernt I. Low Hartmann's procedure for severe anorectal Crohn's disease. Dis Colon Rectum. 1992;35:975–80.

21. Cirincione E, Gorfine SR, Bauer JJ. Is Hartmann's procedure safe in Crohn's disease? Report of three cases. Dis Colon Rectum. 2000;43:544–7.

22. Ritchie JK, Lockhart-Mummery HE. Non-restorative surgery in the treatment of Crohn's disease of the large bowel. Gut. 1973;14:263–9.

23. Brand MI, Milsom JW, Fazio VW. Coloanal or low colorectal anastomosis for severe rectal Crohn's disease. Gastroenterology. 1995;108:A1213.

24. Hull TL, Fazio VW. Surgical approaches to low anovaginal fistula in Crohn's disease. Am J Surg. 1997;173:95–8.

25. Simmang CL, Lacey SW, Huber PJ Jr. Rectal sleeve advancement: repair of rectovaginal fistula associated with anorectal stricture in Crohn's disease. Dis Colon Rectum. 1998;41:787–9.

26. Martin A, Dinca M, Leone L *et al*. Quality of life after proctocolectomy and ileo-anal anastomosis for severe ulcerative colitis. Am J Gastroenterol. 1998;93:166–9.

27. Thirlby RC, Land JC, Fenster LF, Lonberg R. Effect of surgery on health-related quality of life in patients with inflammatory bowel disease. Arch Surg. 1998;133:826–32.

28. Scammell BE, Andrews H, Allan RN, Alexander-Williams J, Keighley MRB. Results of proctocolectomy for Crohn's disease. Br J Surg. 1987;74:671–4.

29. Lock MR, Fazio VW, Farmer RG, Jagelman DG, Lavery IC, Weakley FL. Proximal recurrence and the fate of the rectum following excisional therapy for Crohn's disease of the large bowel. Ann Surg. 1981;194:754–60.

30. Goligher JC. The long-term results of excisional surgery for primary and recurrent Crohn's disease of the large bowel. Dis Colon Rectum. 1985;28:51–5.

31. Andrews HA, Lewis P, Allan RN. Prognosis after surgery for colonic Crohn's disease. Br J Surg. 1989;76:1184–90.

32. Marchesa P, Hull TL, Fazio VW. Advancement sleeve flaps for treatment of severe perianal Crohn's disease. Br J Surg. 1998;85:1695–8.

Section V
Diseases of the anal and perianal region

21
Non-surgical haemorrhoidal therapy

E. A. TROWERS

INTRODUCTION

Over 75% of persons in the United States have haemorrhoids at some time during their lives, and an estimated 50% of those over the age of 50 require some type of conservative or operative therapy[1]. Haemorrhoids are a very common and widespread pathology and a very ancient disease as well[2]. In 83 BC a famous Latin poet, Marziale, was considering how common haemorrhoids were, and he found it prodigious that the disease was common in the poor as well as in the rich, in the young as well as in the old. According to Hippocratic doctrine, in cases of madness and melancholy the bleeding of haemorrhoids was a good thing because the veins to the haemorrhoids carried away melancholic blood, the purported cause of such diseases[3]. The word 'haemorrhoid' is derived from the Greek '*haema*' = blood and '*rhoos*' = flowing, and was originally applied by Hippocrates to the flow of blood from the veins of the anus[4]. In contrast, the term 'piles' is used to denote the swellings produced by the haemorrhoids (Latin '*pila*' – a ball).

During the Middle Ages an integral part of the therapy for certain ailments included supplication to 'patron' saints for possible divine intervention[5]. Through legends surrounding his life, St Fiacre, a 7th-century Irish monk, has become the patron saint for haemorrhoid sufferers. Born around the year AD 600, Fiacrius (or Fevrus) was the first-born son of the King of Scotland, Eugene IV[6].

Major events of history have frequently turned on seemingly trivial matters[7]. One such situation involves Napoleon Bonaparte at Waterloo in 1815. Napoleon was not feeling well on the day of the battle of Waterloo, despite fighting well at Ligny, a few days before the last dramatic June 18 battle. There is considerable indication that Napoleon was bothered by very painful thrombosed haemorrhoids.

The classical role of the gastroenterologist in the care of the patient with haemorrhoidal disease has been limited to providing an appropriate diagnosis, evaluating for possible associated neoplastic or inflammatory bowel disease, initiating conservative non-invasive therapy, and effecting surgical referral for symptomatic refractory patients[8]. Although a number of non-surgical semi-invasive therapeutic modalities, e.g. injection therapy, thermal coagulation, and rubber-band ligation, have been effective and available alternatives to surgery, these have remained within the province of the colorectal surgeon. With the proliferation of a new generation of non-operative techniques for the treatment of haemorrhoidal disease, all of which bear resemblance to forms of therapy that are a part of the gastrointestinal endoscopist's activities, the classical role of the gastroenterologist to these patients may be changing.

There are a number of recent reports concerning the anoscopic use of a variety of probes that deliver heat through either infrared light (IRC), laser light, bipolar current (BC), or with a heater probe coil (HP). The aim of these systems is to effect sclerosis of the vascular root and to fix the mucosa to the underlying submucosa and muscle. This chapter will review the current state of the art concerning the pathophysiology and non-surgical therapy of internal haemorrhoids.

DEFINITION OF HAEMORRHOIDS: ANATOMY AND PHYSIOLOGY

What are haemorrhoids and what is their relationship to the portal venous system[9]? New concepts of the pathophysiology of haemorrhoids have been defined during the past 10 or more years, yet medical education at the undergraduate and graduate levels has not kept pace with the newer concepts. The traditional concepts are being perpetuated in all medical dictionaries and in most textbooks of surgery, medicine, anatomy, and pathology. Haemorrhoids are not varicosities, but rather are vascular cushions composed of arterioles, venules, and arteriolar–venular communications which slide down, become congested, enlarged, and bleed. The pathogenesis begins in the fibromuscular supporting layer of the submucosa, above the vascular cushions. The bright red bleeding, which accompanies haemorrhoidal disease, is arteriolar in origin. Portal hypertension has been shown not to be the cause of haemorrhoids. Haemorrhoids are not just 'varicose veins' since they do not contain valves, as do lower-extremity veins[1]. Haemorrhoids are generally present at the right posterior, right anterior and left lateral positions. Dilated haemorrhoidal veins are found even in neonates and, given the widespread prevalence of haemorrhoids among asymptomatic persons, it has been suggested that haemorrhoids are normal features of the human canal. In 1975 Thomson injected the superior haemorrhoidal vein in 95 cadavers (including 10 infants), and showed that: (1) dilatation of the haemorrhoidal veins is a regular feature of normal anatomy present from birth and (2) in the anal canal are specialized structures which he termed 'anal cushions', that are composed of discrete masses of submucosa containing: (a) veins, or more correctly venous sinusoids, into which small arterioles empty directly; (b) collagenous and elastic connective tissue; and (c) smooth muscle that attaches the mucosa to the muscle wall[8].

Thompson concluded that haemorrhoids were normal features of the human anal canal, forming pads that bulge into the lumen[4]. These anatomical features have been confirmed quite recently by Haas, who went on to describe three major components: (1) the lining which can be mucosa or anoderm; (2) the stroma with blood vessels, smooth muscle elements, and supportive connective tissue – the vessels forming arteriovenous shunts; and (3) the anchoring connective tissue system, which secures the haemorrhoids to the internal sphincter and the conjoined longitudinal coat. Internal haemorrhoids consist of redundant mucus membrane of the anal canal above the dentate line and are the most common cause of bleeding with defaecation. External haemorrhoids usually consist of an epithelial lining and lie below the level of the dentate line.

The use of rubber bands, sclerosing solutions, cryosurgery, or the infrared beam in the early stages of haemorrhoidal disease can take care of prolapse and bleeding and can prevent the development of third- and fourth-degree haemorrhoids[1].

Hence, haemorrhoids can no longer be considered as a simple congestion of a venous plexus; they are also due to anatomical and inflammatory alterations of the mucous membrane, of the anchoring connective tissue system and of the anal sphincter[2].

Generally, the diagnosis of hemorrhoids includes a classification of the disease in four degrees:

1. Haemorrhoids of the first degree are internal and do not move from the anal canal.
2. Haemorrhoids of the second degree are internal. They can move from the anal canal during defaecation and come back spontaneously.
3. In the third degree, haemorrhoids are prolapsed but can be manually reintroduced into the anus.
4. In the fourth degree, haemorrhoids are prolapsed and cannot be reintroduced.

The aetiology of haemorrhoids has been explained in the past based on anatomical principles, but Deutch and co-workers studied the relationship of resting anal pressures to haemorrhoid aetiology in 38 patients with haemorrhoids and 29 controls with no perianal symptoms[10]. Three months after treatment by elastic-band ligation, anal pressures were again measured in the haemorrhoid group. Anal pressures were significantly higher in the haemorrhoid group before treatment $(102 \pm 26.33\,\mathrm{mmHg})$ as compared with the controls $(76.75 \pm 19.56\,\mathrm{mmHg})$ $(p < 0.001)$. Three months following elastic-band ligation there was a small drop in anal pressure $(100 \pm 26.84\,\mathrm{mmHg})$ but it remained significantly higher than in the control group. There was also a significant correlation between symptoms and level of anal pressures. The results indicate that persons with haemorrhoids have higher anal pressures than controls. Elastic-band ligation relieves the symptoms but should not affect the anal sphincter pressure. The fact that the anal pressures remained high after treatment could imply that higher pressures are an aetiological component in the formation of haemorrhoids.

Jacobs et al. studied the relationship of haemorrhoids to portal hypertension[11]. Records of 188 patients with documented portal hypertension were reviewed to determine the incidence of haemorrhoids as well as bleeding complications associated with this condition. The incidence of haemorrhoids among these patients was not increased compared to the normal population. Six of the patients with portal hypertension did, however, bleed massively from haemorrhoids. Elevated portal venous pressure is an important factor in those patients having severe haemorrhoidal bleeding. The presence of coagulation defects may also be of considerable importance.

Anorectal varices (ARVs) and haemorrhoids are separate and distinct entities[12]. They coexist in 30% of cases and both can bleed, but their treatments are different. Therefore, a careful examination is necessary to avoid incorrect diagnosis and inappropriate therapy. ARVs are categorized based on their specific sites: external anal varices, on inspection, appear as perianal swellings that empty of blood by digital pressure and refill within 2 s of release; anal canal varices are grey or blue saccular swellings on proctoscopy; and rectal varices consist of dilated submucosal veins (3–6 mm in diameter) on sigmoidoscopy. Haemorrhoids are vascular cushions composed of venular and arteriolar anastomoses without connection to the portovenous system. At proctoscopy they are purple in colour, usually prolapse into the proctoscope, and do not extend proximal to the dentate line. The prevalence of ARVs ranges from 44% in cirrhotic patients to 59% in patients with bleeding oesophagogastric varices (EGVs). Bleeding ARVs are rare and usually mild, but can be massive and fatal. The risk of bleeding from ARVs is 0.5–5%. As opposed to EGVs, ARVs are deeper than the submucosal layer and have a lower risk of bleeding.

The frequency of bleeding ARVs without haematemesis is rare; and the absence of physical evidence of portal hypertension may mislead physicians to suspect alternative diagnoses. ARVs are described as small if <5 mm in diameter and large if >5 mm. In one study the risk of bleeding ARVs was correlated with their size.

NON-SURGICAL THERAPY

The approach to treatment of external and internal haemorrhoids depends on the patient's symptoms[13]. Haemorrhoidal symptoms may be a manifestation of a myriad of medical conditions and therefore careful evaluation of the patient must be conducted to determine the underlying causes of the patient's complaints. A directed history includes assessment of the patient's coagulation history and the possibility of immunosuppressive disease. If possible, before initiating any therapy, rectosigmoid evaluation and anoscopy should be performed.

The key to differentiating between prolapsed internal haemorrhoids and dilated or thrombosed external haemorrhoids is the simple fact that internal haemorrhoids are covered by mucosa and external haemorrhoids by skin[14]. Internal haemorrhoids, once identified, do not necessarily require treatment. Treatment may be recommended if symptoms are present and other causes have been ruled out. There are three levels of treatment and they are applied based on the degree of internal haemorrhoidal prolapse. First, all patients are placed on a bowel management programme, which is as rigorous as necessary to reduce difficult evacuation as a factor. According to Orkin[14], there is no role for topical agents or suppositories because he believes that commonly available preparations are, at best, soothing placebos and, at worst as in the case of steroids, impediments to healing. It should be noted that haemorrhoids are a mechanical disorder and not an inflammatory one; therefore anti-inflammatory agents have no role in their treatment.

The second level of treatment includes various methods used to fix the loose tissue internally and to reduce blood flow in the enlarged columns. These treatments are performed in the office through a small anoscope and are quick and often very effective. This approach is appropriate for bleeding first-degree internal haemorrhoids and for second- and some third-degree prolapsing haemorrhoids. Rubber-band ligation, infrared coagulation, and sclerotherapy are common techniques. Laser treatment as an office procedure or with operative haemorrhoidectomy is of no proven benefit, is more expensive, and is used mostly for marketing purposes. Ninety per cent of patients with symptomatic haemorrhoids are adequately treated without surgery. Office treatment is easy, well tolerated, and low-risk when performed correctly. However, several visits are often necessary to resolve symptoms. Recurrence is not uncommon but re-treatment is often possible. Adherence to a high-fibre diet will generally reduce the likelihood of further symptoms.

The third level of treatment is an operative haemorrhoidectomy. This approach is necessary in only a few patients. Fourth-degree internal haemorrhoids that are prolapsed and not reducible, and extensive third-degree internal haemorrhoids that are not amenable to office treatment, may be excised surgically. An operative haemorrhoidectomy is not to be undertaken lightly. The indications should be clear, and the patient must be educated about the procedure, perioperative care, recovery, and risks. Patients need to understand that this is an operation and that there is a 3–4-week recovery period afterwards. Most haemorrhoidectomies are now performed in an ambulatory setting. Although only one bundle needs to be removed in an occasional patient, usually three quadrants are addressed. Pain is significant for 1–2 weeks after haemorrhoidectomy, and complete recovery is attained by 4–5 weeks. Recurrence rates are only 2–5%. Complications should be rare and include bleeding, thrombosis of adjacent vessels, wound separation, and stenosis. When a patient is operated on for incarcerated and thrombosed internal haemorrhoids, recovery maybe prolonged but the final result is usually quite good.

Perez-Miranda *et al.* studied 50 patients with bleeding internal haemorrhoids who were randomized into two groups[15]. Patients in the study group were treated with a commercially available preparation of *Plantago ovata* (Metamucil) and those in the control group were treated with a placebo. Endoscopy was performed on every patient before and after treatment to establish: (a) the degree of haemorrhoidal prolapse, (b) the number of congested haemorrhoidal cushions and (c) contact bleeding haemorrhoids. Perez-Miranda and co-workers concluded that the addition of dietary fibre may improve internal bleeding haemorrhoids, although without an effect in under 1 month. Fibre addition should be ensured in patients who refuse invasive treatment, those waiting for a more defined form of treatment, or those with contraindications.

Ligation of internal haemorrhoids was first described by Blaisdell[16]. Barron took Blaisdell's instrument and ingeniously modified it. Rubber-band ligation should be recommended for grade I to grade III internal haemorrhoids and patients treated with rubber-band ligations are less likely to require further therapy as compared with those treated with injection or infrared coagulation.

Jensen and co-workers examined the natural history of symptomatic haemorrhoids[17]. With almost 100% follow-up information in patients who had developed a first episode of second-degree haemorrhoids, they demonstrated that rubber-band ligation was superior to expectant management in affording symptomatic relief, and that the probability of remaining free of symptoms as a function of time up to 4 years was significantly higher in patients treated by rubber-band ligation than in patients randomized to expectant management. It should be noted that 25% of the patients treated expectantly were likely to need no therapy for up to 4 years, either due to spontaneous disappearance or considerable improvement of symptoms.

MacRae and McLeod state that rubber-band ligation is recommended as the initial mode of therapy for grades 1–3 haemorrhoids[18]. Although haemorrhoidectomy showed better response, it is associated with more complications and pain than is rubber-band ligation. Thus, it should be reserved for patients whose haemorrhoids fail to respond to rubber-band ligation.

With modern suction applicators rubber-band ligation can easily be achieved without an assistant to hold the scope[19]. Stonelake and Hendrickse recommend rubber-band ligation as an effective and efficient treatment with advantages for both patients and the providers (and purchasers) of health care.

Trowers *et al.* performed 70 haemorrhoidal ligations during 23 separate endoscopic haemorrhoidal ligation (EHL) sessions[20]. Successful placement of elastic bands was accomplished in all patients. All patients had symptomatic grade 2/3 internal haemorrhoids. At the initial EHL session, two bands were placed in one patient, three bands in 17 patients, and four bands in two patients. Only one banding session was required in 18 of the 20 (90%) patients. One patient underwent two sessions and another three sessions. Bleeding resolved in 18 of 20 (90%), and pain resolved in all seven of the patients who had this additional symptom. In none of the 23 treatment sessions was bleeding precipitated or exacerbated by EHL. Completion of the ligation procedure occurred in less than 15 min in all sessions. Endoscopic examination 3 weeks post-banding revealed superficial healing ulcers similar to those seen with oesophageal variceal banding. Reduction of haemorrhoids by one grade size or more occurred in 19 of 20 (95%) patients. The patients benefited from this method of haemorrhoidal banding as 18 out of 20 (90%) reported alleviation of symptoms. No major complications resulted from endoscopic haemorrhoidal ligation.

Injection therapy for haemorrhoids was only begun in 1869 by Morgan of Dublin, who used iron persulphage[4]. Subsequently, iron perchloride and then carbolic acid were used for this purpose. Injection sclerotherapy via anoscopy was initially popularized by Mitchell in 1871[21].

In a crossover prospective trial no difference could be found between standard medical therapy and direct-current electrotherapy in the treatment of symptomatic haemorrhoidal disease[22].

NEW NON-SURGICAL TREATMENT MODALITIES

The pathogenesis of haemorrhoids is based on a vicious cycle: the vascular submucosal plexus protrudes through the anal canal, the anal canal becomes tighter and the sphincter tonus increases, the plexus becomes more congested, and the protrusion increases[2]. Each therapeutic approach aims at breaking this cycle: reducing the congestion (dietary manipulation, anti-inflammatory agents, phlebotonics, anal dilatation, sphincterotomy), fixing the mucosa to the muscle layer (sclerotherapy, infrared coagulation, bipolar diathermy), reducing the size and vascularization of the haemorrhoidal plexus (rubber-band ligation, surgery, excision of haemorrhoids).

These phlebotonic agents have been used in patients with haemorrhoids with results that have sometimes been striking, especially in the acute haemorrhoidal attack.

Nitric oxide has recently been identified as the chemical messenger of the non-adrenergic, non-cholinergic pathway (NANC) mediating relaxation of the internal anal sphincter[23]. Applying glyceryl trinitrate (GTN), which donates nitric oxide into the pathway that relaxes the anal sphincter, lowers the resting pressure in the anus in both normal people and in patients with various anal conditions. Surgical stretching of the internal sphincter had previously been proposed as treatment for haemorrhoids. Ahmed studied GTN as an agent for biochemical sphincterotomy in the therapy of haemorrhoids with or without surgery[23]. A prospective, non-randomized study design was used in consecutive patients presenting with haemorrhoids, anal fissure, idiopathic anal pain or pain post-perianal surgery from August 1997 to March 1998. An overall improvement was achieved in 70% (21/30) over 6–16 weeks. Four patients needed operative intervention to heal their fissures, i.e. 13.3% (4/30). Two (6.6%) patients had haemorrhoidectomy and three (10%) did not complete the full follow-up schedule.

Fissure-in-ano and acutely thrombosed external haemorrhoids are common, benign anal conditions, usually characterized by severe anal pain[24]. Internal anal sphincter (IAS) hypertonia appears to play a role in the aetiology of this pain. Nitric oxide has recently been identified as the 'novel biological messenger' that mediates the anorectal inhibitory reflex in humans. Gorfine documented a therapeutic role for nitroglycerine, a nitric oxide donor, in the treatment of acutely thrombosed external haemorrhoids and anal fissure[24]. It seems highly probable that the pain relief experienced by patients in this study was caused by NO-mediated relaxation of the IAS.

Acute haemorrhoidal disease is associated with venous dilatation and an acute inflammatory reaction with ulceration of the overlying mucosa[25]. The great majority of venous pathology, probably also the haemorrhoidal pathology, is connected to a reduction of venous tone[2]. Today some phlebotonic agents, such as Daflon 500 mg, a new compound of micronized diosmin and hesperidin, a flavonoid extract, have been developed, that are particularly efficient in increasing venous tone: the exact mechanism of action is not yet known, but a reduction of venous distensibility lasting 4 h after a single dose of Daflon 500 mg has been demonstrated. The beneficial effect of Daflon 500 mg is also believed to be the result of a lymphatic drainage and a decreased inflammatory reaction and capillary leakage. Treatment with Daflon 500 mg is now becoming the method of choice for the early stages of this condition according to Nicolaides[25].

The safety of use of Daflon 500 mg, shown in the experimental animal, has been confirmed clinically in long-term trials lasting 6 months and 1 year[26]. Daflon 500 mg is a well-tolerated drug. Side-effects are rare and mild, being principally of a gastrointestinal and autonomic nature. Their incidence and nature have also been shown to be similar to those found with a placebo in double-blind, controlled trials.

Analysis of Godegere's study results shows that the micronized formulation of the active principle, diosmin, is effective in the symptomatic treatment of internal haemorrhoidal disease at a dose of 900 mg daily[27]. A double-blind approach was essential to validate these results in that, depending on the parameter, 47–59% of the 120 patients improved on placebo. Nevertheless, the active principle was significantly more effective than placebo across all the evaluation criteria used.

Botulinum toxin A (BTA) can be used in the treatment of chronic anal fissure by injection into the internal or external sphincter[28]. BTA reliably relieves sphincter spasm, and sphincter relaxation promotes healing by increasing the blood flow through the posterior anal artery. The minimum basal pressure in patients suffering from haemorrhoids or chronic anal fissure is significantly higher than in healthy individuals. It can be assumed that prolapsing haemorrhoids may obstruct healing, as they create an extra volume (in addition to faeces) dilating the anal sphincters. Madalinski *et al.* reported two cases in which BTA injection was combined with ligation with success[28].

COMPLICATIONS

Local anaesthetics comprise drugs with different chemical structures[29]. Some, like benzocaine, frequently cause allergic dermatitis; others more rarely. Lodi *et al.* reported three cases of contact allergy to caines, caused by antihaemorrhoidal ointments.

Bullock reported three cases of impotence after sclerotherapy for haemorrhoids[30]. The development of pelvic pain at the time of injection, and urinary symptoms within a few hours, was highly suggestive of a misplaced injection into the prostatic or periprostatic tissue. Haematuria, haematospermia, prostatic abscess, epididymitis, urethral stricture, chronic cystitis, urolithiasis, seminal vesicle abscess, and urinary perineal fistula have also been reported after sclerotherapy for haemorrhoids.

The combination of urinary hesitancy, perianal pain, and systemic symptoms shortly after ligation of haemorrhoids should alert the physician to a potentially life-threatening condition requiring immediate evaluation and therapy[31]. Early detection, helped by a high degree of suspicion, seems crucial to a favourable outcome. Physical examination, anoscopy, and proctoscopy, should be performed. Computerized tomography of the pelvis is a non-invasive means of looking for occult abscesses and thickened, oedematous pelvic tissues. Broad-spectrum antibiotics with anaerobic coverage and early aggressive surgical management, including debridement, would seem to be critical.

Brook and Frazier demonstrated the polymicrobial nature and predominance of anaerobic bacteria in infected haemorrhoidal tissue[32]. The predominant isolates recovered in the infected sites were *Bacteroides* spp., *Peptostreptococcus* spp., and Enterobacteriaceae, all known to be part of the normal gastrointestinal flora. Similar flora were isolated in infected pilonidal sinuses and perirectal abscesses and in subcutaneous abscesses of the vulvovaginal areas.

Surgical management, including penicillin-resistant anaerobic bacteria, however, such as the *Bacteroides fragilis* group, may warrant the administration of appropriate antimicrobial agents such as clindamycin, cefoxitin, metronidazole, imipenem, or the combination of a beta-lactamase inhibitor and a penicillin.

Ribbans and Radcliffe reported a case of a patient who underwent submucosal injection sclerotherapy for haemorrhoids[33]. Subsequent necrosis of the underlying tissues produced a rectal perforation and retroperitoneal abscess, which necessitated emergency laparotomy and colostomy. Healing of the perforation allowed later closure of the stoma.

A case of life-threatening retroperitoneal sepsis after injection sclerotherapy for first-degree haemorrhoids has also been reported[34].

Rubber-band ligation is an efficacious and cost-effective alternative to conventional haemorrhoidectomy for symptomatic internal haemorrhoids even though the well-recognized complications of bleeding and thrombosis occur infrequently. Far more serious septic complications have only recently been described[35]. Quevedo-Bonilla *et al.* reported that, in five of their patients, four cases were serious enough to necessitate surgical intervention, and one patient died. Pain followed by urinary dysfunction with or without toxic symptoms should alert the physician to the probability of localized perianal or systemic sepsis. Acute awareness of these rare but potentially life-threatening complications, and immediate aggressive treatment, is mandatory if death is to be prevented. According to Quevedo-Bonilla *et al.*, rubber-band ligation of internal haemorrhoids need not be abandoned; however, the indications should be clear, the technique mastered, and a close patient follow-up maintained.

Buchmann and Seefeld reported a patient with haemorrhoids treated with rubber-band ligation who developed a huge supralevator abscess[36]. A diverting sigmoidostomy had to be established as surgical drainage via the rectum was not adequate. Eventually the patient accepted HIV testing, which proved positive. Six months later the sigmoidostomy was still needed as the abscess cavity remained large. Buchmann and Seefeld concluded that rubber-band ligation in HIV-positive patients should not be used.

CONCLUSIONS

Haemorrhoids are very prevalent in the Western world, with over 75% of persons in the United States experiencing haemorrhoids during their lives, and the majority requiring some type of conservative or operative therapy. New concepts of the pathophysiology of haemorrhoids define haemorrhoids not as varicosities, but rather as vascular cushions composed of arterioles, venules, and arteriolar–venular communications which slide down, become congested, enlarged, and bleed.

The approach to treatment of haemorrhoids depends on the patient's symptoms. A directed history should be performed, which includes an assessment of the patient's coagulation history and, the possibility of immunosuppressive disease. If possible, before initiating any therapy, rectosigmoid evaluation and anoscopy should be performed. Non-surgical therapeutic approaches such as rubber-band ligation, sclerotherapy or bipolar coagulation aims at reducing congestion, fixing the mucosa to the muscle layer, and reducing the size and vascularization of the haemorrhoidal plexus. Rubber-band ligation is recommended as the initial mode of therapy for grades 1 to 3 haemorrhoids. Although haemorrhoidectomy shows a better response, it is associated with more complications and pain than rubber-band ligation. Thus, it should be reserved for the 10% of patients whose haemorrhoids fail to respond to rubber-band ligation or other non-surgical therapeutic approaches.

References

1. Pfenninger JL, Surrell J. Nonsurgical treatment options for internal hemorrhoids. Am Fam Phys. 1995;52:821–34.
2. Arullani A, Gianfranco C. Diagnosis and current treatment of hemorrhoidal disease. Angiology. 1994;45:560–5.
3. Nutton V. Montanus, Vesalius and the haemorrhoidal veins. Clio Med. 1983;18:33–6.
4. Dennison AR, Whitson RJ, Rooney S, Morris DL. The management of hemorrhoids. Am J Gastroenterol. 1989;84:475–81.
5. Bonello JC, Cohen H, Gorlin RJ. Of heliotropes and hemorrhoids. St. Fiacre, patron saint of gardeners and hemorrhoids suffers. Dis Colon Rectum. 1985;28:702–4.
6. Racouchot JE, Petouraud C, Rivoire J. Saint Fiacre. The healer of hemorrhoids and patron saint of proctology. Am J Proctol. 1971;4822:175–9.
7. Weslling DR, Wolff BG, Dozois RR. Piles of defeat. Napoleon at Waterloo. Dis Colon Rectum. 1988;31:303–5.
8. MacLeod JH. Rational approach to treatment of hemorrhoids based on a theory of etiology. Arch Surg. 1983;118:29–32.
9. Bernstein WC. What are hemorrhoids and what is their relationship to the portal venous system. Dis Colon Rectum. 1983;26:829–34.
10. Deutch AA, Moshkovitz M, Nudelman I, Dinari G, Reiss R. Anal pressure measurements in the study of hemorrhoid eitiology and their relation to treatment. Dis Colon Rectum. 1987;30:855–7.
11. Jacobs DM, Bubrick MP, Onstad GR, Hitchcock CR. The relationship of hemorrhoids to portal hypertension. Dis Colon Rectum. 1980;23:567–9.
12. Batoon SB, Zoneraich S. Misdiagnosed anorectal varices resulting in a fatal event. Am J Gastroenterol. 1999;94:3076–7.
13. Anonymous. Practice parameters for the treatment of hemorrhoids. The Standards Task Force American Society of Colon and Rectal Surgeons. Dis Colon Rectum. 1993;36:1118–20.
14. Orkin B, Schwartz AM, Orkin M. Hemorrhoids: what the dermatologist should know. J Am Acad Dermatol. 1999;41:449–56.
15. Perez-Miranda M, Gomez-Cenelilla A, Leon-Colombo T, Pajares J, Mate-Jimenez J. Effect of fiber supplements on internal bleeding hemorrhoids. Hepato-Gastroenterology. 1996;43:1504–7.
16. Salvati EP. Nonoperative management of hemorrhoids. Dis Colon Rectum. 1999;42:989–93.
17. Jensen SL, Harling H, Arseth-Hansen P, Tange G. The natural history of symptomatic hemorrhoids. Int J Colorect Dis. 1989;4:41–4.
18. MacRae HM, McLeod RS. Comparison of hemorrhoidal treatments: a meta-analysis. Can J Surg. 1997;40:14–17.
19. Stonelake PS, Hendrickse CW. Rubber band ligation is effective and efficient. Br Med J. 1997;315:881–2.
20. Trowers EA, Ganga U, Rizk R, Ojo E, Hodges D. Endoscopic hemorrhoidal ligation: preliminary clinical experience. Gastrointest Endosc. 1998;48:49–52.
21. Ponsky JL, Mellinger JD, Simon IB. Endoscopic retrograde hemorrhoidal sclerotherapy using 23.4% saline: a preliminary report. Gastrointest Endosc. 1990;37:155–8.
22. Wright RA, Kranz KR, Kirby SL. A prospective crossover trial of direct current electrotherapy in symptomatic hemorrhoidal disease. Gastrointest Endosc. 1991;37:621–3.
23. Mathur D, Ahmed S, Subramaniam S, Modgill VK, Banerjee AK. Biochemical sphincterotomy is effective treatment for hemorrhoids and associated conditions: an audit. Biochem Soc Trans. 1998;26:S326.
24. Gorfine SR. Treatment of benign anal disease with topical nitroglycerin. Dis Colon Rectum. 1995;38:453–7.
25. Nicolaides AN. Overview: Dalfon 500 mg. Angiology. 1994;45:493–4.

26. Meyer OC. Safety and security of Daflon 500 mg in venous insufficiency and in hemorrhoidal disease. Angiology. 1994;45:579–84.
27. Godegere P. Daflon 500 mg in the treatment of hemorrhoidal disease: a demonstrated efficacy in comparison with placebo. Angiology. 1994;45:574–8.
28. Madalinski M, Labon M, Adrich Z, Kryszewki A. Internal hemorrhoids coexisting with chronic anal fissure: new nonsurgical modalities. Endoscopy. 1998;30:S96.
29. Lodi A, Ambonati M, Coassini A, Kouhdari Z, Palvarini M, Crosti C. Contact allergy to 'caine' caused by antihemorrhoidal ointments. Contact Dermatitis. 1999;41:221–2.
30. Bullock N. Impotence after sclerotherapy of hemorrhoids: case reports. BMJ 1997;314:419.
31. Russell T, Donohue JH. Hemorrhoidal banding a warning. Dis Colon Rectum. 1985;28:291–3.
32. Brook I, Frazier EH. Aerobic and anaerobic microbiology of infected hemorrhoids. Am J Gastroenterol. 1996;91:333–5.
33. Ribbans WJ, Radcliffe AG. Retroperitoneal abscess following sclerotherapy for hemorrhoids. Dis Colon Rectum. 1985;28:188–9.
34. Barwell J, Watkins RM, Lloyd-Davies E, Wilkins DC. Life-threatening retroperitoneal sepsis after hemorrhoid injection sclerotherapy. Dis Colon Rectum. 1999;42:421–3.
35. Quevedo-Bonilla G, Farkas AM, Abcarian H, Hambrick E, Orsay CP. Septic complications of hemorrhoidal banding. Arch Surg. 1988;123:650–1.
36. Buchmann P, Seefeld U. Rubber band ligation for piles can be disatrous in HIV-positive patients. Int J Colorect Dis. 1989;4:57–8.

22
The anal fissure – conventional therapy

J.-U. BOCK and J. JONGEN

An anal fissure is an acute or chronic lesion in the highly sensitive anoderm. It typically occurs in the posterior wall (90%) of the anal canal, possibly due to the anatomy of the oval anus and/or reduced perfusion[1–3]. Fissures are much less common in the anterior midline (upto 10%). The differential diagnosis includes herpes, *Chlamydia*, venereal diseases, Crohn's disease or colitis ulcerosa, especially with atypical fissures located off the midlines. The aetiology of a classic anal fissure is unknown. Hard bowel movements, as well as a diarrhoea or a cryptitis with diminished elasticity of the anoderm in this area can cause a fissure[4]. Depending on the localization the case history is characteristic. Patients with an acute fissure report extreme pain during and after defaecation, which may last several hours, bleeding during and sometimes after bowel movements, blood in the toilet and on the toilet paper as well as dysuria. They often develop constipation from fear of the next bowel movement, or conversely abuse laxatives for the same reason. Pain in a chronic fissure is less intensive. Patients frequently complain of a skin tag externally (the sentinel tag), or pruritus ani due to soiling the perianal skin and underwear. Physical examination supplements the case history as the diagnosis is easily determined by inspection of the anus – a lesion of the anoderm in acute cases and/or a sentinel tag in chronic cases – cautious digital examination (after using a local anaaesthetic) and proctoscopy.

The pathophysiological cycle appears to be as follows: an initial anodermal tear causes pain during and after defaecation; the pain leads to a reactive hypertonus of the internal anal sphincter followed by an increased resting pressure and a relative stenosis[3]. The latter changes diminish perfusion to the anoderm, which impairs fissure healing and the vicious circle starts again with the next hard bowel movement. The acute fissure, which resembles a spindle-like tear, becomes chronic with a variable-sized sentinel tag externally, an ulcer with a fibrotic lateral wall in the anal canal, and a hypertrophied papilla. Over time a chronic fissure can be complicated by an incomplete anal fistula, and later by an abscess followed by a complete fistula.

The aim of therapy is to break the vicious circle already in the acute stage. Local anaesthetics (as ointments or anal tampons – suppositories ascend into the rectum and are not efficient – or as an injection) relieve pain and improve the blood supply by abolishing both the spasm of the sphincter and the relative stenosis. Other topical agents which may diminish spastic anal tone include nitroglycerine, calcium channel blockers, or botulinum toxin (this requires injection into the internal anal sphincter)[5]. Once the patient is pain-free a well formed stool (the best anal dilator) improves the elasticity of the anal canal with or without an anal dilator. The body of the latter should be cylindrical (sizes up to 22 mm in diameter) so it can dilate the full length of the anal canal – conical dilators simply move the spastic anus in front of them without dilating the sphincters. Warm sitz baths may relax the muscles before this therapy[6,7] and make dilation easier. The dilator should be inserted into the anal canal for 2–3 min, the muscles contracted with the bougie inside and this exercise should be repeated frequently within 10–15 min. Laxatives are contraindicated, whereas bulk laxatives such as wheat bran, linseeds or plantago seeds, are recommended. Equally important is a sufficient fluid supply: besides the normal fluid intake for an adult of 2–2.5 L/day, for example, an additional supply of 250 ml is necessary for every spoonful of wheat bran. Even in the case of a chronic anal fissure the same conservative therapy should be employed, with the expectation that 80–90% will completely heal. In the period from 1 January to 30 June 2000 we treated in our office more than 1800 patients. Of these, 103 suffered from an anal fissure. Only 20 need an operation, but in six of these cases the fissure was not the main indication.

If the conservative therapy fails an operation is indicated. The maximal anal stretch was introduced first by Recamier in 1838 and later reported by F. v. Esmarch (a famous surgeon in Kiel at that time) in a manual on the therapy of the 'anal spasm' in 1872:

> In France where hygiene in the hospitals caused the surgeons 'to fear their scalpels' (because of infections) a technique was developed to separate sphincters bloodlessly. The violent dilation recommended by Recamier is done by placing the four fingers of each hand on the buttocks, then inserting both thumbs into the anus and stretching the sphincter rapidly so that the two thumbs touch the tuber ossis ischii on both sides. This technique causes the extended sphincter muscles to rupture under a palpable crack and the fissure tears up to the muscle – then when the thumbs are retracted usually some blood flows out of the anus[8].

The description is self-explanatory, as is the result – faecal incontinence. Just as we reject the 'maximal anal stretch', the more limited Lord's procedure, in which six fingers are inserted into the anal canal, is equally abhorrent because of the uncontrolled rupture of the sphincter[9]. It is possible to demonstrate sphincter diruption even with 'normal' dilation with endoanal ultrasound[10,11]. Using a 'controlled' dilation with the Parks speculum opened up to 5 cm, or a balloon in a similar size, Sohn *et al.* showed success in treating a fissure in more than 90%, with subsequent continence problems in only 2%[12].

Another treatment option is anal sphincterotomy. Eisenhammer was one of the first to recognize the relationship between the fissure and the internal anal sphincter. He described the posterior sphincterotomy of the internal anal sphincter in

1952 as operative therapy[13,14]. This therapy was abandoned in later years because of the resulting 'keyhole deformity'. The technique was modified to an open or semi-closed lateral internal sphincterotomy[15,16], which has become the gold standard in English-speaking countries[5,15–17]. The success rate of this technique approaches 95%; however, there have been reports of incontinence following the procedure. Notaras was one of the first who reported his results of semi-closed lateral internal sphincterotomy in 1969; however 6% of 66 patients complained of anal soiling[18].

Except in cases of sphincter sclerosis, in which a dilatation will disrupt the sphincter, we do not perform a lateral (semi-closed) sphincterotomy because it does not improve the results obtained with the 'controlled' dilatation, it produces a defect in the internal anal sphincter, it may impair anal continence for flatus and soiling in up to 35% and produce stool incontinence in up to 9%[19–22]. These symptoms may progress as the patient ages, which is another of our concerns. Finally, the procedure does not address the sentinel tag or hypertrophied papilla.

If conservative treatment fails we prefer the following technique. Under general anaesthesia a Parks speculum demonstrates the fissure, which allows excision of the sentinel tag externally and the hypertrophied papilla internally. The ulcer, including the fibrotic bed and lateral margins, is then excised so that the fibres of the internal sphincter are exposed and the wound bed is clean and even. Associated fistulas in the distal aspect of the fissure are frequently present and can be managed by simultaneous fistulotomy[23]. Successful treatment is confirmed by the ability to easily open the speculum to 4 or 5 cm without tension on the anal canal. If a significant stenosis is present we attempt to open the speculum under general anaesthesia to 4–5 cm or do a 'controlled' dilatation so that we can insert up to two fingers (depending on the size) of both hands side by side to that diameter. In our opinion it is important that the patient is under full relaxation to avoid reactive lesions in the sphincter muscle resulting in injury to the muscle.

To define the relative advantages of these techniques, we reviewed the outcome of 49 patients (age *now* 54 years on average (20–86 years)) managed with controlled anal dilatation (CAD) in 1990 and compared it with 61 patients (age *now* 58 years on average (35–92 years)) operated a year ago by lateral internal sphincteromy (LIS). The case records of these 110 patients showed no significant differences with respect to hospital stay or time out of work. In the LIS group there was one patient with prolonged wound-healing; in the CAD group there were five; three of these had to be reoperated. In the LIS group only one patient showed prolonged wound-healing. That means an overall success rate of more than 96%. To date 37 patients with CAD (19 male and 18 female) and 43 with LIS (13 male and 30 female) have returned a completed questionnaire. 34 and 41 of these, respectively, could be evalutated. The most important questions regarded episodes of minor or major incontinence. The overall outcome in the two groups was similar: most of these 75 patients (76%) had no episodes of incontinence after treatment of anal fissure; 16% (12) of the LIS group and 8% (six) of the CAD group claimed occasional minor soilage and incontinence for flatus. Major continence problems were reported by one patient (3%) in the group with CAD and two patients (5%) in the LIS group. We are currently evaluating data regarding differences between these two groups based upon transanal ultrasound, anal manometry and the effect of age and sex on the development of incontinence after either treatment of anal fissure. Although further investigations are necessary it seems that there is an advantage for CAD.

A review from 1992 which included cases in which excision of a sentinel tag and hypertrophied papilla (30% of the cases) was performed demonstrated a healing rate of 93–94%, with major incontinence problems in less than 2%[12].

Postoperative care includes use of analgesics, sitz baths, and avoidance of constipation to ensure a well-formed stool and to maintain the re-established elasticity of the anal canal.

References

1. Klosterhalfen B, Vogel P, Rixen H, Mittermayr C. Topography of the inferior rectal artery: a possible cause of chronic, primary anal fissure. Dis Colon Rectum. 1989;32:43–52.
2. Schouten WR, Briel JW, Auwerda JJA. Relationship between anal pressure and anodermal blood flow: the vascular pathogenesis of anal fissure. Dis Colon Rectum. 1994;37:664–9.
3. Schouten WR, Briel JW, Auwerda JJA, De Graf EJR. Ischaemic nature of anal fissure. Br J Surg. 1996;83:63–5.
4. Jensen SL. Diet and other risk factors for fissure-in-ano. Prospective case–control study. Dis Colon Rectum. 1988;31:770–3.
5. Lund JN, Scholefield JH. Aetiology and treatment of anal fissure. Br J Surg. 1996;83:1335–44.
6. Dodi G, Bogoni F *et al*. Hot or cold in anal pain? A study of changes in internal sphincter pressure. Dis Colon Rectum. 1986;29:248–51.
7. Jiang JK, Chiu JH, Lin JK. Local thermal stimulation relaxes hypertonic anal sphincter. Dis Colon Rectum. 1999;42:1152–9.
8. Esmarch F v. Die Krankheiten des Mastdarmes und des Afters. In: Pitha, Billroth, editors. Handbuch der allgemeinen und speciellen Chirurgie. Erlangen: Verlag Ferdinand Enke, 1872:143.
9. Lord PH. A new regimen for the treatment of haemorrhoids. Proc R Soc Med. 1968;61:935–6.
10. Nielsen MB, Rasmussen O, Pedersen JF, Christiansen J. Risk of sphincter damage and anal incontinence after anal dilatation for fissure in ano: an endosonographic study. Dis Colon Rectum. 1993;36:677–80.
11. Speakman CTM, Burnett SJD, Kamm MA, Bartram CI. Sphincter injury after anal dilatation demonstrated by anal endosonography. Br J Surg. 1991;78:1429–30.
12. Sohn N, Eisenberg MM, Weinstein MA *et al*. Precise anorectal sphincter dilatation – its role in the therapy of anal fissures. Dis Colon Rectum. 1992;35:322–7.
13. Eisenhammer S. The surgical correction of chronic internal anal (sphincteric) contracture. S Afr Med J. 1951;25:2486–9.
14. Eisenhammer S. The evaluation of the internal anal sphincterotomy operation with special reference to anal fissure. Surg Gynecol Obstet. 1959;109:583–90.
15. Abcarian H, Lakshmanan S, Read DR, Roccaforte P. The role of internal sphincter in chronic anal fissures. Dis Colon Rectum. 1982;25:525–8.
16. American Society of Colon and Rectal Surgeons, Standards Task Force. Practice parameters for ambulatory anorectal surgery. Dis Colon Rectum. 1991;34:285–6.
17. Khubchandani IT, Reed JF. Sequelae of internal sphincterotomy for chronic fissure in ano. Br J Surg. 1989;76:431–4.
18. Notaras M. Lateral subcutaneous sphincterotomy for anal fissure – a new technique. Proc R Soc Med. 1969;62:713.
19. Abcarian H. Surgical correction of chronic anal fissure: results of lateral internal sphincterotomy vs fissurectomy–midline sphincterotomy. Dis Colon Rectum. 1980;23:31–6.
20. Jensen SL, Lund F, Nielsen OV, Tange G. Lateral subcutaneous sphincterotomy versus anal dilatation in the treatment of fissure in ano in outpatients: a prospective randomised study. Br Med J. 1984;289:528–30.
21. Nyam DCNK, Pemberton JH. Long-term results of lateral internal sphincterotomy for chronic anal fissure with particular reference to incidence of fecal incontinence. Dis Colon Rectum. 1999;42:1306–10.

22. Pernikoff BJ, Eisenstat TE, Rubin RJ, Oliver GC, Salvati EP. Reappraisal of partial lateral internal sphincterotomy. Dis Colon Rectum. 1994;37:1291–5.
23. Dörner A, Winkler R. Diagnostik und Behandlungsprinzipien der Analfissur. Langenbecks Arch Chir Suppl II Verh Dtsch Ges Chir. 1989;785–8.

23
Treatment of anal fissure
with botulinum toxin-A

W. H. JOST

INTRODUCTION

Use of botulinum toxin in anal fissure may be considered an effective procedure, since the toxin interferes with the pathogenic mechanisms of chronification. Compared with other indications the effect is not limited to symptomatology alone, but the injection also effects healing in the majority of patients.

PATHOGENESIS AND CLINICAL PICTURE

Next to haemorrhoids, anal fissure is the most frequent ailment in proctology[1]. It is defined as a longitudinal ulcer of the dry, sensitive anoderm, between the linea dentata and linea anocutanea. It is localized at the posterior median line in about 90% of cases[1]; followed by involvement of the anterior commissure in about 9% of cases. Atypical localization is rare and suggestive of specific inflammation. Distribution between the sexes is about even[1].

The aetiology of this disorder has not yet been elucidated. Based on the common incidence in the posterior commissure, some researchers maintain that the rigidity and hypoperfusion of the anal canal caused by Y-shaped clefting of the external anal sphincter muscle with adhesion to the coccygeal bone are to blame[1,2]. Another approach focuses on the frequent hypertension of the sphincter seen with anal fissure, which is why this condition had earlier been referred to as anal cramp. We still do not know whether this is the cause or sequela of severe pain. A spasm of the internus muscle is apparently not the sole cause of fissure[3,4]. Relations with cryptitis, papillitis and haemorrhoids, with anal glands and embryonal malformations, are also being studied[1]. A multifaceted/multifactorial genesis of this disease seems most likely.

The vicious circle with its factors of inflammation–pain–sphincter spasm is the main reason for the development of 'chronic' anal fissure (Fig. 1).

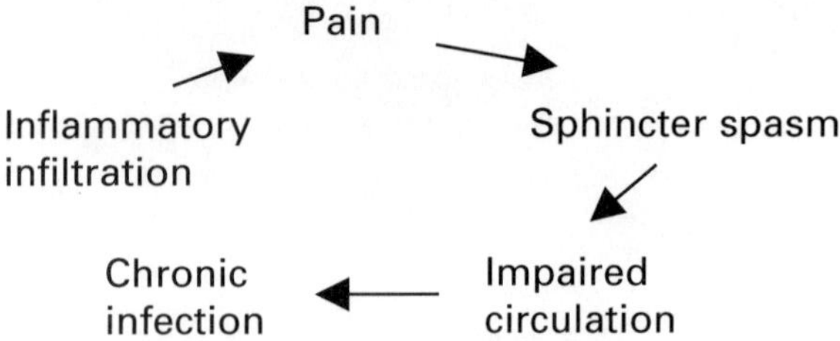

Figure 1 The vicious circle in the development of anal fissure

The disease is marked by severe anal pain on defaecation, which may last for hours afterwards. Burning sensations, oozing and bleeding are additional complaints. Constipation is not rare either, owing to painful bowel evacuation.

The diagnosis is made on the grounds of a typical history and the findings on inspection. The fissure is visualized on mild spreading of the anus, frequently presenting with an inflammatory border at its inferior margin, the so-called sentinel tag. Proctoscopy and rectoscopy are advised for differential diagnosis.

TREATMENT TO DATE

Therapeutic interventions all start at one point of the vicious circle. Conservative treatment, for instance, with its unguents, suppositories, anal plugs and sitzbaths is mainly directed towards inflammation and pain (including the spasm).

Depression of the sphincter tonus seems to make more sense, especially in view of its long-standing tradition in the management of anal fissure.

By the beginning of the last century various therapeutic approaches had already been described in the French-speaking linguistic area[5-7].

Various drug therapies are currently being pursued, topical application of nitroglycerine unguents in particular, which help to reduce sphincter tone[8-11]. The anal dilator is still in use, not only to widen the anal canal but also to lower sphincter tone. Excessive anal expansion, e.g. by spreader or intraoperatively, will damage the sphincter. Lateral sphincterotomy is still performed in chronic uncomplicated fissures[12,13]. Sphincter spasm is reduced by splitting the internal sphincter muscle, in this way helping the fissure to heal. It must be stressed, though, that the incontinence rate associated with lateral sphincterotomy is substantial, not just initially but above all on a long-term basis[14].

In younger patients this deficit is often asymptomatic, with further damage to continence mechanisms; however, the defect will become symptomatic, albeit with some delay.

In chronic complicated fissures the fissure is excised along with removal of the ulcer and the secondary lesions with the effect of consecutive depression of sphincter tonus. In the past, fissurectomy was quite frequently combined with posterior sphincterotomy, but this practice has increasingly been abandoned. Fissurectomy without sphincterotomy seems to be much superior to lateral sphincterotomy[14].

Possible later incontinence apart, the surgical methods are burdened by the operation *per se*, by hospitalization, pain and the likelihood of complicated wound healing[14].

BOTULINUM TOXIN IN ANAL FISSURE

In 1990, botulinum toxin to treat anal fissure was injected for the first time[15,16]. Meanwhile, more than 10 studies on the treatment of anal fissure with botulinum toxin have been completed worldwide, all of them with comparable success (refs 17–24, among others).

Initially we injected into the internal anal sphincter, as plays a major role in sphincteral hypertension. We discovered that diffusion of the toxin results in paralysis of both sphincters. Since the external anal sphincter in easier to puncture, in due course we decided to apply the toxin to the externus. Moreover, our examinations showed that both the internal and external sphincter muscles are involved in sphincter hypertension[26].

Many other work groups continue to inject into the internal sphincter (e.g. refs 20, 22, 23) although it cannot be punctured precisely. This procedure carries the risk of the toxin getting into the intersphincteral cleft.

PATIENT SELECTION

Patients referred for botulinum toxin therapy are in need of detailed proctological evaluation. Fistulas, abscesses or underlying disease must be excluded. An injection should be administered only after spontaneous remission[27], or if healing under topical applications has not resulted.

The rate of spontaneous remission appears to be considerably higher than previously assumed[27]. Patients should present with increased sphincter tonus since elimination of sphincteral hypertension is the objective; reduced tonus and additional paralysis of the sphincters carry the risk of incontinence of faeces. Manometry is not mandatory since the values recorded are falsified because of the pain.

Coagulation disorders, treatment with marcumar and complicated fissures, with formation of fistulas, constitute the only relative contraindications. The patient should be informed in detail about the favourable and possibly undesired side-effects. Since we are dealing with an approved agent for an indication not approved, it is advisable to have patients sign a paper of written information and consent.

PRACTICAL APPLICATION OF BT-A INJECTION

What it takes; patient preparation; dosage and points of injection

One vial of Botox®, for instance, can be dissolved in 4 ml of isotonic saline solution, or one vial of Dysport® in 2.5 ml. Injections are made via a so-called insulin syringe and a fine needle (27 gauge), pierced about 1 cm into the external anal sphincter on both sides laterally and distally of the fissure, and slightly laterally off the anocutaneous line. The clinician should avoid injecting too deeply, to prevent diffusion of the toxin into the puborectal muscle, which would increase the incontinence hazard.

Quantities used per injection site are: 0.1 ml (2.5 U) to 0.2 ml (5 U) of Botox[®] or 0.05 ml (10 U) to 0.1 ml (20 U) of Dysport[®]. Different dilutions produce different volumes.

No data have yet been published on botulinum toxin B (Neurobloc[®]) or botulinum toxin F. The dose depends on muscle tone, indicating that the dose must be increased in cases of very high muscle tone. Local anaesthesia is not called for. The injection technique is simple, and can be acquired in a one-off instruction class. No specific measures are mandatory after the injection. We merely tell patients to use proper anal hygiene (showering with lukewarm water after bowel motion).

We do not feel that the higher doses, quoted by some authors, are necessary, as we were able to produce an adequate effect using the doses quoted above. Higher doses will increase costs, and contribute to the incidence of undesired effects. A third injection site, below the fissure, is not necessary.

The fact that the Italian work group in particular obtained better results by applying higher doses[22,23] might be related to their patient recruitment. In our studies the indication for injection was made only after surgery had been suggested by the proctologist.

Onset of action – duration of action

The effect in patients can usually be seen within a few days, with the empirical observation that pain relief comes first, frequently within the first 2 days. Paralysis is of maximum intensity after 4–7 days, lasting for about 4 weeks, and then gradually remitting. Patients should be clearly informed that they cannot expect any effect immediately after the injection. The period of maximal action may be associated with marked paralysis and atrophy of the injected sphincters. On inspection this looks like a funnel, since the puborectal muscle still continues to contract.

Undesired effects

Significant adverse effects are not be expected when using the above doses. We have never seen relevant local haematomas or similar phenomena. The 300 patients treated and published worldwide did not develop infections. In individual cases we initially found perianal thrombosis[28], which was no longer observed in the 200 consecutive cases.

The only possible undesired effect is incontinence of faeces. Patients must be fully informed about this possible consequence. The probability of anal incontinence is increased with reduced tonus, and is higher in females, in advanced age and after several deliveries. The incontinence rate in our collective was found to be <5% with the above doses, and this incontinence was transitory, lasting for 2 weeks at maximum, and limited to incontinence of flatus and faecal spotting. To date we have noted no incontinence of solid stools. Remission of paralysis is complete. Systemic effects are not to be expected with the lower dose.

RESULTS OF HEALING

There is marked alleviation of pain in 75% of cases within the first few days. Significantly reduced sphincter tonus is found in most patients. Relevantly reduced puborectal tone with the above dosage[29,30] was detected in only a few cases. The cure rate in our collective of patients after first therapy is slightly below 80% (Tables 1 and 2). No relevant differences between the two substances (Tables 1 and 2) were revealed in the literature. Even higher cure rates are described in the literature. We screened our patients carefully to rule out spontaneous remission, and to make sure that the possibilities of conservative management had been exhausted. The higher cure rate of the other authors could be due to their patient selection.

It first therapy fails to produce the desired outcome, reinjection is possible after the effect of the toxin has worn off. Reinjection is also advised in the event of recidivation[31].

We were able to achieve analgesia within the first week in most cases (95%), in a patient group presenting with relapse. Healing was confirmed in 70% at 3 months later (Table 3). Undesired effects were not reported[31]. Among patients

Table 1 Symptoms, course and undesired effects in 100 patients treated with Botox®, $2 \times 2.5\,U^{29}$

	1 week later	After 3 months	After 6 months
Pain-free	78/100	82/82	79/79
Reduced sphincter tone	89/100	0/82	0/79
Reduced tone of the puborectal muscle	4/100	0/82	0/79
Continence maintained	93/100	82/82	79/79
Healing without surgery	—	82/100	79/100
Relapse	—	5/100	8/100
Surgery	—	18/100	21/100
Undesired effects	0/100	0/82	0/79

Table 2 Results and undesired effects following a Dysport® injection[29]: group 1 receiving $2 \times 10\,U$ ($n = 25$), group 2 receiving $2 \times 20\,U$ ($n = 25$)[30]

	Time after Dysport® injection			
	1 week		3 months	
Dose	$2 \times 10\,U$	$2 \times 20\,U$	$2 \times 10\,U$	$2 \times 20\,U$
Healing without surgery	—	—	19/25	20/25
Relapse	—	—	1/25	2/25
Analgesia	20/25	21/25	19/19*	20/20*
Reduced sphincter tone	22/25	25/25	0/19*	0/20*
Reduced puborectal tone	0/25	3/25	0/19*	0/20*
Temporary incontinence	1/25	3/25	0/19*	0/20*

*Results in patients with healed fissure

Table 3 Data on the course of the patients studied[31] with relapse ($n = 30$) and incomplete healing, respectively ($n = 20$)

Non-responders	Relapses		Non-responders	
	1 week after BT-A	3 months after BT-A	1 week after BT-A	3 months after BT-A
Pain-free	22/30	19/19	19/20	14/14
Reduced tone	29/30	0/19	17/20	0/14
Reduced puborectal	3/30	0/19	0/20	0/14
Continence maintained	28/30	19/19	14/20	14/14
Undesired effects	0	0	0	0

not responding to the primary injection[31] 73.3% were pain-free within the first week. Mild transitory incontinence was seen in solitary cases (6.7%). After 3 months, healing was evident in 70% of patients (Table 3). Our results confirm a positive therapeutic effect of repeat BT-A injection on both relapse and defective healing.

We can also recommend applying the toxin prior to fissurectomy without sphincterectomy, the objective being to decrease muscle tone and to improve healing.

COMPARISON WITH NITROGLYCERINE PREPARATIONS

Shortly after publication of the first therapeutic successes due to BT-A, positive experiences with the topical application of gylceryl trinitrate preparations were also described. Many studies on that topic have been published in the meantime (refs 9, 32 and 33, among others). The theoretical approach is quite similar to that of botulinum toxin therapy. This alternative method is above all disadvantaged by headaches as a side-effect. The disadvantage compared with BT-A consists in the continuous application of nitroglycerine unguent, which is mandatory several times a day for some weeks. Most patients tend to carry on treatment until they are pain-free, subsequently forgetting to apply the ointment. The effect of a BT-A injection, however, will last for several weeks. Active patient cooperation is not required; systemic effects do not occur. A comparative study proved the superiority of BT-A over the nitroglycerine preparation[34]. In another comparative study, lateral sphincterotomy was found to be superior to nitroglycerine application[13].

In view of their unnecessary systemic effect, use of oral nifedipine preparations does not appear to be a sensible alternative.

FURTHER USE OF BOTULINUM TOXIN

Postoperatively increased sphincter tone due to pain is found in a large number of patients who underwent proctological surgery – patch grafts in fistulas, conventional haemorrhoidectomies and sphincteral reconstruction, to name just a few. This kind of reflex raised sphincter tone frequently leads to impaired wound healing, thereby prolonging the period of hospitalization and increasing costs.

Re-surgery is also required, on occasion. Transitory paralysis of the muscles responsible for increased sphincter tone might be the solution to this problem, and this effect can be accomplished by a BT-A injection.

Circular injections are advised preoperatively in four sites of the external anal sphincter muscle. By diffusion the internal muscle is also paralysed. Minor paralysis of the puborectal muscle is the result of deeper injection. The dose is determined according to the degree of paralysis desired. If mild to moderate paralysis is desired, $4 \times 2.5\,U$ of Botox® or, alternatively $4 \times 10\,U$ of Dysport®, will suffice. By injecting $4 \times 2.5\,U$ of Botox®, or alternatively $4 \times 10\,U$ of Dysport®, we are able to produce significant paralysis. Higher doses make no sense, as incontinence of several weeks duration would be the consequence. The injection is logically done preoperatively since there will be no adequate appreciable action until some days later. Abscesses in the area of injection are a definite contraindication. Coagulation disorders and intake of anticoagulants constitute a relative contraindication. Patients should be informed about possible temporary incontinence. Over the past 3 years we have treated several patients preoperatively. So far, from these studies, our patients indicate less pain postoperatively, impaired healing is less common, and the rate of relapse is significantly reduced. Undesired effects have not been observed. Incontinence has been quite rare; if any it will last for only a few days to a maximum of 2 weeks, and will be only in the form of flatulence and thin stools.

RISK–BENEFIT CONSIDERATIONS

The hazards involved with BT-A injection are minimal and temporary. The possible benefit in anal fissure is healing, first of all, and secondly avoidance of surgery with possible incontinence. The sphincteral system is maintained. This therapy should thus be tried prior to any operation. All patients who are likely candidates for surgery should be informed not only about the risks involved, but also about this alternative therapeutic option.

References

1. Jost WH. Die Analfissur. Z Allg Med. 1990;66:652–6.
2. Blaisdell PC. Pathogenesis of anal fissure and implications as to treatment. Surg Gynecol Obstet. 1937;65:672–7.
3. Braun J, Raguse T. Zur pathophysiologischen Rolle des inneren Analsphinkters bei der chronischen Analfissur. Z Gastroenterol. 1985;23:565–72.
4. Jost WH, Schimrigk K, Mlitz H. The riddle of the sphincters in anal fissure (letter). Dis Colon Rectum. 1995;38:555.
5. Boyer A. Remarques et observations sur quelques maladies de l'anus. J Compl Dict Sc Med. 1818;2:24–44.
6. Dupuytren G. Leçons orales de clinique chirurgale. Paris: Germer Bailliére, 1839.
7. Récamier JCA. Recherches sur le traitement du choléra-morbus. Augmentées d'un premier supplément. Paris: Gabon, 1832.
8. Cook TA, Humphreys MM, Mortensen McC NJ. Oral nifedipine reduces resting anal pressure and heals chronic anal fissure. Br J Surg. 1999;86:1269–73.
9. Loder PB, Kamm MA, Nicholls RJ, Phillips KS. 'Reversible chemical sphincterotomy' by local application of glyceryl trinitrate. Br J Surg. 1994;81:1386–9.
10. Pitt J, Craggs MM, Henry MM, Boulos PB. Alpha-1-adrenoceptor blockade: potential new treatment for anal fissures. Dis Colon Rectum. 2000;43:800–3.

11. Zielanwoski MM. Topical ketanserin gel for anal fissure: an open-label, prospective study. Adv Ther. 2000;17:27–33.
12. Argov S, Levandovsky O. Open lateral sphincterotomy is still the best treatment for chronic anal fissure. Am J Surg. 2000;179:201–2.
13. Richard CS, Gregoire R, Plewes EA *et al.* Internal sphincterotomy is superior to topical nitroglycerin in the treatment of chronic anal fissure. Dis Colon Rectum. 2000;43:1048–58.
14. Jost WH, Raulf F, Müller-Lobeck H. Anal fissures: results of surgical treatment. Colo-Proctology. 1991;13:110–13.
15. Jost WH, Schimrigk K. Use of botulinum toxin in anal fissure. Dis Colon Rectum. 1993;36:974.
16. Jost WH, Schimrigk K. Therapy of anal fissure using botulin toxin. Dis Colon Rectum. 1994;37:1321–4.
17. Espi A, Melo F, Mínguez M *et al.* Therapeutic effects of different doses of botulinum toxin in chronic anal fissure. Dis Colon Rectum. 1998;41:A16(abstract).
18. Mínguez M, Melo, F, Espí A *et al.* Therapeutic effects of different doses of botulinum toxin in chronic anal fissure. Dis Colon Rectum. 1999;42:1016–21.
19. Fernandez Lopez F, Conde Freire R, Rios Rios A, Garcia Iglesias J, Cainzos Fernandez M, Potel Lesquereux J. Botulinum toxin for the treatment of anal fissure. Dig Surg. 1999;16:515–18.
20. Gui D, Caessetta E, Anastasio G, Bentivoglio AR, Maria G, Albanese A. Botulinum toxin for chronic anal fissure. Lancet. 1994;344:1127–8.
21. Hasler WL. The expanding spectrum of clinical uses for botulinum toxin: healing of chronic anal fissures. Gastroenterology. 1999;116:221–3.
22. Maria G, Brisinda G, Bentivoglio AR, Caessetta E, Gui D, Albanese A. Botulinum toxin injections in the internal anal sphincter for the treatment of chronic anal fissures: long-term results after two different dosage regimens. Ann Surg. 1998;228:664–9.
23. Maria G, Cassetta E, Gui D, Brisinda G, Bentivoglio AR, Albanese A. A comparison of botulinum toxin and saline for the treatment of chronic anal fissure. N Engl J Med. 1998;338:217–20.
24. Mason PF, Watkins MJG, Hall HS, Hall AW. The management of chronic fissure-in-ano with botulinum toxin. J R Coll Surg Edinb. 1996;41:235–8.
25. Phillips RKS. Botulinum toxin promoted healing and relieved symptoms of chronic anal fissure. Gut. 1998;43:601.
26. Jost WH, Mlitz H, Kaiser T, Schimrigk K. The importance of sphincters in anal fissure. Int J Surg Sci. 1997;4:22–4.
27. Jost WH. Incidence of anal fissure in nonselected neurological patients. Dis Colon Rectum. 1999;42:828.
28. Jost WH, Schanne S, Mlitz H, Schimrigk K. Perianal thrombosis following injection therapy into the external anal sphincter using botulin toxin (letter). Dis Colon Rectum. 1995;38:781.
29. Jost WH. One hundred cases of anal fissure treated with botulin toxin: early and long-term results. Dis Colon Rectum. 1997;40:1029–32.
30. Jost WH, Schrank B. Chronic anal fissures treated with botulinum toxin injections: a dose-finding study with Dysport®. Colorectal Dis. 1999;1:26–8.
31. Jost WH, Schrank B. Repeat botulin toxin injections in anal fissure: in patients with relapse and after insufficient effect of the first treatment. Dig Dis Sci. 1999;44:1588–9.
32. Gorfine SR. Topical nitroglycerin therapy for anal fissures and ulcers. N Engl J Med. 1995;333:1156–7.
33. Oettlé W. Glyceryl trinitrate vs. sphincterotomy for treatment of chronic fissure-in-ano. Dis Colon Rectum. 1997;40:1318–20.
34. Brisinda G, Maria G, Bentivoglio AR, Cassetta E, Gui D, Albanese A. A comparison of injections of botulinum toxin and topical nitroglycerin ointment for the treatment of chronic anal fissure. N Engl J Med. 1999;341:65–9.

24
Fistula-in-ano

T. C. HICKS

INTRODUCTION

A fistula is an abnormal communication between any two epithelial-lined surfaces. A fistula-in-ano is an abnormal communication between the anal canal and the perineal skin. Fistulas represent a relatively small part of most surgeons' practice, and complex fistulas usually do not compromise more than 10% of their practice. Most fistulas (90–95%) are simple, meaning that the fistula is easy to treat. This definition implies that the fistula tract is easily identifiable and that after surgical intervention anorectal function is not significantly impaired. Complex fistulas refer to those clinical situations where the fistula's anatomy or the patient's co-morbidities alter the routine surgical approach of simple fistulotomy. Complex fistulas may have more than one opening, more than one tract, a horseshoe configuration, a high internal opening or a high extension. Co-morbid factors that may affect healing include Crohn's disease, hidradenitis suppurativa, tuberculosis, lymphogranuloma, HIV disease and neoplasms. The goal in the treatment of all fistulas is to achieve a cure while minimizing the loss of sphincter control[1,2].

ANATOMY

Familiarity of the surgeon with the anatomy of the anorectal area, and with pathogenesis and classifications of fistulas, is essential for their adequate management. The sphincter mechanism is composed of two cylinders of muscles, an inner cylinder of smooth muscle (the internal sphincter), which is continuous with the circular muscle of the rectum, and the outer cylinder of striated muscle (the external sphincter). The external sphincter is inseparable from the lower muscular margin of the levator muscle, the puborectalis muscle. The *intersphincteric space* is the term that denotes the potential space between the internal sphincter and the external sphincter. The *ischiorectal space* is the space that is lateral to the external sphincters. The *supralevator space* is bounded superiorly by the peritoneum, laterally by the pelvic wall, medially by the rectal wall and inferiorly by the levator ani muscles. The *perianal space* is located near the anal verge, and it becomes fused with the ischiorectal fat laterally while it extends into the lower portion of the anal canal medially. Posterior to the anus a potential space is termed the *deep post-anal space* which extends from the coccyx to the posterior margin of the external sphincter.

The encircling sphincter muscles form the anal canal which is divided in half by the dentate line. The dentate line separates the anal mucosa and the anoderm. On the proximal side of the dentate line is the site where the mucosa contains the crypts. In the depths of these crypts is a duct and gland system, which is a site felt to be the nidus of infection and abscess that leads to the majority of fistulas (the cryptoglandular origin theory) (Fig. 1).

CLASSIFICATION

A well-accepted classification scheme of anal fistulas was proposed by Parks *et al.* in 1976 (Fig. 2)[3]. This classification system is based upon the relationships to spaces around the sphincter muscles. There are four groups utilized in this classification: intersphincteric, trans-sphincteric, supersphincteric and extrasphincteric. Trans-sphincteric and intersphincteric fistulas account for more than 90% of all fistulas. The fistulas are labelled according to the relationship with the external sphincter, as essentially all anal fistulas involve a portion of the internal sphincter beyond the dentate line. Fistulas can become complicated when they

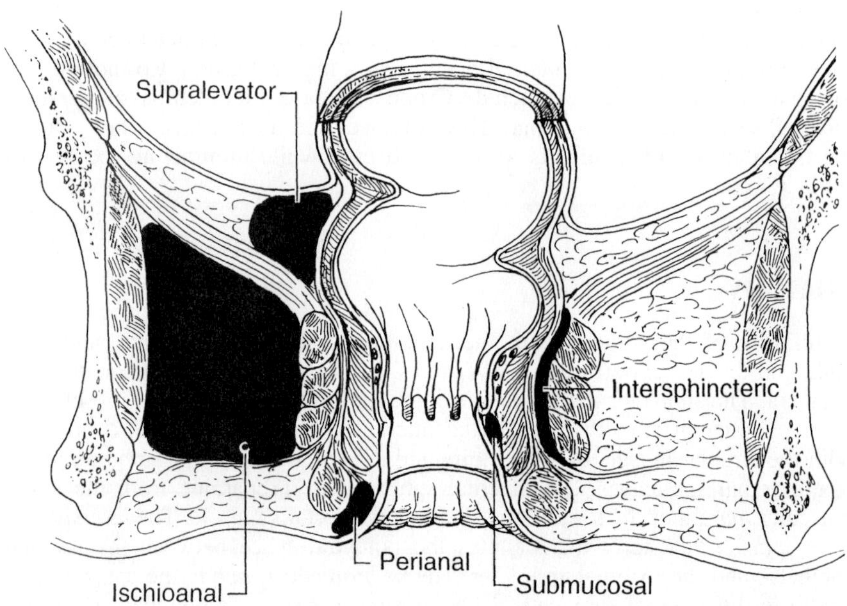

Figure 1 Anorectal spaces

have coexistent extensions high along the sphincter muscles, hidden openings, multiple tracts, and horseshoe configurations.

Intersphincteric fistula-in-ano

This is the most common type of fistula and accounts for approximately 70% of all fistulas[3]. The tract in this fistula passes between the sphincters with possible extension cephalad as a high blind intersphincteric tract. Additionally, it may originate as a pelvic abscess or may extend into the supralevator spaces as a high blind tract. There is no downward extension to the anal margin, and thus no external opening is present. It is also important to note that an intersphincteric fistula may originate in the pelvis as a pelvic abscess but manifest itself in the perianal area.

Trans-sphincteric fistula-in-ano

This is an unusual type of fistula and it results from an ischiorectal abscess. In Parks' study it represented only 23% of fistulas seen. The fistula tract passes from the internal opening through the internal and external sphincters to the ischiorectal fossa (see Fig. 2). A high blind tract may also occur in this situation in which the upper arm of the tract may pass into the levator ani muscles and thereby into the pelvis[3].

Supersphincteric fistula-in-ano

This fistula accounts for only 5% of fistulas in most series and results from a supralevator abscess. The tract arises as an intersphincteric abscess and then

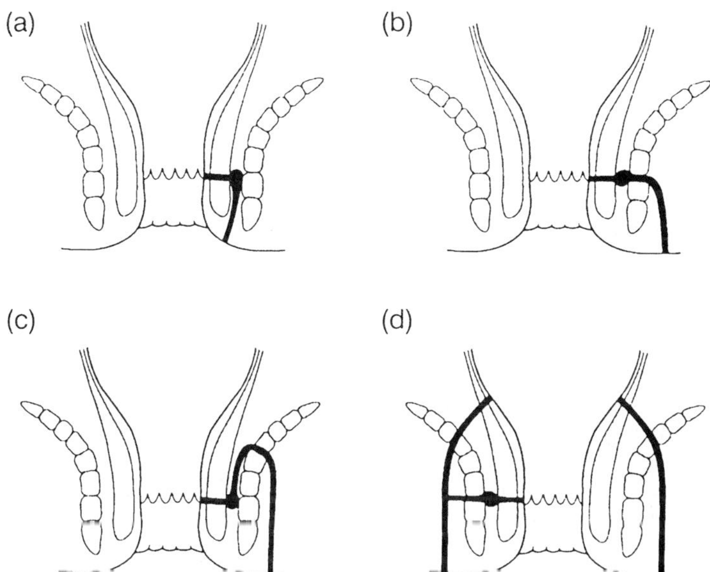

Figure 2 Classification of fistula-in-ano: (a) intersphincteric, (b) trans-sphincteric, (c) suprasphincteric, (d) extrasphincteric

passes above the puborectalis. The tract curves downwards lateral to the external sphincter in the ischiorectal space to the perirectal skin. When a supersphincteric fistula-in-ano forms a high blind tract, it may result in a horseshoe extension[3].

Extrasphincteric fistula-in-ano

Only 2% of patients will present with this type of fistula. The fistula tracts from the rectum to a site above the levators and descends through the levator muscles to the perineal skin via the ischiorectal space. This fistula has been attributed to foreign body perforation of the rectum with subsequent drainage through the levators, to rectal cancer, or to Crohn's disease. It is felt that the most common cause is probably iatrogenic, secondary to vigorous probing during fistula surgery[3].

DIAGNOSIS

The majority of patients with fistula-in-ano will have a history of abscess development and drainage. The abscess that precedes the fistula is recognized as a red, hot, swollen, painful site on the anus. This site may be less obvious if it is a supralevator or deep post-anal abscess. The chronic form of the abscess is the fistula and sometimes the fistula openings will close over, and the abscess will re-form. The external openings may be open and draining, or may be seen as a dimple or scar. A physical examination performed in the office will generally reveal an external opening which on gentle probing will support the diagnosis of fistula-in-ano. Palpation may reveal a tract as an indurated linear structure extending from the external opening. Often a bi-digital examination with a finger in the anus will allow the examiner to follow the course of the tract. Anoscopy should be performed although the actual internal opening is rarely identifiable in the office. Goodsall's rule suggests that the external fistula opening posterior to the line drawn transversely across the perineum will cure posteriorly to open at the dentate line in the posterior midline, while anterior fistula tracts tract radially directly to the anal canal (Fig. 3)[4].

As an adjunct to fistula tract identification the utilization of dyes or peroxides injected into the tract may be helpful in finding the elusive internal opening. Radiological techniques are often employed to help delineate the complexity of tracts, the number of the tracts or the site of the internal opening[5]. Fistulograms utilizing water-soluble contrast material may be helpful, and it may be helpful to the radiologist if a steel clip is applied to the posterior midline and anteriorly as well[6]. This allows the radiologist a reference point. Some authors have suggested that anal ultrasound may be useful when the tracts are filled with peroxide prior to the examination. The selective use of anal manometry is championed by those physicians who feel that significant risk factors are present. These factors have been identified as those patients suspected of needing substantial portions of their external sphincter divided for a fistula cure; patients with suspected preoperative sphincter impairment and those women who have a history of multiparity or difficult deliveries. The utilization of CT scans and MRIs has been reported to be useful in situations in which complex fistulas occur, but their expense is often prohibitive[7].

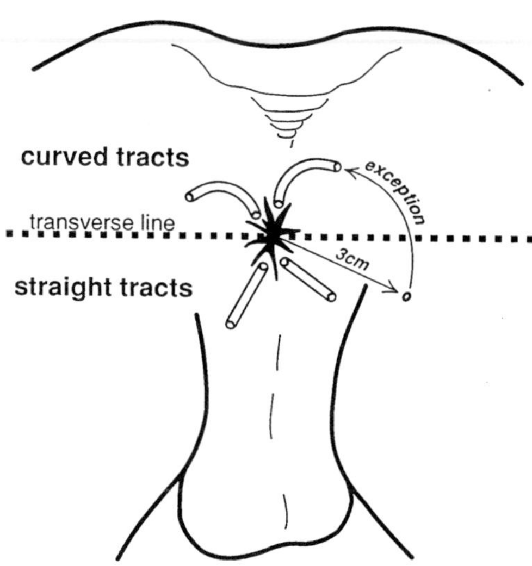

Figure 3 Goodsall's rule

Prior to examining the patient under anaesthesia and selecting appropriate fistula-in-ano treatment, the physician should be suspicious of any underlying disease processes such as Crohn's disease or immune suppression. If these clinical conditions exist, an appropriate preoperative evaluation should be undertaken.

TREATMENT

The three major goals of fistula surgery are[8]:

1. To cure the fistula (prevent recurrence).
2. To preserve anorectal function (avoid incontinence).
3. To optimize healing time (return to normal activities and enhance the quality of life).

Prior to any surgical intervention for fistula-in-ano the physician should carefully explain to the patient potential early and possibly permanent alteration of anatomical contour and faecal continence. The patient should be reassured that in most cases the potential for permanent loss of control of gas or stool is small, but that the ultimate outcome in fistula surgery cannot always be predicted. Patients should also be informed that in most reported series the potential for recurrence ranges from 1% to 18%. Fazio suggests that four major surgical principles should be observed during any operative intervention for fistula-in-ano disease[5]:

1. The internal and external opening of the tract must be identified.
2. The relationship of the tract to the anorectal ring (puborectalis) must be established.

3. Sphincter preservation or minimization of sphincter sectioning is attempted but not at the risk of significant chance of recurrence of the fistula.
4. Perineal deformity is minimized. That is, preserve perianal skin as much as possible, avoid contour defects which may allow escape of mucus from the anus, and minimize the production of perianal scar tissue.

At surgery there are several methods available for determining the fistula tract.

1. Probing the tract. After the patient has been appropriately anaesthetized (caudal, spinal or general anaesthesia), the patient is placed in the jack-knife position. The surgeon should always be cognizant of gently probing the tract so as to avoid the creation of a false passage. Periodic adjustment of the curve of the probe may facilitate its passage. In those cases where the internal opening is easily seen, as well as the external opening, but the probe cannot be passed without causing trauma to the tract, two probes may be utilized, entering at opposite ends of the tract and being passed until they meet (metal on metal). This process may allow the surgeon to dissect the external tract down into the point of the internal probe, thus identifying the tract without causing undue trauma.
2. If the internal opening is not easily discovered, a number of agents have been inserted into the external fistula opening with a syringe and an angio-catheter. Surgeons have utilized milk, dilute methylene blue or hydrogen peroxide to assist in targeting the internal opening.
3. In those occasions when the complete fistula tract is not identified, the surgeon may choose to curette that portion of the tract that is identifiable and then discontinue the examination in an effort to avoid leading to more complications.
4. Should the fistula persist, the surgeon may choose to use transanal ultrasound or a fistulogram or CT scan prior to re-exploration[9].

OPERATIVE MANAGEMENT

Fistulotomy (The lay-open technique)

This technique has served as the gold standard of treatment for most fistulas. After the patient has received adequate anaesthesia he/she is placed in the prone jack-knife position (Fig. 4). The surgeon then carefully passes a probe along the full extent of the tract. An electrocautery is used to incise the tissues directly over the probe. Once the probe is completely exposed, many surgeons will curette the base of the primary tract and any extensions that exist, to aid in wound healing. Some authors also support marsupialization on either edge of the incision tract but this often proves to be unnecessary. A simple non-adhesive dressing is applied to the operative site. The patient is usually treated on an out-patient basis, is given adequate analgesia on discharge from the hospital and is instructed to take sitz baths two or three times a day for appropriate patient comfort and perineal toilet.

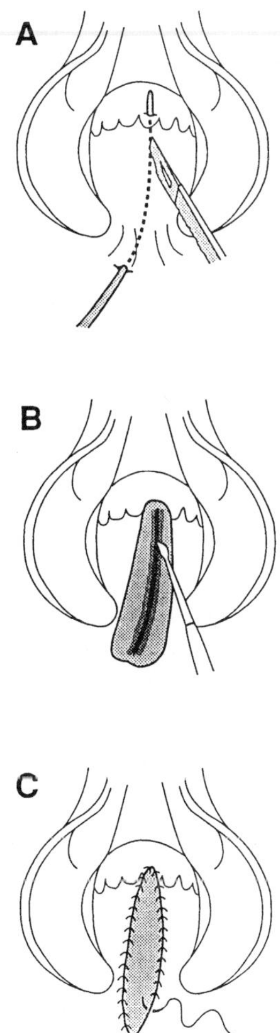

Figure 4 Fistulotomy – the lay-open technique: A: insertion of probe and incision of tissue overlying probe, B: curettage of granulation tissue, C: marsupialization of wound edges

Fistulectomy

Fistulectomy or excision of the fistula tract is no longer felt to be an appropriate treatment for fistula-in-ano. These larger wounds have significantly delayed healing time and put the patient at greater risk for incontinence secondary to excising underlying muscle.

Setons

A seton is any foreign substance which can be inserted into the fistula tract to encircle the sphincter muscles (Fig. 5). Surgeons commonly utilize silk or other non-absorbable suture material, Penrose drains, rubber bands, vessel loops and

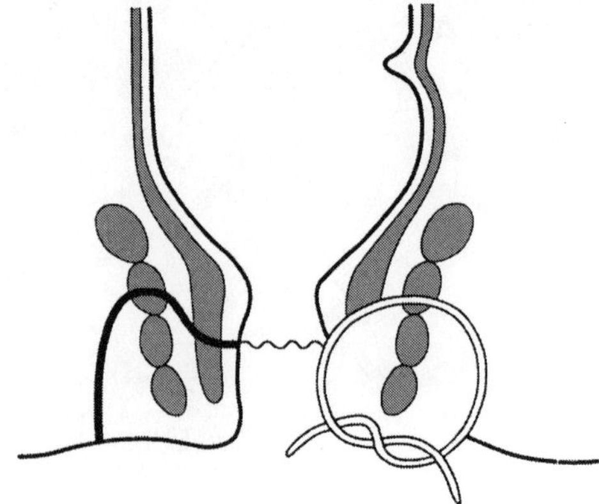

Figure 5   Anal seton

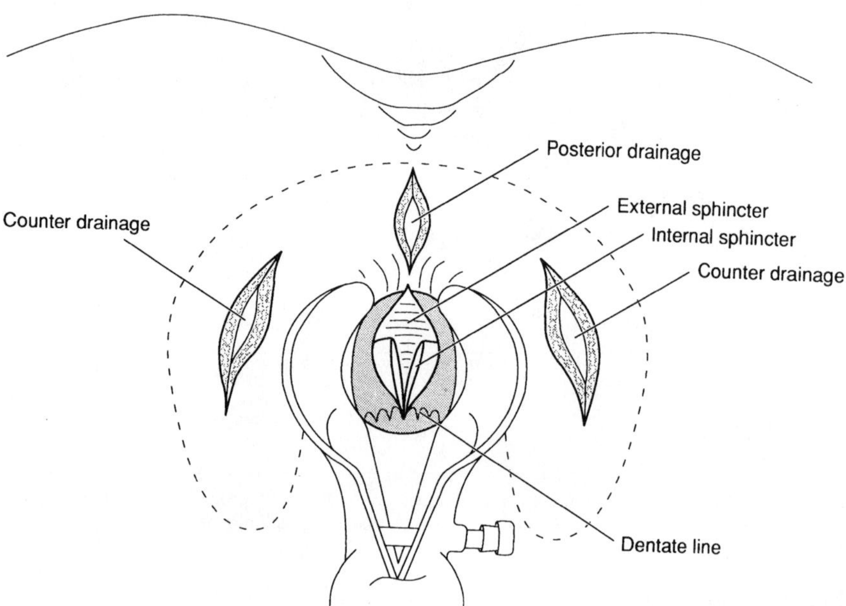

Figure 6   Surgical approach to a 'horseshoe' abscess

Silastic catheters[10]. The utilization of a seton is an adjunct to a staged fistulo-tomy (Fig. 6). When patients develop high intersphincteric fistulas anal conti-nence may be compromised by strictly using a lay-open technique. With this technique the inferior portion of the internal sphincter is carefully divided along with skin so that the surgeon can reach the external opening. Then a seton is inserted circumferentially through the fistula tract. The surgeons then at subse-quent office visits can tighten the seton so that it slowly cuts through the sphincter muscle allowing for scarring, to keep the continuity of the anorectal ring intact. Some surgeons utilize this technique to convert a high trans-sphincteric fistula into a low fistula, and can perform a second-stage fistulotomy of any remaining sphincter muscle at approximately 8–10 weeks after seton placement. Another role for the seton has been as a drain to be used in complex fistulas. In these cases a small Penrose drain serves as an excellent non-absorbable material. Pearl *et al.*, in their 1993 article in *Diseases of the Colon and Rectum*[11], identified several specific indications for the utilization of setons, which included:

1. To identify and promote fibrosis around the complex anal fistula that encircles the lowest or all of the sphincter mechanism.
2. The anterior, high trans-sphincteric fistulas in women. Since the puborectalis is absent in this area, and the external sphincter is quite tenuous, primary fistulotomy may result in incontinence.
3. For those patients who are immunocompromised, and in whom poor healing is felt to be a major factor.
4. To promote long-term drainage in patients with Crohn's disease.
5. For patients who have had multiple fistula repairs, and in any patients in whom there is a fear that the surgery may result in incontinence.

When a supersphincteric fistula presents as a 'horseshoe' the surgeon is faced with multiple external openings a great distance from the cryptoglandular source. The surgical approach to this problem includes the appropriate drainage of the post-anal space with identification of the internal openings and adequate counterdrainage for the horseshoe fistula extension[12].

Anorectal advancement flap

Patients with multiple or complex fistulas, along with patients with inflammatory bowel disease, high trans-sphincteric or suprasphincteric fistulas or anterior fistulas in women, may not be good candidates for the standard fistulotomy technique. The anorectal advancement flap offers the advantages of no additional damage to the sphincter muscles (as they are not divided), less deformity of the anal canal and a reported reduction in the duration of healing (Fig. 7). Preoperatively the patients are given a mechanical and antibiotic bowel preparation. After obtaining adequate regional anaesthesia the patient is placed in the prone jackknife position and the fistula tract is identified and either curetted or cored out. The surgeon then injects an epinephrine solution (1–200 000) under the submucosa to obtain haemostasis and then develops a full-thickness flap that can be advanced below the internal opening. The tip of the mucosal flap which contains the fistulous opening is excised and then the remaining tissue is sutured back in appropriate anatomical position. As with all flaps, it is important for the surgeon to make sure that the flap is twice the width of the apex in order to ensure an adequate blood supply. Kodner, in his article in *Surgery* in 1993, noted that most series report a 40–70% success rate[5,10,13,14].

Recurrence

Recurrence rates following fistula surgery range from 0% to 18%[15] (Table 1). Authors report that the most common causes of failure are related to the inability

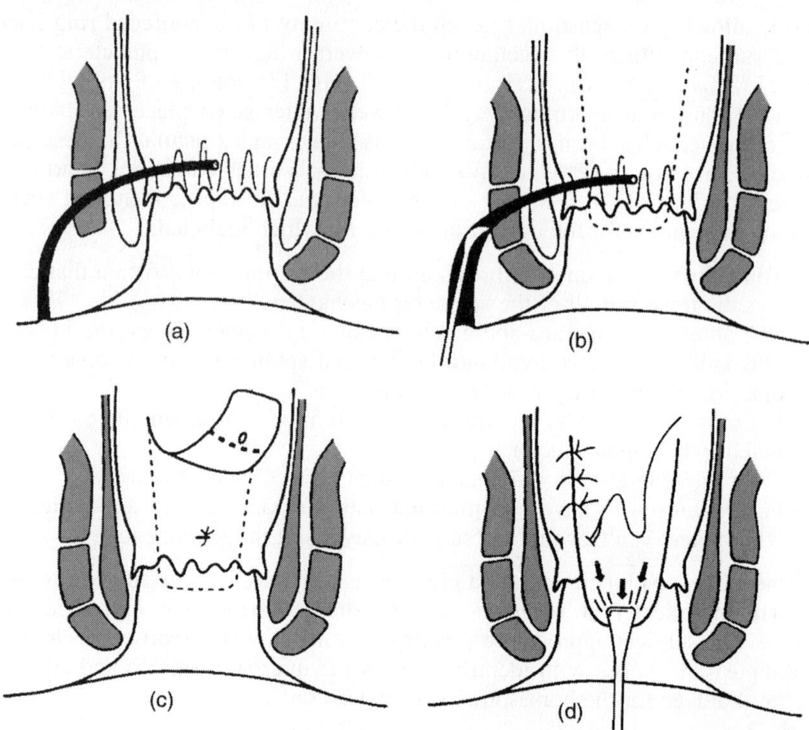

Figure 7 Anorectal advancement flap: (a) anotomy of trans-sphincteric fistula-in-ano, (b) curetting of fistula tract, (c) anorectal advancement flap construction, (d) flap advancement and suturing

Table 1 Results of fistula surgery

Author	Year	No. of patients	Recurrence (%)	Incontinence (%)
Bennett	1962	108	2.0	36.0
Hill	1967	626	1.0	4.0
Lilius	1968	150	5.5	13.5
Mazier	1971	1000	3.9	0.001
Ani and Solanke	1976	82	17.0	1.0
Marks and Ritchie	1977	793	—	3,17,25*
Ewerth *et al.*	1978	143	2.8	3.5
Adams and Kovalcik	1981	133	3.8	0.8
Kuijpers	1982	51	4.0	10.0
Sainio and Husa	1985	199	11.0	34.0
Vasilevsky and Gordon	1985	160	6.3	0.7,2.0,3.3[†]
Fucini	1991	99	3.0	0,0.2,0.5[‡]
Van Tets	1994	19	—	33.0
Sangwan	1994	461	6.5	2.8
Garcia-Aguilar *et al.*	1996	293	7.0	42.0

* 3% solid stool, 17% liquid stool, 25% flatus.
[†] 0.7% solid stool, 2.0% liquid stool, 3.3% flatus.
[‡] 0% solid stool, 0.2% liquid stool, 0.5% flatus.

Table 2 Results of staged fistulotomy using a seton

Author	Year	Recurrence (%)	Incontinence (%)
Ramanujam	1983	1/45 (2)	1/45 (2)
Kuijjpers	1984	0/10 (0)	1/10 (10)
Culp	1984	0/20 (0)	0/20 (0)
Christensen	1986	0/21 (0)	6/21 (29)
Held	1986	0/7 (0)	0/7 (0)
Fasth	1990	0/7 (0)	0/7 (0)
Williams	1991	2/28 (8)	1/24 (4)
Pearl	1993	3/116 (3)	5/116 (5)
Van Tets	1994	—	15/29 (54)
Graf	1995	2/25 (8)	11/25 (44)
Garcia-Aguilar	1996	6/63 (9)	39/61 (64)

to identify a primary opening or failure to recognize extensions of the fistula. Interestingly, recurrence rates following staged repairs which utilized a seton range from 0% to 8% (Table 2). As mentioned earlier, failure rates with anorectal advanced flaps may be as high as 30%[16].

Incontinence

Following fistula surgery different degrees of continence complaints may range as high as 50%[17]. Significant incontinence findings are related to patients with complex fistulas. Impaired continence was also associated with increasing age and with female patients. For major faecal incontinence, most series report from 5% to 6.7%, and the authors describe factors to be considered, such as complexity of the fistula, the patient's preoperative continence state, as well as the patient's wound-healing response to surgical intervention[11].

Special considerations

Patients with Crohn's disease and anal fistulas have often challenged the surgeon. It has been reported that 38% of such fistulas will heal spontaneously, although a significant number of fistulas require surgical intervention[18]. Prior to the late 1980s surgeons took a conservative approach to patients with Crohn's fistulas secondary to a fear of leaving the patient incontinent. Sir Alexander-Williams stated that 'incontinence is likely to be the result of aggressive surgeons, not of aggressive disease'[19]. Surgeons have reported the best results when patients receive appropriate medical management. This includes the utilization of steroids or 5-ASA compounds. Some important concepts about Crohn's fistulas include the idea that asymptomatic fistulas do not necessarily require interventional treatment, draining setons can be used to control fistula tracts and prevent further abscess formation, and maximizing the patient's medical condition prior to attempting the fistulotomy should be the standard of care. In Crohn's disease patients it has been reported that, after drainage of perirectal abscesses, up to 73% of patients will develop a fistula[20]. However, it is important that the surgeon does not perform a primary fistulotomy because of the risk of incontinence. Low fistulas with simple tracts have been managed successfully with a lay-open technique, but complex fistulas with high rectal openings must be managed conservatively with a seton technique in order to prevent incontinence.

The HIV patient

Surgeons should carefully assess the severity of the illness of HIV patients prior to embarking on a surgical procedure. Recent data by Consten and colleagues[21] found that low CD4 lymphocyte counts in patients with perianal sepsis are at risk for disturbed wound-healing. For patients who have asymptomatic fistulas no surgical treatment is required, but in those cases that require surgical intervention discretion should be utilized so as not to create large wounds or to injure the sphincter muscle. It has also been recommended in the perioperative period that these patients should receive an appropriate antibiotic course. For HIV patients who have high complex fistulas the utilization of draining setons is recommended, while patients with low fistulas may undergo fistulotomy.

WHAT'S NEW?

Repair of fistula-in-ano using fibrin adhesive

In 1998 the Food and Drug Administration (FDA) gave their approval for the utilization of fibrin sealant for use in the operating room. Many investigators have used fibrin adhesives to repair fistula tracts. Initial studies showed success rates between 60% and 80%, but unfortunately these studies lacked adequate sample sizes and appropriate long-term follow-up data[22–24]. The University of Illinois, Department of Colon and Rectal Surgery reported on 79 patients with an 18-month follow-up[25]. Twenty-six of their patients were treated with autologous fibrin tissue adhesive made from their own blood, and 53 were treated with commercial fibrin sealant. They examined each patient under anaesthesia and curetted the fistula tract; then the fibrin adhesive was injected into the secondary fistula tract opening until adhesive was seen to arise from the primary opening. The patients then had a petroleum jelly gauze placed on both the primary and secondary openings, and were discharged. The authors noted that in 1 year 26 (54%) of the patients treated with autologous fibrin tissue adhesive from their own blood had complete closure of their fistulas, whereas 34 of 53 patients (64%) treated with commercial fibrin sealant had closure of their fistulas. The authors conclude that the fibrin tissue adhesive offers a unique mode of managing fistulas which is surgically less invasive, but recurrence can occur up to 1 year. They also note that success with fibrin adhesive materials is dependent upon an adequate curettage of the fistula tracts.

References

1. Shouler PJ, Grimley RP, Keighley MR *et al.* Fistula-in-ano is usually simple to manage surgically. Int J Colorect Dis. 1986;1:113–15.
2. Gordon PH. Anorectal abscess and fistula-in-ano. In: Gordon PH, Nivatvongs S, editors. Principles and Practice of Surgery for the Colon, Rectum and Anus. St Louis: Quality Medical Publishing, 1992:221–65.
3. Parks AG, Gordon PH, Hardcastle JD. A classification of fistula-in-ano. Br J Surg. 1976;63:1–12.

4. Goldberg SM, Nivatvongs S. Principles of Surgery. New York: McGraw-Hill, 1979:12431.
5. Fazio VW. Complex anal fistula. Gastrointest Clin N Am. 1987;16:101.
6. Parks AG, Gordon PH. Fistula-in-ano perineal fistula of intra-abdominal or intrapelvic origin simulating fistula-in-ano: report of seven cases. Dis Colon Rectum. 1976;19:50.
7. Rafal RB, Nicholls JN, Cennerezzo WJ *et al*. MRI for the evaluation of perianal inflammation. Abdom Imaging. 1995;20:248–52.
8. Vasilevsky CA. Fistula-in-ano and abscess. In: Beck DE, Werner SD, editors. Fundamentals of Anorectal Surgery. Philadelphia: W. B. Saunders, 1998;153.
9. Law PJ, Talbot RW, Bartram CI, Northover JMA. Anal endosonography in the evaluation of perianal sepsis and fistula-in-ano. Br J Surg. 1989;76:752–5.
10. Seow-Choen F, Nicholls RJ. Anal fistula. Br J Surg. 1992;79:197–205.
11. Pearl RK, Andrews JR, Orsay CP *et al*. Role of the seton in the management of anorectal fistulas. Dis Colon Rectum. 1993;36:573–9.
12. Parks AG, Stitz RW. The treatment of high fistula-in-ano. Dis Colon Rectum. 1976;19:487–499.
13. Gordon PH. Management of anorectal abscess in fistulous disease. In: Kodner IJ, Frye RD, Roe JP, editors. Colon, Rectum and Anal Surgery. St Louis; CV Mosby, 1985;91–107.
14. Kodner IJ, Mazor A, Shemesh EI, *et al*. Endorectal advancement flap repair of rectovaginal and other complicated anorectal fistulas. Surgery. 1993;114:632–9.
15. Sangwan YP, Rosen L, Riether RD *et al*. Is simple fistula-in-ano simple? Dis Colon Rectum. 1994;37:885–9.
16. Aguilar PS, Plasencia G, Hardy TG *et al*. Mucosal advancement in the treatment of anal fistula. Dis Colon Rectum. 1985;28:496–8.
17. van Tets WF, Kuijpers HC. Continence disorders after anal fistulotomy. Dis Colon Rectum. 1994;37:1194–7.
18. Buchmann P, Keighley MRB, Allan RN *et al*. Natural history of perianal Crohn's disease: 10 year follow up. A plea for conservatism. Am J Surg. 1980;140:642–4.
19. Alexander-Williams J, Buchmann P. Perianal Crohn's disease. World J Surg. 1980;4:203–8.
20. Williams JG, Rothenberger DA, Nemer FD, Goldberg SM. Fistula-in-ano in Crohn's disease. Results of aggressive surgical treatment. Dis Colon Rectum. 1991;34:378–84.
21. Consten CJ, Siors FJM, Noten HJ *et al*. Anorectal surgery in human immunodeficiency virus-infected patients. Dis Colon Rectum. 1995;38:1169–75.
22. Abel ME, Chiu YS, Russell TR, Volpe PA. Autologous fibrin glue in the treatment of rectovaginal and complex fistulas. Dis Colon Rectum. 1993;36:447–9.
23. Kirkegaard P, Madsen PV. Perineal sinus after removal of the rectum: occlusion with fibrin adhesive. Am J Surg. 1983;145:791–4.
24. Hjortrup A, Moesgaard F, Kjaergard J. Fibrin adhesive in the treatment of perineal fistulas. Dis Colon Rectum. 1991;34:752–4.
25. Cintronn JR, Park JJ, Orsay CP. Repair of fistula-in-ano using fibrin adhesive: Long-term follow up. Dis Colon Rectum. 2000;43:994–50.

25
Therapy of perianal fistulas associated with Crohn's disease

J. SCHMIDT, P. KIENLE and C. HERFARTH

INTRODUCTION

Since the observation by Alexander-Williams[1] that incontinence in patients with perianal Crohn's disease is frequently the consequence of aggressive surgery, and less due to the progression of the disease itself, surgical therapy remains a matter of constant debate. Perianal fistulas represent a difficult problem in the management of Crohn's disease[2]. These fistulas can range from short submucosal anocutaneous to complex fistulas involving the upper or mid rectum, the vagina, the bladder, the urethra, the colon and the small intestine. They can have one or multiple internal and external openings or end as a blind tract. Frequently they originate from other parts of diseased bowel and travel down into the small pelvis where they can penetrate the pelvic floor and discharge through the skin. Perianal fistulas sometimes resolve when Crohn's disease in other parts of the gastrointestinal tract is treated successfully. Furthermore, these fistulas do not always cause symptoms, but may remain oligosymptomatic for long periods of time. Hence surgical therapy should be restricted to symptomatic fistulas or those that threaten the integrity of the sphincter apparatus. Medical treatment can be achieved by anti-inflammatory drugs (corticosteroids, 6-mercaptopurine)[3,4], antibiotics (metronidazole, ciprofloxacin)[5] or specific antibodies (anti-TNF etc.)[6]. Especially the latter should be used only within clinical trials as its long-term effectiveness and side-effects are not yet fully understood and abscess rates are high.

When treating a perianal fistula associated with Crohn's disease one should always attempt to obtain adequate histology to rule out specific inflammation or carcinoma[7]. In our experience we had three cases of fistula-associated carcinoma in patients with perianal fistula secondary to Crohn's disease.

SURGICAL MANAGEMENT

The following recommendations are based on the experience with 327 perianal operations for Crohn's disease performed at our institution since 1982, most of them due to perianal fistulas.

It was shown that 5–10% of all patients with Crohn's disease and 15–60% of surgical patients, demonstrate perianal fistulas. As mentioned previously, aggressive therapy should be restricted to symptomatic fistulas because many fistulas in Crohn's disease tend to reoccur and the integrity of the sphincter may be at risk if repair is attempted using inappropriate techniques. If an abscess is present, primary incision and drainage should be performed until the inflammation has settled. Frequently a seton is sufficient for continuous drainage and the fistula then remains asymptomatic. If symptoms are present, repair should be undertaken only if the rectum and anus are free of inflammation and after exact diagnosis of the fistula morphology, which can be done by thorough clinical examination, endosonography (Fig. 1)[8] and/or MRI (Fig. 2)[9]. If sphincter destruction is imminent by the septic-fistulizing process, we prefer to create a protective loop ileostomy or colostomy to transfer the problem into an elective setting[10]. For the surgical treatment of Crohn's associated fistulas it is imperative to identify the anatomical structures involved. The classification of perianal and perirectal fistulas according to Parks *et al.*[11] can easily be applied to Crohn's disease-associated fistulas (Table 1, Fig. 3).

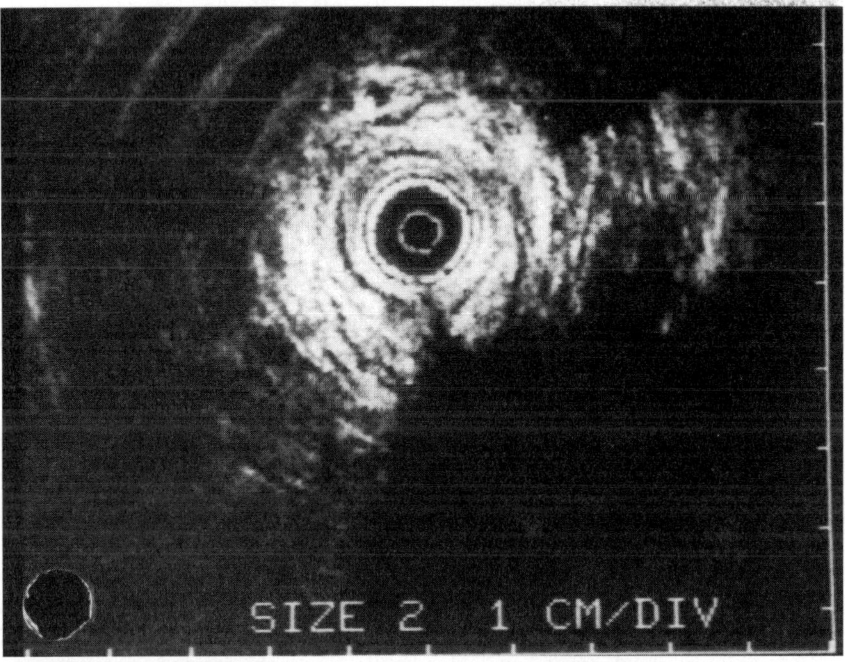

Figure 1 Endosonographic image of a trans-sphincteric fistula in a patient suffering from Crohn's disease. There is a penetration of both the internal and external sphincter at 5 o'clock. Treatment consisted of eradication of the local inflammation by local corticosteroids and metronidazole and a seton. In a second step mucosa advancement flap, in combination with careful excision of the external fistula tract, was performed. The sphincter penetration site was sutured using 4/0 PDS

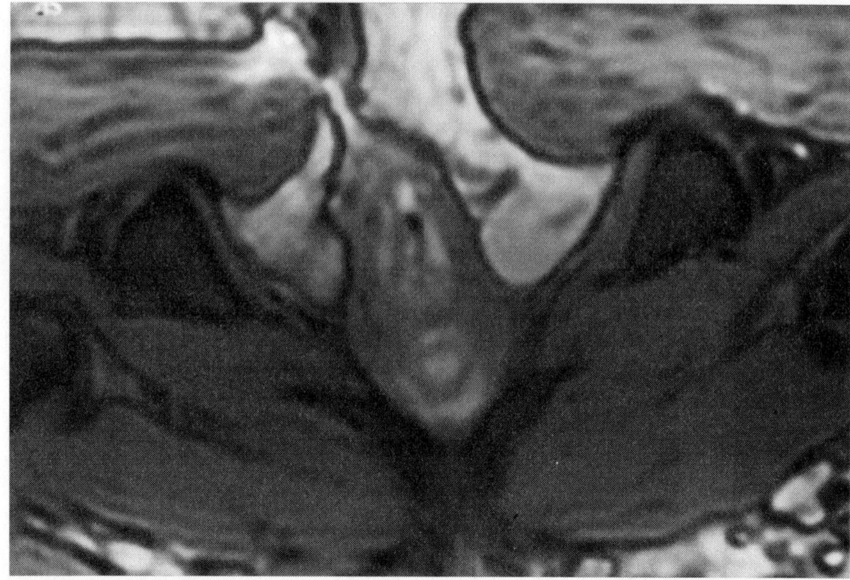

Figure 2 MR imaging of a similar trans-sphincteric fistula in Crohn's disease as in Fig. 1. The fistula penetrates both the internal and external sphincter at 11 o'clock and leads to some distortion of the anal canal. Treatment was identical to that in Fig. 1

Table 1 Fistula in ano according to Parks *et al.* (1976)[11]

Intersphincteric	Simple low tract, high blind tract, high tract with rectal opening, extrarectal extension, extrarectal genesis
Trans-sphincteric	Uncomplicated, high blind tract
Suprasphincteric	Uncomplicated, high blind tract
Extrasphincteric	Following anal fistulas, secondary to trauma, secondary to anorectal diseases, secondary to pelvic inflammation

INFRASPHINCTERIC OR SUBCUTANEOUS FISTULAS

Fistulas, that travel down from the dentate line without involving the sphincter ani are easy to treat. In most cases a simple 'open-lay' technique is sufficient to obtain secondary healing[12,13]. It is important that all fistula tracts are unroofed and potential perineal, scrotal or labial fistula tracts are drained. The unroofed fistula tracts can then be marsupialized to speed epithelialization. This local therapy must be accompanied by adequate perianal hygiene and systemic and/or local drug therapy, for example corticosteroids and antibiotics (e.g. metronidazole).

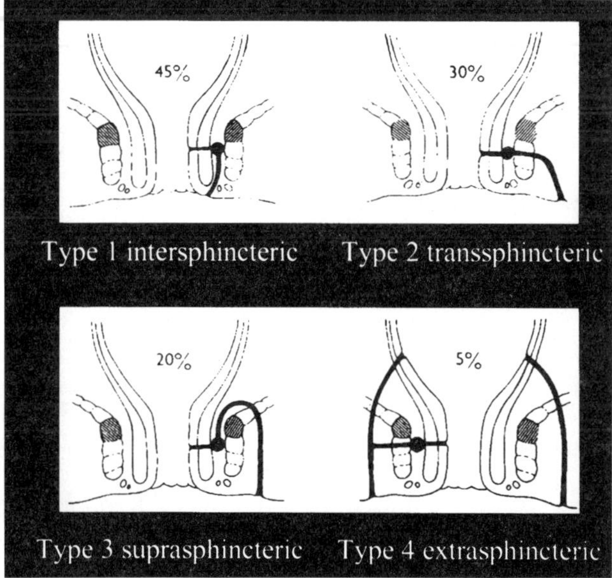

Figure 3 Parks classification of fistula in ano (see also Table 1)

INTERSPHINCTERIC FISTULAS

If the internal sphincter is penetrated, but the external sphincter is intact, and if the fistula tract is low (dentate line and below) surgical treatment is identical to that for subcutaneous fistulas. If there is a high intersphincteric fistula tract with or without internal opening treatment may be much more difficult, and there is no general rule for treatment. Depending on preoperative sphincter function, the extent of rectal involvement, the severity of symptoms and other factors, either the lay-open technique or drainage and mucosal advancement flap may be indicated[2,14]. In selected cases, especially in cases of recurrence, temporary stool deviation may be necessary.

TRANS-SPHINCTERIC FISTULAS

Fistulas that affect the internal and external sphincter, and originate within the anal canal, are much more difficult to treat (Figs 1 and 2). Low trans-sphincteric fistulas can also be treated by the lay-open technique ($>65\%$). The concept of treating all other (high) trans-sphincteric fistulas includes careful excision of the fistula tract (left open), suture of the excised sphincter penetration site (PDS 4/0) and a mucosa advancement flap[2,15]. In cases of high trans-sphincteric fistulas a temporary stool deviation is frequently necessary. In all cases, prior to repair, one should attempt to achieve an inflammation-free state by local and systemic therapy.

Table 2 Surgical procedures of the Department of Surgery University of Heidelberg in Crohn's disease (1982–2000)

Resection		Reconstruction	
Fistula procedures			
Small bowel	224	Stricturoplasty	175
Interenteric	216		
Ileocaecal resection	254	Fistula closure	159
Enterocutaneous	84		
Anastomotic resection	207	Omentoplasty	83
Enterogenital	67		
Colon segment	53	Reconstruction of continuity	14
Enterovesical	35		
Hemicolectomy	95	Closure of ileostomy	111
Retroperitoneal	35		
Subtotal colectomy	99	Closure of colostomy	6
Anal	260		
Proctocolectomy/proctectomy	64	Pouch construction	4
Deviation		*Other*	
Ileostomy	251	Abscess	156
Colostomy	39	Ureterolysis	20
Hartmann procedure	19	Explorative laparotomy	22
Intestinal bypass	3	Lavage	29
Gastroenterostomy	6	Endoscopic intervention	36
		Other	178

SUPRASPHINCTERIC AND EXTRASPHINCTERIC FISTULAS

These fistulas almost never heal without temporary stool deviation[16,17], the reason probably being the suprasphincteric high-pressure zone in the rectal ampulla, from where the fistula finds its way down if the rectum is inflamed (Figs 4 and 5). Our concept includes primary incision and drainage if a localized abscess is present. Subsequently we perform an exact diagnosis of the fistula type, and then stoma deviation, mostly by loop ileostomy. After an interval of at least 12 weeks, and after systemic and/or local therapy of the rectum (free of inflammation), and if the fistula origin is low in the anal canal, excision of the fistula tract, together with excision and suture of muscular rectal wall and mucosa (two-layer) is performed. If the fistula originates high in the anal canal, especially if the puborectal loop is involved, deep anterior resection of the rectum, possibly with coloanal anastomosis, may be necessary provided the neorectum is free of inflammation. In some cases, when the fistula system is complex and rectal involvement is severe, a Miles procedure with sphincter resection becomes necessary to obtain local control.

RECTOVAGINAL FISTULAS

A special example of extrasphincteric fistulas are rectovaginal fistulas. These fistulas originate typically just above the sphincter and drain into the introitus

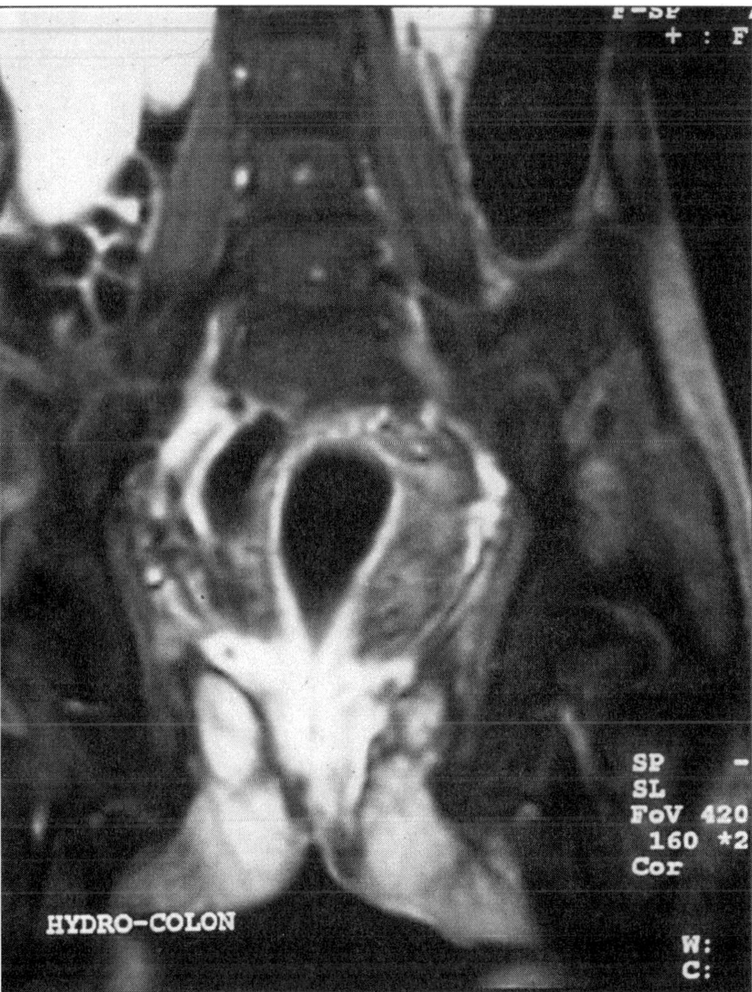

Figure 4 MR imaging of a translevatoric fistula associated with Crohn's disease. There is oedema and penetration of the left levator muscle by a fistula with a supralevatoric origin in the rectum which was heavily inflamed. Treatment consisted of deviation by loop ileostomy and secondary repair by mucosa advancement flap, excision and suture of the rectal wall and excision of the fistula tract below the levator muscle (left open for secondary healing). These fistulas have a tendency to recur mainly influenced by recurrence of rectal inflammation

vaginae. In our experience the therapy described in the literature[18,19] with simple excision and mucosa advancement flap without stoma is usually insufficient. Whenever possible, we perform a temporary deviation by loop ileostomy. After local inflammation has subsided, careful excision of the fistula tract, a mucosa advancement flap of the rectum, and levatorplasty, by joining both levators in the rectovaginal septum followed by suture of the vaginal epithelium, is performed.

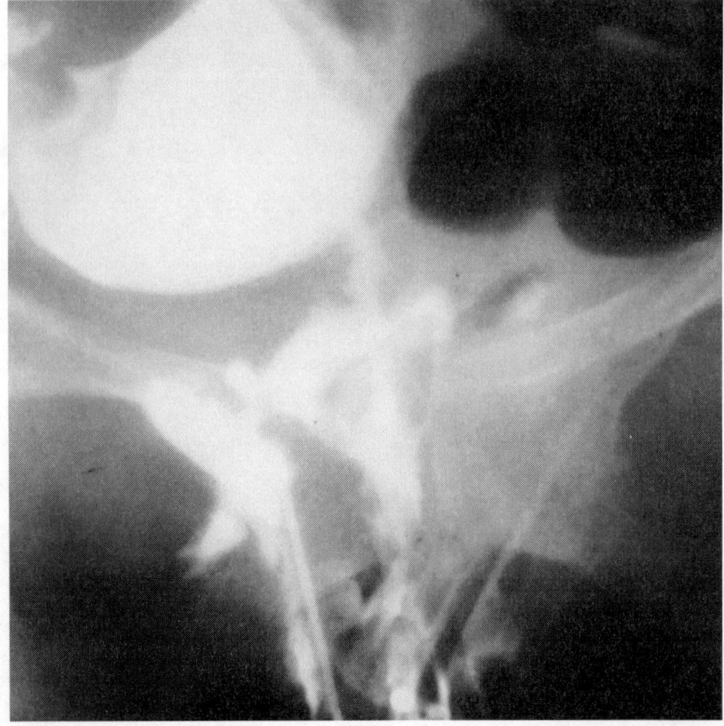

Figure 5 Scarring and narrowing of the rectum in a patient with rectal Crohn's disease. There is a complex trans-sphincteric and supralevatoric fistula system delineated by water-soluble contrast enema. Removal of the rectum and sphincter with permanent terminal colostomy was necessary for healing

After an interval of at least 3–6 months continuity can be restored. In our hands the latter technique led to no recurrences after 24 months in 15 cases of rectovaginal fistulas due to Crohn's disease[20].

FOLLOW-UP

The fact that Crohn's disease *per se* has a defined risk of recurrence makes a thorough follow-up mandatory. In our patient population we identified early onset of disease, proximal jejunal involvement and fistulas (interenteric and perianal) as independent risk factors for recurrence[21]. This is the reason why all patients with perianal fistulas require clinical follow-up, either in the outpatient department or by local gastroenterologists or surgeons with special expertise in this field. Regular mailing of IBDQ questionnaires[22] may be helpful in that regard, as this can reveal recurrent fistulas by a decrease in the quality of life with subsequent check-up and throrough examination and treatment.

References

1. Alexander-Williams J. Fistula in ano. Management of Crohn's fistula. Dis Colon Rectum. 1976; 19:518.
2. Athanasiadis S, Köhler A, Weyand G, Nafe M, Kuprian A, Oladeinde I. Endoanal and transperineal sphincter saving techniques in the surgical treatment of Crohn fistulas. A prospective longterm study in 186 patients. Chirurg 1996;67:59–71.
3. Present DH, Korelitz BI, Wisch N, Glass JL, Sachar DB, Pasternacle BS. Treatment of Crohn's disease with 6-mercaptopurine. A longterm, randomized, double blind study. N Engl J Med. 1980;302:981–7.
4. Pearson DC, May GR, Fick GH, Sutherland LR. Azathioprine and 6-mercaptopurine in Crohn's disease. A meta-analysis. Ann Intern Med. 1995;123:132–42.
5. Schneider MU, Laudage G, Guggenmoos-Holzmann I, Riemann JF. Metronidazole in the treatment of Crohn's disease. Results of controlled randomized prospective trials. Dtsch Med Wochenschr. 1985;110:1724–30.
6. Present DH, Rutgeerts P, Targan S et al. Infliximab for the treatment of fistulas in patients with Crohn's disease. N Engl J Med. 1999;340:1398–405.
7. Vernava AM 3rd. Cancer in chronic perianal fistulas of Crohn's disease. Dis Colon Rectum. 1999;42:282–3.
8. El Mouaaouy A, Tolksdorf A, Starlinger M, Becker HD. [Endoscopic sonography of the anorectum in inflammatory rectal diseases]. Z Gastroenterol. 1992;30:486–94.
9. Hansmann HJ, Kosa R, Düx M et al. Hydro-MRT chronisch entzündlicher Darmerkrankungen. Fortschr Roentgenstr. 1997;167:132–8.
10. Yamamoto T, Allan RN, Keighley MR. Effect of fecal diversion alone on perianal Crohn's disease. World J Surg. 2000;24:1258–63.
11. Parks AG, Gordon PH, Hardcastle JE. A classification of fistula in ano. Br J Surg. 1976;63:1–12.
12. Bayer I, Gordon PH. Selected operative management of fistula-in-ano in Crohn's disease. Dis Colon Rectum. 1994;37:760.
13. Bernard D, Morgan S, Tasse D. Selective surgical management of Crohn's disease of the anus. Can J Surg. 1986;29:318.
14. Hyman N. Endoanal advancement flap repair for complex anorectal fistulas. Am J Surg. 1999;178:337–40.
15. Berman IR. Sleeve advancement anorectoplasty for complicated anorectal/vaginal fistula. Dis Colon Rectum. 1991;34:1032.
16. Givel JC, Hawker P, Allan RN, Alexander-Williams J. Enterovaginal fistulas associated with Crohn's disease. Surg Gynecol Obstet. 1982;155:494.
17. Harper PH, Kettlewell MG, Lee EC. The effect of split ileostomy on perianal Crohn's disease. Br J Surg. 1982;69:608.
18. Rothenberger DA, Christenson CE, Balcos EG. Endorectal advancement flap for treatment of simple rectovaginal fistula. Dis Colon Rectum. 1981;25:297.
19. Radcliffe AG, Ritchie JK, Hawley PR, Lennard-Jones JE, Northover JMA. Anovaginal and rectovaginal fistulas in Crohn's disease. Dis Colon Rectum. 1988;31:94.
20. Herzog L, Herzog A, Glaser F, Herfarth C. Rektovaginale Fisteln bei Patienten mit Morbus Crohn: Therapie und Prognose. Langenbecks Arch Chir Suppl. 1998;II:1002–3.
21. Post S, Herfarth C, Böhm E, Timmermanns G, Schumacher H, Schürmann G, Golling M. The impact of diseases pattern, surgical management, and individual surgeons on the risk for relaparotomy for recurrent Crohn's disease. Ann Surg. 1996; 223:253–60.
22. Irvine EJ, Feagan B, Rochon J et al. Quality of life: a valid and reliable measure of therapeutic efficacy in the treatment of inflammatory bowel disease. Gastroenterology. 1994;106:287–96.

26
Perianal eczema

V. WIENERT

DEFINITION

Anal eczema is one of the most frequent proctological diseases. It is not a discrete disease entity *sui generis*, but is a concomitant manifestation of various different dermatological, allergological, microbiological or proctological processes.

AETIOPATHOGENESIS

The anal region is characterized by special anatomical features which favour the development of perianal eczema: the almost continuously closed anal cleft on the one hand and the retention of the excretion of the eccrine and apocrine sudorific glands which lead to the 'moist chamber' on the other hand. The following forms of eczema are distinguished:

Irritative toxic or cumulative toxic eczema

This form of eczema is the response of the skin to external irritants without development of specific immune reactions. In long-maintained exposure to the noxae the irritative toxic eczema gradually transforms into cumulative toxic eczema. The irritative toxic factors are, for example, ammoniacal or feculant secretions occurring as a result of proctological diseases which impair the fine closure of the anus (haemorrhoidal disease, prolapse) and reduce the muscular capacity to retain faeces (sphincter failure), but also conditions due to direct secretion into the perianal region affecting the perianal region (fistulas, condylomas). It is also a possible consequence of skin damage from irritant substances such as metal salts (cobalt, mercury, cadmium, zinc) or mechanical trauma (e.g. abrasive toilet paper). The extent of skin damage depends on the concentration, the duration of action of the noxae and the individual predisposition of the skin (e.g. atopic diathesis).

First, proctological diseases such as prolapse, incontinence, haemorrhoids, fistulas, chronic inflammatory intestinal diseases, condylomas, multiple or excessively large skin tags should be ruled out. Potentially irritative substances such as metal salts or toilet paper can be identified in the 'rub test' on the forearm.

If identified, the irritant is eliminated immediately. Definitive treatment of concomitant proctological conditions is urgently necessary.

Atopic eczema

The perianal region is a typical predilection site for this eczema that is closely related to atopic diathesis. The term 'atopy' designates a genetic predisposition to develop certain diseases. Atopic eczema of the anal region arises gradually on the basis of hypersensitivity reactions of the skin and mucosa to environmental antigens (type I allergy) associated with IgG formation.

The diagnosis is easy when other predilection sites such as the poplietal fossa and angle of the elbow are affected. If the condition is manifested only in the region of the anus, the clinical diagnosis becomes more difficult. Further investigation techniques must be used. Atopic diathesis of the skin can be diagnosed using the Erlangen point schedule for detecting a raised risk of eczema[1]. This schedule registers positive data in the patient's history and that of the family with regard to atopic diseases, as well as skins associated with atopy such as white dermatographism, sebostasis, palmar hyperlinearity, Hertoghe's sign, pilar keratosis or double infraorbital fold. The induction of white dermatographism has proved to be a helpful and reliable marker in diagnosis of atopic eczema. Almost 80% of all atopic patients show this sign, in contrast to 7% of the normal population[2]. The 'atopy patch test' can also provide a crucial indication: after epicutaneous application of IgE-inducing aeroallergens such as pollen and house dust mites, there is a dose-dependent eczematous reaction[3].

Initial short-term local application of a corticosteroid and subsequently coal tar preparation is recommended. In many cases irradiation with high-energy UVA light also causes this eczema to heal. Owing to the chronic recurrent course the patient must be instructed about interval therapy.

Allergic contact eczema

In this form of eczema the skin reacts to external foreign substances with a specific immunologically mediated inflammation (type IV allergy). These foreign substances are mostly constituents of skin-care preparations, sprays applied to the external genitals, proctological preparations and some types of moist toilet paper which have sometimes been used for years. The allergens chiefly detected are scents, cinchocaine HCl, mafenide, hexylresorcinol, lidocaine HCl, Albothyl®, chamomile extract, quinine sulphate and menthol. Allergic reaction is rare when dry toilet paper is used; possible eczematogens are cathon C6 and euxyl K 400[4,5].

The cause of the allergy is clarified with the epicutaneous test carried out with standard substances, the ointment bases, 'anal block' and if appropriate with suspect substances. After contact of the foreign substance with the epidermis the characteristic test reaction develops within 48–72 h.

If there is a suspicion of contact allergy all topically applied medications should be discontinued. Only indifferent topical products such as soft zinc paste (DAB 10) and aqueous emulsifying ointment should be applied up to time of allergological testing. If appropiate, topical corticosteroids (without preservatives) can also be applied for a short time.

DIFFERENTIAL DIAGNOSIS

The following diseases must be considered in terms of differential diagnosis: psoriasis inversa, anal candidiasis, erythrasma, perianal streptococcal dermatitis, Bowen's disease, Paget's disease, lichen ruber planus and lichen sclerosus et atrophicus.

Inversa or intertriginous psoriasis

This is manifested in the anal region as an itching, highly erythematous, rarely desquamating dermatitis often accompained by the pathognomonic rhagade in the anal cleft. Certain factors (secretion containing faeces, sweat) provoke psoriasis; they trigger the 'isomorphic' irritant effect.

The diagnosis is especially difficult when the manifestations of psoriasis such as dandruff beyond the hairline, affection of the elbow or knee, or stippled nails are absent. The diagnosis may be validated by histological investigation. Therapy consists in application of calcipotriol ointment or strength I Farber–Harris paste or dyes. Corticosteroid preparations should be applied for only a short time.

Anal candidiasis

Intestinal candidiasis with detection of *Candida albicans*, *tropicalis* or *glabrata* can lead to secondary *Candida* infection and thus to exacerbation of the anal eczema very much more frequently on predamaged skin in incontinent or immunosupressed patients than in healthy subjects.

The condition is appropriately detected by faecal investigation and perianal skin smear, by microscopic examination of the unincubated preparation and by culture.

Treatment is necessary only in unequivocal anal findings in conjunction with detection of intestinal pathogens.

Paste or lotions containing nystatin are applied, clearing the gastrointestinal tract if appropriate.

Erythrasma

Erythrasma is an infection of the perianal skin with a pigment-producing *Corynebacterium*. There is mostly an extensive, dry, desquamating sharply circumscribed focus that is light to dark brown in colour and sometimes even of reddish colour. After erythrasma has been present for some time, maceration, excoriation and lichenification are found owing to constant scratching. Erythrasma often causes pruritus or burning. If untreated, the skin changes spread continuously over months and years. Under the Wood lamp (UVA light, 366 nm), there is characteristic coral or salmon-red fluorescence of the porphyrin of the skin. In patients with thorough anal hygiene the fluorescence may be absent because the water-soluble porphyrins have been washed out[6].

The treatment consists in applying a gel containing erythromycin twice a day for 7 days[7,8]. In the event of recurrence, systemic administration of 250 mg erythromycin four times a day for 14 days is recommended.

Perianal streptococcal dermatitis (perianal cellulitis, perianal streptogenic dermatitis)

This is manifested as a perianal, sharply delimited erythema that is sometimes exudative and accompanied by formation of pustules in the periphery. It is caused by beta-haemolytic streptococci of group A (detection of the causative organism in culture). Symptoms are a burning or pain in defaecation and itching. In contrast to erysipelas, the patients' general well-being is not affected. Penicillin V (100 000 IU/kg body weight administered systemically per os for 10–14 days) is the therapy of choice. Erythromycin is indicated in penicillin allergy.

Bowen's disease

The disease is an obligatory precancer, an epidermal in-situ carcinoma. Unclearly delimited brownish-red non-prominent or only slightly raised erosive weeping foci of a few centimetres diameter are seen perianally. Intra-anally, Bowen's disease appears as a sharply delimited red velvety lesion, often interspersed with leukoplakia-like deposits. As a rule the disease occurs as a solitary lesion; yet multiple foci are also seen. In the focus itself, human papillomaviruses HPV 16/18/58 are found[9]. Bowen's disease occurs at every age, but is more frequent in women than in men. Patients report pain, pruritus and bleeding[10]. The course is always chronic, but in the long term a prickle-cell carcinoma arises. There are indications that Bowen disease patients develop secondary carcinomas (cutaneous, visceral)[11]. An unequivocal diagnosis is made on the basis of an exploratory biopsy with subsequent histological investigation. The treatment of choice is excision far into healthy tissue, possibly with covering of the defect.

Paget's disease

Paget's disease is a rather rare epidermotropic apocrine carcinoma of the sudorific glands which occurs in elderly patients. It is manifested perianally, intra-anally and intrarectally. Perianally, a sharply delimited pink to reddish slightly infiltrated area is shown which is partly covered with scales and partly shows erosions. Paget's disease (type 1) associated with rectal carcinoma is distinguished from Paget's disease (type 2), which only spreads cutaneously around the anus. The majority of patients complain of persistent itching[12]. In the presence of eczema-like lesions which are resistant to therapy, a Paget's disease must be considered. Ultimately the diagnosis can be made only on the basis of an exploratory excision with subsequent histological investigation. In positive findings, endoscopy is urgently necessary to rule out rectal carcinoma. The therapy of choice is extensive excision far into healthy tissue with histological checks of the excision margins, since as a rule the focus is very much more extensive than can be discerned clinically.

MORPHOLOGICAL FINDINGS

Perianal eczema is manifested around the anus and intra-anally. It is only occasionally confined to one segment of perianal skin. Depending on its acuity (acute, subacute, chronic) erythema, papules, seropapules, vesicles, erosions, lichenification but almost never scales are shown. Differential diagnosis of perianal eczema is not really possible on the basis of morphology alone.

CLINICAL PICTURE

The main symptom of all perianal eczemas is persistent and excruciating anal itching. Further symptoms are burning, soreness and weeping. As a rule, the condition is more intensive at night, so that patients are unable to sleep.

COURSE AND PROGNOSIS

The occurrence of perianal eczema for different lengths of time requires clinical differentiation between acute, subactue and chronic eczema. The longer a perianal eczema has been present, the more likely is its cause to be polyaetiological. For example, if an irritative toxic or atopic eczema occurs primarily, an allergic contact eczema easily superimposes itself as a result of sensitization in reduced barrier function, or anal candidiasis is manifested secondarily.

References

1. Diepgen TL, Fartasch M, Hornstein OP. Kriterien zur Beurteilung der atopischen Hautdiathese. Dermatosen. 1991;39:79–83.
2. Wein S, Blecher P, Ruzicka T. Die Rolle der Atopie in der Pathogenese des Analekzems. Hautkrht. 1994;69:113–19.
3. Darsow U, Vieluf D, Ring J. Atopy patch test with different vehicles and allergen concentrations – an approach to standardisation. J Allergy Clin Immunol. 1995;95:677–84.
4. Blecher T, Korting HC. Tolerance to different toilet paper preparations: toxicological and allergological aspects. Dermatology. 1995;191:299–304.
5. De Groot AC, Baar TJM, Terpstra H et al. Contact allergy to moist toilet paper. Contact Dermatitis. 1991;24:135–6.
6. Sindhuphak KW, Mac Donald E, Smith EB. Erythrasma. Overlooked or misdiagnosed? Int J Dermatol. 1995;24:95–6.
7. Paradisi M, Cianchini G, Angelo C et al. Efficacy of topical erythromycin in treatment of perianal streptococcal dermatitis. Pediatr Dermatol. 1993;10:297–8.
8. Paradisi M, Cianchini G, Angelo C et al. Perianal streptococcal dermatitis. Two familial cases. Cutis. 1994;54:341–2.
9. Uezato H, Hagiwara K, Munruno M et al. Detection of human papilloma virus type 58 in a case of perianal Bowen's disease coexistent with T-cell leukemia. J Dermatol. 1999;26:160–3.
10. Kreydon OP, Herzog U, Ackermann C et al. 11 cases of Bowen's disease. Schweiz Med Wochenschr. 1996;126:1536–40.
11. Graham JH, Helwig EB. Bowen's disease and its relationship to systemic cancer. Arch Derm Syph (Chicago). 1959;80:133–6.
12. Jensen SL, Sjölin KE, Shokoneh Amiri MH et al. Paget's disease of the anal margin. Br J Surg. 1988;75:1089–92.

27
Diagnosis and non-surgical treatment of faecal incontinence in the proctological practice

D. GEILE, I. ZINNER, F. ERBEL, M. SCHÄFER
and G. OSTERHOLZER

DIAGNOSTICS IN THE PROCTOLOGICAL PRACTICE

According to a study published by Pehl in the *Deutsches Ärzteblatt* in May 2000, incorporating the evaluations of seven authors, the prevalence of stool incontinence is between 0.3% and 1.5% of the population[1]. Estimates from 10 and more years ago indicated a prevalence of 10% of the adult population in the Federal Republic of Germany and in France[2]. The first evaluations, as far back as in 1984, of patient data in proctological practice indicated a frequency of manifest incontinence, in an initial examination of new patients, of 14.1%[3]; this order of magnitude has remained until today, as shown by the evaluations from between July 1999 and June 2000 (13.1% of patients in the practice).

By far the greatest proportion of patients suffer from an idiopathic incontinence; this term comprises several pathogeneses such as occult sphincter injuries, neurogenic and muscular degenerations, geriatric degenerative changes, reduced rectum compliance[4], and morphological deformations such as internal rectum prolapse.

Neurological conditions, iatrogenic damage (postnatal or resulting from operations) and gastroenterological conditions occur with a roughly equal frequency of 10.5%. The remaining 5% are a result of other causes, such as congenital deformations.

The above represents a greatly simplified breakdown – as a rule the different groups overlap in every direction and there are coincidences within the groups, as with idiopathic incontinence. For this reason several points should be considered with respect to making a basic practical diagnosis:

1. A multifactorial genesis is to be assumed in the case of faecal incontinence – in 80% of patients the condition has several causes[1].

2. The diagnosis of faecal incontinence is still made as a result of a carefully and precisely conducted *anamnesis*. It should be assumed that patients rarely comment on their complaints and symptoms of their own accord[5,6].
3. Continence and incontinence scores, and quality-of-life scores, should be regarded as precise aids not only for performing diagnoses but also for making evaluations and for population checks[7].
4. The type and extent of the damage, and a statement on the structures involved, are supplied through additional examinations, such as are to be discussed in the following.

The proctological examination procedure to be applied in diagnosing faecal incontinence can be divided into a general and a specific section. The basic diagnosis always consists of the five steps of proctological examination: anamnesis, inspection, digital examination, proctoscopy and rectoscopy.

The valency of the individual stages of the examination is known; what is interesting here is the categorization of digital examination as a specific diagnostic method for faecal incontinence. According to the study by Pehl, mentioned previously, digital examination is highly sensitive when it comes to judging pressure at rest (median 74%) and contraction pressure (median 78%). These values are derived from four studies comprising a total of 647 patients. The high specificity continues with respect to diagnosing a sphincter defect, whereby the median value is 85% (taken from six studies of a total of 289 patients). It is recommended that the person conducting the examination adheres to a plan of digital examination at rest in contraction function and in press function. An experienced examiner can thus gain extensive indications relating to pressure at rest, contraction pressure, asymmetries, morphological changes, rectoceles, prolapse form and also sensitivity and reflex behaviour in the anal region.

It must be emphasized that a 'normal' digital examination which does not produce any conspicuous findings can in no way exclude the existence of incontinence.

Coloscopy plays a particularly important role in the basic diagnosis of faecal incontinence. The figures from the practice show that in incontinent patients a disproportionately high frequency of sigmoid diverticuloses with motility changes occur in the region of the sigma possibly accompanied by signs of inflammation (see Table 1). Precisely how the pathogenic mechanism leads here to a decompensation of a just-about-adequate continence function still has to be clarified, but the conclusion that can definitely be drawn from these figures is that every time a 'new' instance of incontinence occurs, a coloscopy should be conducted. This applies in particular to older people; not only sigmoid diverticuloses

Table 1 Role of diverticulosis of the sigmoid in the diagnosis of faecal incontinence, 1 July 1999–30 June 2000

Number of patients	3960
With diverticula	472 (11.9%)
Patients with faecal incontinence	518
With diverticula	97 (18.7%)

Proktologisches Zentum München-Ost, 10/2000

but also tumours in this region, as well as, in rare cases, caecum tumours have a negative effect on anal function.

Additional methods of standard functional diagnosis are: endoanal sonography, manometry, and neurophysiological examinations such as EMG and nervus pudendus latency period measurement.

There is clear evidence of the valency of endo-anal sonography in sphincter lesions and post-partum injuries, from the Pehl study and also from many other authors, making it unnecessary to do likewise in this chapter.

Anal manometry can provide additional information regarding the pathophysiology of continence disorders[1]; it is particularly important in the practice for objectifying and quantifying changes in continence function. However, it is not able to deliver information regarding the aetiology of faecal incontinence. According to the Pehl study it has the highest valency in the detection of pathological functions, with a median of 88%, composed of five studies with a total of 471 patients. It appears just as high in the reduction of the function of the musculus sphincter ani externus, or contraction pressure, with a median value of 74%, taken from seven studies with 1160 patients. For all other functions the valency should be looked upon with a degree of doubt.

In the practice a number of simple and therefore only relatively evaluable methods of examination have proven worthwhile; for instance the microtip transducer can produce a good relationship to normal conditions, using the same method of examination applied by the same examiner each time. Table 2 shows the norm value attained in practice for the machine used there (Pelvicheck, Medicheck Company – Standard Instruments). The first 120 patients to be examined with this system in a proctological practice show significant deviations in all measured parameters (median values – Table 3).

A surface EMG is used to take sum potentials of sphincter contractions as a measure of sphincter strength, again only in relation to measurements to be evaluated. Both norm values and function values are given in Tables 2 and 3.

Table 2 Normal values of anal manometry in patients with no faecal incontinence ($n = 178$)

MARP	59.06 mmHg (SD 13.46)
MASP	100.53 mmHg (SD 19.13)
Difference amplitude	46.71 mmHg (SD 10.27)
Strength of contraction	16.09 μV (DS 3.04)

Table 3 Pathological values of anal manometry in patients with faecal incontinence ($n = 120$)

MARP	42.9 mmHg (SD 22.1)	$\alpha < 0.1\%$
MASP	70.6 mmHg (SD 22.2)	$\alpha < 0.1\%$
Differential amplitude	26.0 mmHg (SD 21.0)	$\alpha < 0.1\%$
Strength of contraction	13.5 μV (SD 4.9)	$\alpha < 0.1\%$

Table 4 Nerve damage in needle EMG in patients with clinically supposed neuropathy, 1999 ($n = 134$)

Without any findings	19
Only local muscle damage	23
Neurogenic damage	90

Proktologisches Zentum München-Ost, 10/2000

The surface EMG represents an excellent parameter of presenting contraction capability and contraction strength, and is used in treatment checking.

Why are neurophysiological examinations important in a practical diagnosis? Nearly half of all patients with a muscle disorder additionally display a neuropathy of the sphincter and pelvic floor muscles[8-11]. The prognosis not only of performing operative treatment but of conducting any treatment at all is dependent on the strength and actuality of the neurogenic degeneration[12,13]. The choice of treatment can also be determined in this way; for instance, whether to apply active or passive training.

Since the pudendus latency period measurement is relatively cost-intensive, in practice the needle EMG should be applied in cooperation with a neurologist. The indication to do so should present itself from previous history and from complaints, should really serious nerve damage be suspected. Table 4 shows the electromyographic findings taken from 134 patients with clinically suspected severe neuropathy . Nearly a third of the patients (31.3%) showed no kind of involvement of nerve function in faecal incontinence (Table 4).

In summary, it can be said that the needle EMG process, although also cost- and time-intensive, and unpleasant for the patient, does in certain cases provide indispensable information about the type and extent of nerve damage with respect to prognosis and treatment.

NON-SURGICAL TREATMENT OF FAECAL INCONTINENCE – TRAINING TREATMENT

Alongside such measures as regulating colon function, thickening the stool, skin care and counselling, all of which are well known by every doctor operating in this field, the various aspects of training are in the foreground of all forms of treatment. In the end only between 5% and 10% of patients are sent for immediate operative treatment and, even then, perioperative training treatment is often appropriate.

Methods which can be considered include: pelvic floor gymnastics, active sphincter training by way of biofeedback (electromyographically controlled nerve and muscle training), passive training by way of electrostimulation, and a combination of both methods.

It is important to be clearly aware of what cannot be trained:

1. Lack of a central function.
2. A completely destroyed nerve.
3. The musculus sphincter ani internus.

4. The musculus sphincter ani externus with a complete separation and dehiscence of more than a few millimetres.
5. A high levator deficiency.

All other patients can profit from training, not least those patients suffering from postoperative incontinence following extensive surgery in the rectal–anal region.

Both in the evaluation by Pehl (20 studies[1]) and in the statistics in the literature shown by Enck (25 studies, personal speech at the 118th Falk Symposium)[20], it is biofeedback training with a median valency of 73% positive results at the end of treatment which is the most successful type of training treatment. On the other hand there is a lack of targeted studies regarding pelvic floor gymnastics; in the end it is not possible for the doctor to check what the patient is in fact contracting!

Although the latest anatomical study indicates that there is indeed a connection between the gluteal muscles and the pelvic floor muscles in the rear anal circumference – as announced by Fritsch at the 118th Falk Symposium, 1 and 2 October 2000, this is in no way sufficient to apply an alternative training of the gluteal muscles to counter incontinence (the principle of 'overflow' does not work!).

The most effective methods so far are, for example, the 'New Callanetics' by B. Cantieni, as described in the book *Tiger Feeling*. In this book the patient is shown ways of controlling the contraction of individual sections of the pelvic floor.

However it is the biofeedback training method which affords better control. Biofeedback means that the patient can control, both qualitatively and quantitatively, his or her activity by means of light and tone signals. In the particular case of faecal incontinence the contractions of the striated sphincter and pelvic floor muscles can be converted into electrical or pressure signals.

Surface electromyography has continued to be an excellent control method for use in the practice, since it reacts separately to sphincter and levator contractions and, with respect to the gluteal muscles, it does not absorb any signals, in contrast to the pressure-controlled sensor. Via two surface electrodes mounted on an anal sensor, at the 3 and 9 o'clock lithotomy positions, the sum activity potentials are registered and converted into a voltage; the unit corresponds to 1 'μV' (Pelvi Plus machine from Medicheck – Standard Instruments). The patient is taught the training technique in monitored sessions in the practice. This is followed by a period of further training at home, between 15 and 20 min, twice a day. The training should be continued for at least 6 months – this figure should be considered the norm value. The latter does not apply to those patients who, after a very short space of time, have learnt to produce sufficient sphincter contractions. The following must therefore be considered in the course of the training:

1. For some patients the learning process itself is of prime importance. Once learnt, the muscle functions of the musculus sphincter ani externus and levator are sufficient. This applies in particular to children and young adults (Figs 1 and 2).
2. A weariness phase should be expected after 8–12 weeks. As a rule the first check-up examination after 3 months falls within this period, and it is often the case that the patient has resigned himself or herself to giving up the training, describing it as pointless. Experience shows, however, that the real rebuilding training begins after this weariness phase (Fig. 3).

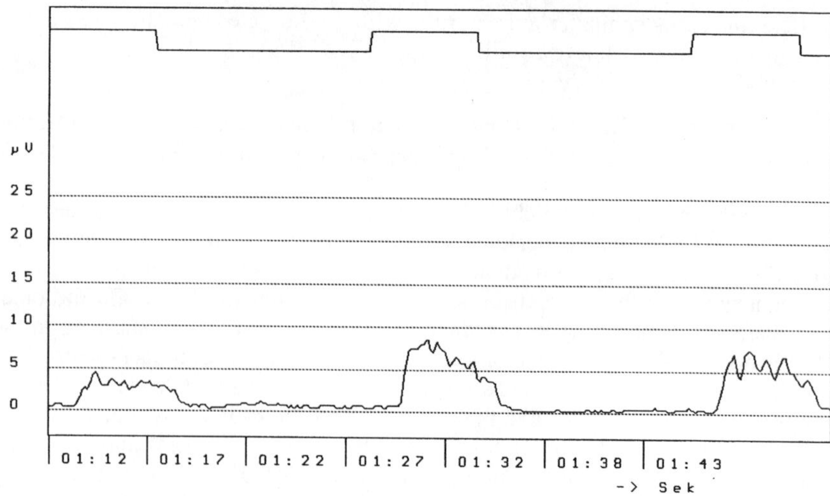

Figure 1 Patient SA, Contraction strength at the beginning of biofeedback therapy (age 36 y)

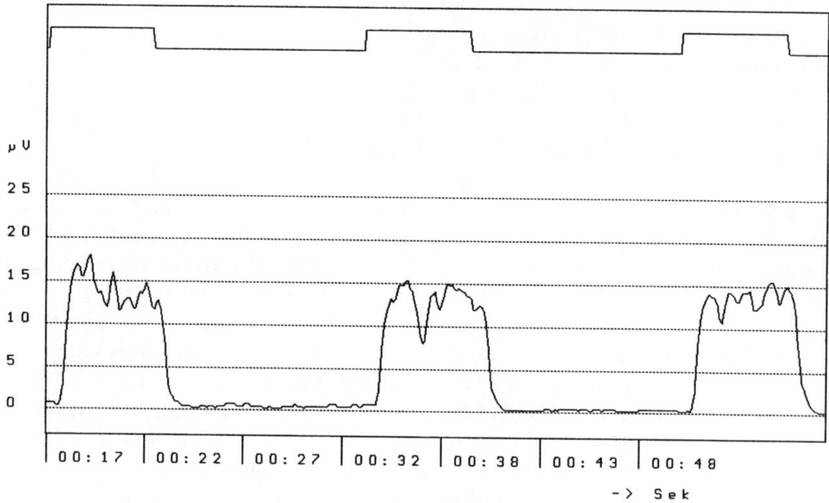

Figure 2 Patient SA: Contraction strength after 2 months of training

3. The rebuilding and strengthening phase of the striated muscles is longer in older patients.

The short-term results of some patients following the end of the controlled treatment are shown in Table 5; it is possible to provide help to nearly 80% of all patients.

The long-term results are, however, significantly poorer. For instance, Jensen and Lowry[14] describe a reduction of the success rate from 80% to 41% after a

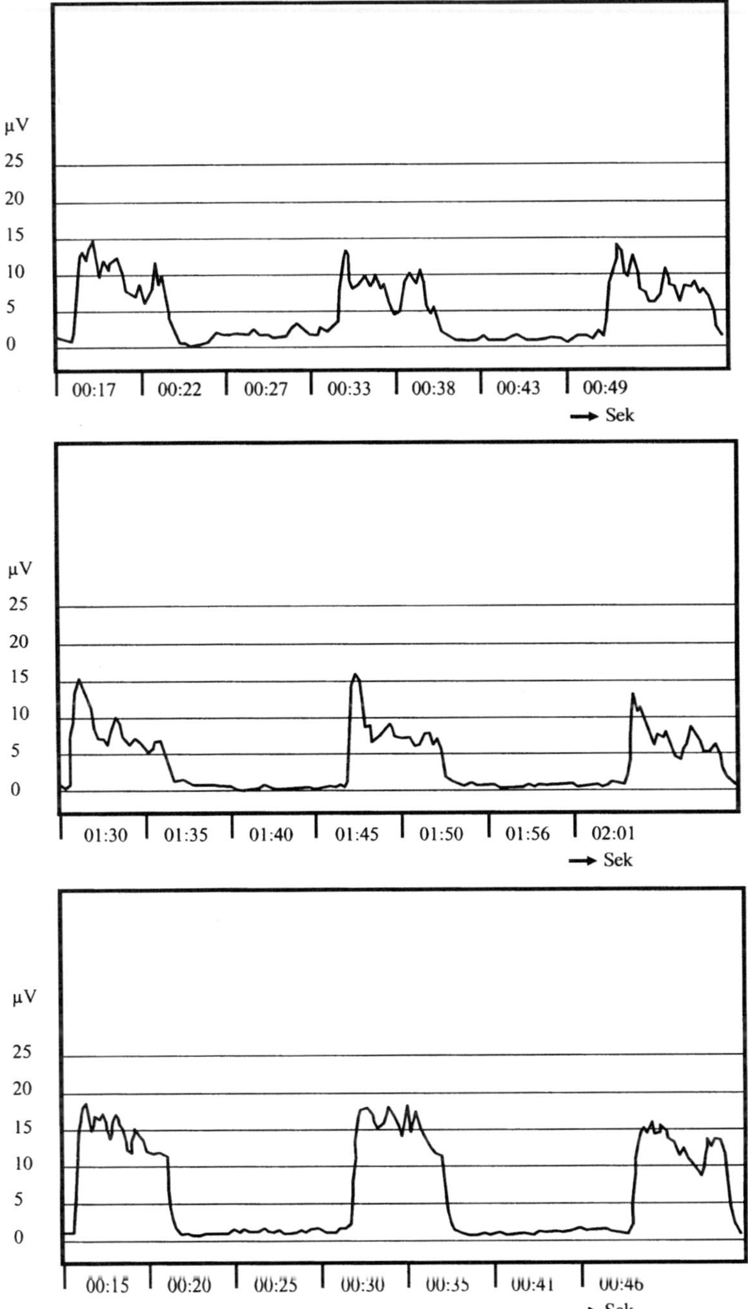

Figure 3 Patient born 21.11.34. Contraction strength at the beginning of therapy, after 7 weeks and after 16 weeks of training

Table 5 Biofeedback short-term results in proctological practice, 1990–June 2000 ($n = 301$)

Without any complaints	181 (60.1%)
Improved	65 (21.6%)
No improvement	25 (8.3%)
Therapy stopped precociously	30 (10%)

Proktologisches Zentum München-Ost, 10/2000

Table 6 Significant difference in CACP continence score 2–4 years after the end of biofeedback therapy ($n = 35$)

	Median score							
Before therapy	1.3 ± 0.7	1.1 ± 0.7	1.3 ± 0.7	0.9 ± 0.7	0.9 ± 0.7	1.8 ± 1.4	0.5 ± 0.6	0.5 ± 0.5	**8.3 ± 4.2**
2–4 years after therapy	1.6 ± 0.6	1.6 ± 0.5	1.8 ± 0.4	1.3 ± 0.7	1.3 ± 0.7	2.7 ± 1.3	0.9 ± 0.5	0.4 ± 0.5	**11.6 ± 3.3**

period of 30 months. An evaluation of a study by Enck from 1994 (12 studies)[15] quotes a return or improvement of continence 2 years after training in 41–63% of cases. This worsening seems to be dependent on the following factors: the duration of the training, ending the domestic further training with no machine, age (!), severity of the neuropathy. However, long-term success seems to be independent both of the cause and severity of the incontinence and of the parameters of the functional diagnosis. The interval does not seem to lead to an increase in the number of failures – after 4 years the proportion of successfully treated patients is approximately at the same level as after 2 years following the end of the training[15]. Table 6 shows one of our own long-term evaluations, using a continence score (CAP after Herold) 2–4 years after ending treatment on 35 evaluable patients. The improvement to the score after this time is significant. Figure 4 is evidence of the dependency of age on long-term success, among the same group of patients. The group of over 60-year-olds shows this worsening.

It is still difficult to judge the effectiveness of electrostimulation as a method of passive training for the striated muscles. The relatively euphoric estimates by Melzer and Knoch[16] cannot yet be proved. However, animal experiments can show a significant increase in pressure at rest after passive stimulation of the striated musculus sphincter ani externus[17]. According to research by Jost, contraction intensity and continence score can be considerably improved[18]. The study by Österberg et al.[19], conducted in 1999, shows an increase in sensitivity for the recto-anal inhibition reflex along with an improvement of the retention capability.

Within our own patient group studied, an indication for passive stimulation has so far been taken very strictly. Only the most severe denervation or extensive nerve damage in the presence of a certain residual sensitivity are subjected to training. Table 7 shows the results of the – only recently integrated – treatment,

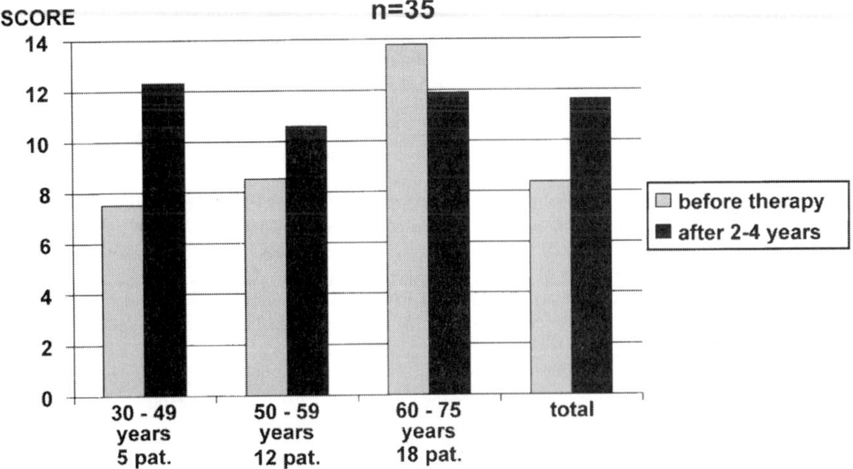

Figure 4   Influence of age on long-term result after biofeedback therapy

Table 7   Electrostimulation in severe denervation – results of anal manometry after 3–6 months of therapy ($n = 6$)

Patient	MAR (mmHg)		MAS (mmHg)	
	Initial	Post-therapy	Initial	Post-therapy
L.M.	41	51	48	75
H.J.	13	41	40	50
R.E.	35	50	40	59
B.J.	34	45	51	65
P.M.	87	90	41	79
L.A.	34	55	104	184

Proktologisches Zentum München-Ost, 10/2000

after 2–6 months. For six out of seven patients both pressure qualities are considerably improved. The number of patients is too small, and the results of the evaluation of the clinical data are still awaited.

In summary, the following can be said about passive electrostimulation:

1. It can sometimes replace the damaged nerve connection by direct muscle stimulation.
2. It may therefore have to be continued for the patient's whole life.
3. It can be used for a shorter period as initial training for creating awareness of the correct muscle groups and the desired function.

In combination with active biofeedback training, this leads to the possibility of non-surgical incontinence treatment, whose promising results should be able to put an end to the negative attitude of doctors and patients towards such treatment of faecal incontinence.

References

1. Pehl C, Birkner B, Bittman W *et al*. Stuhlinkontinez, Diagnostisches und therapeutisches Stufenschema. Deutsche Ärzteblatt. 2000;19:A-1302–8.
2. Denis P, Bercroff E, Bizien MF *et al*. Prevalence of anal incontinence in adults. Gastroenterol Clin Biol. 1992;16:344–50.
3. Geile D, Hauck R, Hörbrand F. Inkontinenz in der Proktologie: Symptomatik und konservative Therapie. Kontinenz. 1995;4:74–7.
4. Mitrani C, Chun A, Desautels S, Wald A. Anorectal manometric charateristics in men and women with idiopathic fecal incontinence. J Clin Gastroenterol. 1998;26:175–8.
5. Abramowitz L, Sobhani I, Ganansia R *et al*. Are sphincter defects the cause of anal incontinence after vaginal delivery? Results of a prospective study. Dis Colon Rectum. 2000;43:590–8.
6. Sultan AH, Kamm MA, Bartram CI, Hudson CN. Anal sphincter trauma during instrumental delivery. A comparison between forceps and vacuum extraction. Int J Gynaecol Obstet. 1993;43:263–70.
7. Rockwood TH, Church JM, Fleshman JW *et al*. Fecal incontinence quality of life scale: quality of life instrument for patients with fecal incontinence. Dis Colon Rectum. 2000;43:9–16.
8. Aubert A, Mosnier H, Amarenco G *et al*. Postsurgical or traumatic anal incontinences. Prospective study in 40 patients explored by endorectal ultrasonography and electromyography. Gastroenterol Clin Biol. 1995;19:598–603.
9. Cheong DM, Vaccaro CA, Salanga VD, Wexner SD, Phillips RC, Hanson MR. Electrodiagnostic evaluation of fecal incontinence. Muscle Nerve. 1995;18:612–19.
10. Felt-Bersma RJ, van Baren R, Koorevaar M, Strijers RL, Cuesta MA. Unsuspected sphincter defects shown by anal endosonography after anorectal surgery. Dis Colon Rectum. 1995;38:248–53.
11. Venerva III AM, Longo WE, Daniel GL. Pudendal neuropathy and the importance of EMG evaluation of fecal incontinence. Dis Colon Rectum. 1993;36:23–7.
12. Roig JV, Villoslada C, Lledo S *et al*. Prevalence of pudendal neuropathy in fecal incontinence. Dis Colon Rectum. 1995;38:952–8.
13. Snooks SJ, Barnes PR, Swash M, Henry MM. Damage to the innervation of the pelvic floor musculature in chronic constipation. Gatroenterology. 1985;89:977–81.
14. Jensen LL, Lowry AC. Biofeedback improves functional outcome after sphincteroplasty. Dis Colon Rectum. 1997;40:197–200.
15. Enck P, Däublin G, Lübke HJ, Strohmeyer G. Long term efficacy of biofeedback training for fecal incontinence. Dis Colon Rectum. 1994;37:997–1001.
16. Melzer B, Knoch HG. Die Elecktrotherapie bei analer Inkontinenz. Zbl Chirurgie. 1985;110:699–704.
17. Lorenz D, Karaorman M, Wipfler G, Junemann P, Richter A, Rumstadt B. Verbesserung der analen Kontinenz durch selektive Stimulation des M. sphincter ani externus. Langenbecks Arch Chir. 1997;382:311–18.
18. Jost WH. Electrostimulation in fecal incontinence: relevance of the sphincteric compound muscle action potential. Dis Colon Rectum. 1998;41:590–2.
19. Österberg A, Graf W, Eeg-Olofsson K, Hallden M, Phalman L. Is electrostimulation of the pelvic floor an effective treatment for neurogenic fecal incontinence. Scand J Gastroenterol. 1999;34:319–24.
20. Enck P. Biofeedbeck treatment of fecal incontinence. Z Gastroenterol. 1990;25:123–6.

Index

Falk Symposium Series

43. Reutter W, Popper H, Arias IM, Heinrich PC, Keppler D, Landmann L, eds.: *Modulation of Liver Cell Expression*. Falk Symposium No. 43. 1987   ISBN: 0-85200-677-2*

44. Boyer JL, Bianchi L, eds.: *Liver Cirrhosis*. Falk Symposium No. 44. 1987
     ISBN: 0-85200-993-3*

45. Paumgartner G, Stiehl A, Gerok W, eds.: *Bile Acids and the Liver*. Falk Symposium No. 45. 1987   ISBN: 0-85200-675-6*

46. Goebell H, Peskar BM, Malchow H, eds.: *Inflammatory Bowel Diseases – Basic Research & Clinical Implications*. Falk Symposium No. 46. 1988   ISBN: 0-7462-0067-6*

47. Bianchi L, Holt P, James OFW, Butler RN, eds.: *Aging in Liver and Gastrointestinal Tract*. Falk Symposium No. 47. 1988   ISBN: 0-7462-0066-8*

48. Heilmann C, ed.: *Calcium-Dependent Processes in the Liver*. Falk Symposium No. 48. 1988   ISBN: 0-7462-0075-7*

50. Singer MV, Goebell H, eds.: *Nerves and the Gastrointestinal Tract*. Falk Symposium No. 50. 1989   ISBN: 0-7462-0114-1

51. Bannasch P, Keppler D, Weber G, eds.: *Liver Cell Carcinoma*. Falk Symposium No. 51. 1989   ISBN: 0-7462-0111-7

52. Paumgartner G, Stiehl A, Gerok W, eds.: *Trends in Bile Acid Research*. Falk Symposium No. 52. 1989   ISBN: 0-7462-0112-5

53. Paumgartner G, Stiehl A, Barbara L, Roda E, eds.: *Strategies for the Treatment of Hepatobiliary Diseases*. Falk Symposium No. 53. 1990   ISBN: 0-7923-8903-4

54. Bianchi L, Gerok W, Maier K-P, Deinhardt F, eds.: *Infectious Diseases of the Liver*. Falk Symposium No. 54. 1990   ISBN: 0-7923-8902-6

55. Falk Symposium No. 55 not published

55B. Hadziselimovic F, Herzog B, Bürgin-Wolff A, eds.: *Inflammatory Bowel Disease and Coeliac Disease in Children*. International Falk Symposium. 1990 ISBN 0-7462-0125-7

56. Williams CN, eds.: *Trends in Inflammatory Bowel Disease Therapy*. Falk Symposium No. 56. 1990   ISBN: 0-7923-8952-2

57. Bock KW, Gerok W, Matern S, Schmid R, eds.: *Hepatic Metabolism and Disposition of Endo- and Xenobiotics*. Falk Symposium No. 57. 1991   ISBN: 0-7923-8953-0

58. Paumgartner G, Stiehl A, Gerok W, eds.: *Bile Acids as Therapeutic Agents: From Basic Science to Clinical Practice*. Falk Symposium No. 58. 1991   ISBN: 0-7923-8954-9

59. Halter F, Garner A, Tytgat GNJ, eds.: *Mechanisms of Peptic Ulcer Healing*. Falk Symposium No. 59. 1991   ISBN: 0-7923-8955-7

60. Goebell H, Ewe K, Malchow H, Koelbel Ch, eds.: *Inflammatory Bowel Diseases – Progress in Basic Research and Clinical Implications*. Falk Symposium No. 60. 1991
     ISBN: 0-7923-8956-5

61. Falk Symposium No. 61 not published

62. Dowling RH, Folsch UR, Löser Ch, eds.: *Polyamines in the Gastrointestinal Tract*. Falk Symposium No. 62. 1992   ISBN: 0-7923-8976-X

63. Lentze MJ, Reichen J, eds.: *Paediatric Cholestasis: Novel Approaches to Treatment*. Falk Symposium No. 63. 1992   ISBN: 0-7923-8977-8

64. Demling L, Frühmorgen P, eds.: *Non Neoplastic Diseases of the Anorectum*. Falk Symposium No. 64. 1992   ISBN: 0-7923-8979-4

64B. Gressner AM, Ramadori G, eds.: *Molecular and Cell Biology of Liver Fibrogenesis*. International Falk Symposium. 1992   ISBN: 0-7923-8980-8

*These titles were published under the MTP Press imprint.

Falk Symposium Series

Falk Symposium Series

82B. Paumgartner G, Beuers U, eds.: *Bile Acids in Liver Diseases*. International Falk Workshop. 1995
ISBN 0-7923-8891-7

83. Dobrilla G, Felder M, de Pretis G, eds.: *Advances in Hepatobiliary and Pancreatic Diseases: Special Clinical Topics*. Falk Symposium 83. 1995.
ISBN 0-7923-8892-5

84. Fromm H, Leuschner U, eds.: *Bile Acids – Cholestasis – Gallstones: Advances in Basic and Clinical Bile Acid Research*. Falk Symposium 84. 1995
ISBN 0-7923-8893-3

85. Tytgat GNJ, Bartelsman JFWM, van Deventer SJH, eds.: *Inflammatory Bowel Diseases*. Falk Symposium 85. 1995
ISBN 0-7923-8894-1

86. Berg PA, Leuschner U, eds.: *Bile Acids and Immunology*. Falk Symposium 86. 1996
ISBN 0-7923-8700-7

87. Schmid R, Bianchi L, Blum HE, Gerok W, Maier KP, Stalder GA, eds.: *Acute and Chronic Liver Diseases: Molecular Biology and Clinics*. Falk Symposium 87. 1996
ISBN 0-7923-8701-5

88. Blum HE, Wu GY, Wu CH, eds.: *Molecular Diagnosis and Gene Therapy*. Falk Symposium 88. 1996
ISBN 0-7923-8702-3

88B. Poupon RE, Reichen J, eds.: *Surrogate Markers to Assess Efficacy of TReatment in Chronic Liver Diseases*. International Falk Workshop. 1996
ISBN 0-7923-8705-8

89. Reyes HB, Leuschner U, Arias IM, eds.: *Pregnancy, Sex Hormones and the Liver*. Falk Symposium 89. 1996
ISBN 0-7923-8704-X

89B. Broelsch CE, Burdelski M, Rogiers X, eds.: *Cholestatic Liver Diseases in Children and Adults*. International Falk Workshop. 1996
ISBN 0-7923-8710-4

90. Lam S-K, Paumgartner P, Wang B, eds.: *Update on Hepatobiliary Diseases 1996*. Falk Symposium 90. 1996
ISBN 0-7923-8715-5

91. Hadziselimovic F, Herzog B, eds.: *Inflammatory Bowel Diseases and Chronic Recurrent Abdominal Pain*. Falk Symposium 91. 1996
ISBN 0-7923-8722-8

91B. Alvaro D, Benedetti A, Strazzabosco M, eds.: *Vanishing Bile Duct Syndrome – Pathophysiology and Treatment*. International Falk Workshop. 1996
ISBN 0-7923-8721-X

92. Gerok W, Loginov AS, Pokrowskij VI, eds.: *New Trends in Hepatology 1996*. Falk Symposium 92. 1997
ISBN 0-7923-8723-6

93. Paumgartner G, Stiehl A, Gerok W, eds.: *Bile Acids in Hepatobiliary Diseases – Basic Research and Clinical Application*. Falk Symposium 93. 1997
ISBN 0-7923-8725-2

94. Halter F, Winton D, Wright NA, eds.: *The Gut as a Model in Cell and Molecular Biology*. Falk Symposium 94. 1997
ISBN 0-7923-8726-0

94B. Kruse-Jarres JD, Schölmerich J, eds.: *Zinc and Diseases of the Digestive Tract*. International Falk Workshop. 1997
ISBN 0-7923-8724-4

95. Ewe K, Eckardt VF, Enck P, eds.: *Constipation and Anorectal Insufficiency*. Falk Symposium 95. 1997
ISBN 0-7923-8727-9

96. Andus T, Goebell H, Layer P, Schölmerich J, eds.: *Inflammatory Bowel Disease – from Bench to Bedside*. Falk Symposium 96. 1997
ISBN 0-7923-8728-7

97. Campieri M, Bianchi-Porro G, Fiocchi C, Schölmerich J, eds. *Clinical Challenges in Inflammatory Bowel Diseases: Diagnosis, Prognosis and Treatment*. Falk Symposium 97. 1998
ISBN 0-7923-8733-3

98. Lembcke B, Kruis W, Sartor RB, eds. *Systemic Manifestations of IBD: The Pending Challenge for Subtle Diagnosis and Treatment*. Falk Symposium 98. 1998
ISBN 0-7923-8734-1

Falk Symposium Series

99. Goebell H, Holtmann G, Talley NJ, eds. *Functional Dyspepsia and Irritable Bowel Syndrome: Concepts and Controversies.* Falk Symposium 99. 1998
ISBN 0-7923-8735-X

100. Blum HE, Bode Ch, Bode JCh, Sartor RB, eds. *Gut and the Liver.* Falk Symposium 100. 1998
ISBN 0-7923-8736-8

101. Rachmilewitz D, ed. *V International Symposium on Inflammatory Bowel Diseases.* Falk Symposium 101. 1998
ISBN 0-7923-8743-0

102. Manns MP, Boyer JL, Jansen PLM, Reichen J, eds. *Cholestatic Liver Diseases.* Falk Symposium 102. 1998
ISBN 0-7923-8746-5

102B. Manns MP, Chapman RW, Stiehl A, Wiesner R, eds. *Primary Sclerosing Cholangitis.* International Falk Workshop. 1998.
ISBN 0-7923-8745-7

103. Häussinger D, Jungermann K, eds. *Liver and Nervous System.* Falk Symposium 102. 1998
ISBN 0-7924-8742-2

103B. Häussinger D, Heinrich PC, eds. *Signalling in the Liver.* International Falk Workshop. 1998
ISBN 0-7923-8744-9

103C. Fleig W, ed. *Normal and Malignant Liver Cell Growth.* International Falk Workshop. 1998
ISBN 0-7923-8748-1

104. Stallmach A, Zeitz M, Strober W, MacDonald TT, Lochs H, eds. *Induction and Modulation of Gastrointestinal Inflammation.* Falk Symposium 104. 1998
ISBN 0-7923-8747-3

105. Emmrich J, Liebe S, Stange EF, eds. *Innovative Concepts in Inflammatory Bowel Diseases.* Falk Symposium 105. 1999
ISBN 0-7923-8749-X

106. Rutgeerts P, Colombel J-F, Hanauer SB, Schölmerich J, Tytgat GNJ, van Gossum A, eds. *Advances in Inflammatory Bowel Diseases.* Falk Symposium 106. 1999
ISBN 0-7923-8750-3

107. Špičák J, Boyer J, Gilat T, Kotrlik K, Mareček Z, Paumgartner G, eds. *Diseases of the Liver and the Bile Ducts – New Aspects and Clinical Implications.* Falk Symposium 107. 1999
ISBN 0-7923-8751-1

108. Paumgartner G, Stiehl A, Gerok W, Keppler D, Leuschner U, eds. *Bile Acids and Cholestasis.* Falk Symposium 108. 1999
ISBN 0-7923-8752-X

109. Schmiegel W, Schölmerich J, eds. *Colorectal Cancer – Molecular Mechanisms, Premalignant State and its Prevention.* Falk Symposium 109. 1999
ISBN 0-7923-8753-8

110. Domschke W, Stoll R, Brasitus TA, Kagnoff MF, eds. *Intestinal Mucosa and its Diseases – Pathophysiology and Clinics.* Falk Symposium 110. 1999
ISBN 0-7923-8754-6

110B. Northfield TC, Ahmed HA, Jazwari RP, Zentler-Munro PL, eds. *Bile Acids in Hepatobiliary Disease.* Falk Workshop. 2000
ISBN 0-7923-8755-4

111. Rogler G, Kullmann F, Rutgeerts P, Sartor RB, Schölmerich J, eds. *IBD at the End of its First Century.* Falk Symposium 111. 2000
ISBN 0-7923-8756-2

112. Krammer HJ, Singer MV, eds. *Neurogastroenterology: From the Basics to the Clinics.* Falk Symposium 112. 2000
ISBN 0-7923-8757-0

113. Andus T, Rogler G, Schlottmann K, Frick E, Adler G, Schmiegel W, Zeitz M, Schölmerich J, eds. *Cytokines and Cell Homeostasis in the Gastrointestinal Tract.* Falk Symposium 113. 2000
ISBN 0-7923-8758-9

114. Manns MP, Paumgartner G, Leuschner U, eds. *Immunology and Liver.* Falk Symposium 114. 2000
ISBN 0-7923-8759-7

115. Boyer JL, Blum HE, Maier K-P, Sauerbruch T, Stalder GA, eds. *Liver Cirrhosis and its Development*. Falk Symposium 115. 2000	ISBN 0-7923-8760-0

116. Riemann JF, Neuhaus H, eds. *Interventional Endoscopy in Hepatology*. Falk Symposium 116. 2000	ISBN 0-7923-8761-9

116A. Dienes HP, Schirmacher P, Brechot C, Okuda K, eds. *Chronic Hepatitis: New Concepts of Pathogenesis, Diagnosis and Treatment*. Falk Workshop. 2000
	ISBN 0-7923-8763-5

117. Gerbes AL, Beuers U, Jüngst D, Pape GR, Sackmann M, Sauerbruch T, eds. *Hepatology 2000 – Symposium in Honour of Gustav Paumgartner*. Falk Symposium 117. 2000
	ISBN 0-7923-8765-1

117A. Acalovschi M, Paumgartner G, eds. *Hepatobiliary Diseases: Cholestasis and Gallstones*. Falk Workshop. 2000	ISBN 0-7923-8770-8

118. Frühmorgen P, Bruch H-P, eds. *Non-Neoplastic Diseases of the Anorectum*. Falk Symposium 118. 2001	ISBN 0-7923-8766-X

119. Fellermann K, Jewell DP, Sandborn WJ, Schölmerich J, Stange EF, eds. *Immuno-suppression in Inflammatory Bowel Diseases – Standards, New Developments, Future Trends*. Falk Symposium 119. 2001	ISBN 0-7923-8767-8

120. van Berge Henegouwen GP, Keppler D, Leuschner U, Paumgartner G, Stiehl A, eds. *Biology of Bile Acids in Health and Disease*. Falk Symposium 120. 2001
	ISBN 0-7923-8768-6

121. Leuschner U, James OFW, Dancygier H, eds. *Steatohepatitis (NASH and ASH)*. Falk Symposium 121. 2001	ISBN 0-7923-8769-4